Post-Traumatic Stress Disorder
FOR
DUMMIES®

by Mark Goulston, MD

BICENTENNIAL
1807
WILEY
2007
BICENTENNIAL

Wiley Publishing, Inc.

Post-Traumatic Stress Disorder For Dummies®

Published by
Wiley Publishing, Inc.
111 River St.
Hoboken, NJ 07030-5774
www.wiley.com

Copyright © 2008 by Wiley Publishing, Inc., Indianapolis, Indiana

Published simultaneously in Canada

No part of this publication may be reproduced, stored in a retrieval system, or transmitted in any form or by any means, electronic, mechanical, photocopying, recording, scanning, or otherwise, except as permitted under Sections 107 or 108 of the 1976 United States Copyright Act, without either the prior written permission of the Publisher, or authorization through payment of the appropriate per-copy fee to the Copyright Clearance Center, 222 Rosewood Drive, Danvers, MA 01923, 978-750-8400, fax 978-646-8600. Requests to the Publisher for permission should be addressed to the Permissions Department, John Wiley & Sons, Inc., 111 River Street, Hoboken, NJ 07030, (201)748-6011, fax (201)748-6008, <u>or</u> online at http://www.wiley.com/go/permissions.

Trademarks: Wiley, the Wiley Publishing logo, For Dummies, the Dummies Man logo, A Reference for the Rest of Us!, The Dummies Way, Dummies Daily, The Fun and Easy Way, Dummies.com and related trade dress are trademarks or registered trademarks of John Wiley & Sons, Inc. and/or its affiliates in the United States and other countries, and may not be used without written permission. All other trademarks are the property of their respective owners. Wiley Publishing, Inc., is not associated with any product or vendor mentioned in this book.

LIMIT OF LIABILITY/DISCLAIMER OF WARRANTY: THE CONTENTS OF THIS WORK ARE INTENDED TO FURTHER GENERAL SCIENTIFIC RESEARCH, UNDERSTANDING, AND DISCUSSION ONLY AND ARE NOT INTENDED AND SHOULD NOT BE RELIED UPON AS RECOMMENDING OR PROMOTING A SPECIFIC METHOD, DIAGNOSIS, OR TREATMENT BY PHYSICIANS FOR ANY PARTICULAR PATIENT. THE PUBLISHER AND THE AUTHOR MAKE NO REPRESENTATIONS OR WARRANTIES WITH RESPECT TO THE ACCURACY OR COMPLETENESS OF THE CONTENTS OF THIS WORK AND SPECIFICALLY DISCLAIM ALL WARRANTIES, INCLUDING WITHOUT LIMITATION ANY IMPLIED WARRANTIES OF FITNESS FOR A PARTICULAR PURPOSE. IN VIEW OF ONGOING RESEARCH, EQUIPMENT MODIFICATIONS, CHANGES IN GOVERNMENTAL REGULATIONS, AND THE CONSTANT FLOW OF INFORMATION RELATING TO THE USE OF MEDICINES, EQUIPMENT, AND DEVICES, THE READER IS URGED TO REVIEW AND EVALUATE THE INFORMATION PROVIDED IN THE PACKAGE INSERT OR INSTRUCTIONS FOR EACH MEDICINE, EQUIPMENT, OR DEVICE FOR, AMONG OTHER THINGS, ANY CHANGES IN THE INSTRUCTIONS OR INDICATION OF USAGE AND FOR ADDED WARNINGS AND PRECAUTIONS. READERS SHOULD CONSULT WITH A SPECIALIST WHERE APPROPRIATE. THE FACT THAT AN ORGANIZATION OR WEBSITE IS REFERRED TO IN THIS WORK AS A CITATION AND/OR A POTENTIAL SOURCE OF FURTHER INFORMATION DOES NOT MEAN THAT THE AUTHOR OR THE PUBLISHER ENDORSES THE INFORMATION THE ORGANIZATION OR WEBSITE MAY PROVIDE OR RECOMMENDATIONS IT MAY MAKE. FURTHER, READERS SHOULD BE AWARE THAT INTERNET WEBSITES LISTED IN THIS WORK MAY HAVE CHANGED OR DISAPPEARED BETWEEN WHEN THIS WORK WAS WRITTEN AND WHEN IT IS READ. NO WARRANTY MAY BE CREATED OR EXTENDED BY ANY PROMOTIONAL STATEMENTS FOR THIS WORK. NEITHER THE PUBLISHER NOR THE AUTHOR SHALL BE LIABLE FOR ANY DAMAGES ARISING HEREFROM.

For general information on our other products and services, please contact our Customer Care Department within the U.S. at 877-762-2974, outside the U.S. at 317-572-3993, or fax 317-572-4002.

For technical support, please visit www.wiley.com/techsupport.

Wiley also publishes its books in a variety of electronic formats. Some content that appears in print may not be available in electronic books.

Library of Congress Control Number: 2007936459

ISBN: 978-0-470-04922-8

10 9 8 7 6 5 4 3

WILEY

About the Author

Mark Goulston, MD, received his medical degree from Boston University, completed his psychiatry training at the UCLA Neuropsychiatric Institute, and is a Fellow of the American Psychiatric Association.

He has been a UCLA Assistant Clinical Professor of Psychiatry for more than 20 years, and in 2004–05, he was selected as one of America's Top Psychiatrists by the Washington, D.C.–based Consumers' Research Council. He is the co-author of *Get Out of Your Own Way: Overcoming Self-Defeating Behavior* (Perigee, 1996) and *The 6 Secrets of a Lasting Relationship: How to Fall in Love Again . . . and Stay There* (Perigee, 2002). He's also the author of *Get Out of Your Own Way at Work . . . and Help Others Do the Same* (Perigee, 2006).

Dr. Goulston has written the nationally syndicated *Knight Ridder/Tribune* college newspaper column "Relationships 101" and regular columns for *EMMY Magazine* and *Fast Company.* In addition, he served as the Parenting Coach and Couples Coach at Time Warner's ParentTime site and iVillage and was the lead life-skills coach at LifeScape. He has taught or lectured at UCLA, USC, and Pepperdine University. Dr. Goulston has also served on the boards of Free Arts for Abused Children and the American Foundation of Suicide Prevention.

Because of his special interest in suicide prevention and teenage violence, Dr. Goulston has trained FBI and police hostage negotiators and has been frequently called upon to address these and other issues on CNN, ABC, NBC, CBS, Fox, and BBC news programs and in the print media, including the *New York Times, Los Angeles Times, Newsweek, Time* magazine, *Wall Street Journal, Harvard Business Review,* and *USA Today.*

For more information, please visit his Web site at www.markgoulston.com.

Dedication

To the soldiers, firefighters, and police officers and their families who have sacrificed so much to create peace on Earth, that this book may help them regain peace of mind.

Author's Acknowledgments

I am fortunate to have been taught, influenced, and inspired by some of the brightest and most caring individuals in the field of mental health, including Drs. Wilfred Bion, Herbert Linden, Lars Lofgren, Karl Menninger, Robert Pynoos, Robert Stoller, Louis Jolyon West, Carl Whitaker, and Peter Whybrow. Their collective wisdom serves as the magnetic north on my compass, and I feel blessed that I could turn to them in person and later on in memory to guide me in trying to ease the suffering of the thousands of people I have seen in my career.

I am especially grateful to Dr. Edwin Shneidman, one of the pioneers in the study of suicide and founder of the American Association of Suicidology. From this teacher, mentor, and now dear friend, I learned more about bringing hope to the hopeless than from any other individual.

On a different note, I am eternally grateful to the late Dr. William MacNary, who as Dean of Students at Boston University School of Medicine safely shepherded me during my medical school training through one of the most difficult and traumatic times in my professional life. My subsequent career and dedication to helping those in difficulty have been an effort to pass on to my patients the kindness that Dean MacNary showed me when I most needed it.

With regard to this book, I am thankful for the enthusiastic support of my agents Bill Gladstone and Ming Russell of Waterside Productions, the steadfast input of my acquisitions editor Tracy Boggier and my project editor Kristin DeMint at Wiley, the polishing done by copy editor Danielle Voirol, and deft assistance with this manuscript by Alison Blake.

I also appreciate the patience and support (and tolerance, especially during those tight deadlines) of my wife, Lisa; my three children, Lauren, Emily, and Billy; and my business partners, Keith Ferrazzi and Peter Winick at the consulting company Ferrazzi Greenlight, through which I do much of my consulting and coaching work.

Finally, I am indebted to the individuals, families, and couples who have entrusted me with the hurt and horror from their lives and in doing so enabled me to help them walk out of the darkness and into the light.

Publisher's Acknowledgments

We're proud of this book; please send us your comments through our Dummies online registration form located at www.dummies.com/register/.

Some of the people who helped bring this book to market include the following:

Acquisitions, Editorial, and Media Development

Project Editor: Kristin DeMint

Acquisitions Editor: Tracy Boggier

Copy Editor: Danielle Voirol

Technical Editor: Merrill Sparago, MD

Senior Editorial Manager: Jennifer Ehrlich

Editorial Assistants: Leeann Harney, Erin Calligan Mooney, Joe Niesen

Cover Photos: © Larry Mulvehill/Corbis, © Ryan McVay/Getty Images, © Edmond Van Hoorick/Getty Images, © Larry Mayer/Jupiter Images

Cartoons: Rich Tennant (www.the5thwave.com)

Composition Services

Project Coordinator: Patrick Redmond

Layout and Graphics: Claudia Bell, Stacie Brooks, Reuben Davis, Barbara Moore, Christine Williams

Illustrations: Kathryn Born, MA

Anniversary Logo Design: Richard Pacifico

Proofreaders: Cynthia Fields, Joni Heredia

Indexer: Cheryl Duksta

Special Help

Carrie A. Burchfield, Kathy Simpson, Sarah Westfall

Publishing and Editorial for Consumer Dummies

Diane Graves Steele, Vice President and Publisher, Consumer Dummies

Joyce Pepple, Acquisitions Director, Consumer Dummies

Kristin A. Cocks, Product Development Director, Consumer Dummies

Michael Spring, Vice President and Publisher, Travel

Kelly Regan, Editorial Director, Travel

Publishing for Technology Dummies

Andy Cummings, Vice President and Publisher, Dummies Technology/General User

Composition Services

Gerry Fahey, Vice President of Production Services

Debbie Stailey, Director of Composition Services

Contents at a Glance

Table of Contents

Introduction

*L*ife is an unpredictable adventure, and it can slip you some pretty big shocks now and then. Often these jolts are exciting, and although they may rattle you briefly, they make for great stories and add richness to your life. But sometimes events can pull the rug out from under you, leaving you feeling shocked, terrified, unsheltered, and alone. These experiences can shake you to your core, altering your feelings about yourself, other people, and the world around you. Consider these people's words:

> A combat survivor says, "The old me died in that war. I don't recognize the person I am now."

> A woman who survived a rape says, "People say I'm cold and unfeeling now. They don't know that inside, I'm falling apart."

> A heart attack survivor says, "I feel so lost. It's like I see my old life in the distance, but I can't find my way back to it."

All these people have post-traumatic stress disorder (PTSD). They're scared, angry, and sad — and they have every reason to be. A traumatic life event turned their lives upside down, transforming their once safe and happy world into a terrifying and alien place they fear they'll never escape.

The most important message of this book is this: *There is a road out of this terrible place.* The fact that you're still afraid doesn't mean you're in any danger. It just takes the will and the way for your heart and soul to accept what the logical part of your mind already knows. I've been treating patients with PTSD for more than two decades, and the vast majority of them make the journey back to wellness. Often, it's not an easy journey — or a short one. But there is help, there is hope, and there is a better future ahead. In short, there's life after PTSD — and a good one, I might add. In this book, I explain how to set your course for that brighter future.

About This Book

I have piles of academic books on PTSD, but they're pretty dry reading. My goal in this book is to cut through all those fancy words and give you the basic facts you really need about what PTSD is and how you can overcome it. I also lighten these pages with a few jokes because I figure you have a sense of humor and can use a good laugh — even though you and I both know that PTSD is a very serious matter.

If you're a trauma survivor with PTSD, this book clearly lays out the steps you can take to reclaim your life and your future. In addition to giving you info about a wide range of therapy approaches, I offer advice on self-help steps that can aid in taming your PTSD symptoms.

If you're caring for a person fighting PTSD, you can find the tools you need to play an active part in your loved one's recovery. Because partners and parents play an especially powerful role in helping a person heal from PTSD, I cover the roles of these very important people in depth. In addition, I offer helpful advice for extended family members and friends.

Whether you're battling PTSD yourself or caring for someone who's facing this challenge, you can begin these pages with a sense of hope — because the fight against PTSD is a battle you can win.

Conventions Used in This Book

If you have PTSD (or are struggling to cope along with someone who does) you're probably feeling more than a little frazzled. To make the process of gathering information as simple as possible for you, I use the following tools throughout the book to help you navigate through the text quickly and easily.

✔ When I introduce a new term, I put it in *italics* to highlight it — and if it's medical jargon (which I avoid as much as possible), I offer a plain-English explanation.

✔ I use **boldface** to set off important keywords and numbered steps.

✔ I use `monofont` to indicate useful Web sites. If a Web address breaks across two lines of text, I don't add an extra hyphen or any spaces, so just type exactly what you see.

What You're Not to Read

I hope you find every part of this book valuable — but don't feel like you need to read every word. Instead, pick and choose the material that suits your needs.

For instance, if you're not into the scientific nitty-gritty about PTSD, you can skip any text marked with the Technical Stuff icon. You can also pass over the sidebars if you're pressed for time — but consider giving these gray boxes a quick glance because they contain lots of useful advice and inspiring stories about others who've walked the path that you or your loved one is on. And of course, feel free to ignore sections that don't have anything to do with your life; for instance, skip the chapter on PTSD in children if you're interested only in adult PTSD.

Foolish Assumptions

In writing this book, I kept a clear picture of you, the reader, in mind. Therefore, I had to assume a few things about you and your needs:

- ✔ You're relatively new to PTSD. Maybe you're newly diagnosed or wondering whether you have the disorder — or maybe you're a relative or friend who's hoping to help a person who's struggling with PTSD.
- ✔ If you have PTSD, you want to know all your options so you can have an active say in your treatment plan.
- ✔ You're willing to face your problem head-on and seek help if you do have PTSD.
- ✔ You want to know that there's real help for the pain you're suffering. (And yes — there is!)

How This Book Is Organized

Post-Traumatic Stress Disorder For Dummies is organized into six parts and 18 chapters. Here's a quick look at each part.

Part 1: The Basics of PTSD

In Chapter 1, you find a quick overview of the history of PTSD, the major causes of this disorder, and the numbers of people it affects. Chapter 2 gives you the lowdown on what *trauma* is and describes the factors that can put you at extra risk for developing PTSD. Next, in Chapter 3, I describe the key symptoms of PTSD and talk about other disorders — such as depression and substance abuse problems — that often complicate the PTSD picture. In addition, I describe the very different symptoms that kids with PTSD can show.

Chapter 4 tackles a very different topic: what experts know (and don't know) about *preventing* PTSD. In this chapter, I talk about what does and doesn't help when you're trying to stop PTSD before it starts. I also offer info about new drug treatments that show promise in short-circuiting the brain changes that can trigger PTSD symptoms.

Part II: Getting a Diagnosis and Drafting a Plan

Maybe you're wondering whether you have PTSD — or maybe you already have a diagnosis but you're not sure where to go from here. Either way, you can find answers to your questions in this part.

In Chapter 5, I offer a self-test to help you determine whether your symptoms point to PTSD, and I provide advice on getting a diagnosis if they do. Chapter 6 describes how and where to locate good therapists and tells you the questions you should ask before deciding whether a particular therapist is right for you. And Chapter 7 talks about the steps you can take *before* therapy to make sure you get optimal results when you start treatment.

Part III: Choosing the Right Treatment Approach

Today's treatments are highly effective in reducing the pain of PTSD, but a treatment that works like a charm for one person can miss the mark with another. When you know the range of treatments available for PTSD, you can choose the approach that works best for you.

In this part, I describe a wide variety of approaches to treating PTSD. Chapter 8 talks about cognitive behavioral therapy (CBT), the most widely used therapy for PTSD. Chapter 9 describes the drug treatments that sometimes play an important role in recovery, and Chapter 10 describes a host of additional therapies and offers some stats on how helpful they are.

Part IV: Healing and Rebuilding during and after Treatment

The most important person on your recovery team is *you* — and in this part, I describe the steps you can take to keep your progress on track. First, I talk about what you can expect from therapy and how to maximize your results. Next, I offer a cornucopia of ways to enhance your mental and physical health, stop stress in its tracks, erase the hidden agendas that hold you back, and enjoy life's pleasures (including intimacy and sexuality) again. I also talk about how to get back into the stream of life — jobs, friendships, life goals — when you get PTSD under control.

However, you're not the only important person involved in your recovery. That's why I also talk about the ways in which PTSD strains family ties — and the steps you can take to make those bonds strong again.

Part V: Stepping In: When You're Not the One Who's Suffering

Maybe you're reading this book because you're worried about a child who's showing signs of PTSD. If so, you can find a wealth of information in Chapter 15 about the treatments you can call on to help your child heal. You can also get tips on making family and friends a part of your child's recovery plan.

On the other hand, you may be reading this book because you're a good friend of a person with PTSD and you want to find ways to help. If so, check out Chapter 16 for practical advice about the do's and don'ts of supporting someone who's struggling to break free from PTSD's grip.

Part VI: The Part of Tens

Knowing the facts about PTSD can help you dispel false ideas that can get in the way of healing. That's why Chapter 17 outlines the ten most common myths about PTSD and gives you the true story about each one. In Chapter 18, I clue you in on some of the subtle and not-so-subtle signs of healing that you can anticipate as time goes by.

Following the Part of Tens, you can find a helpful appendix listing Web sites, books, documentaries, and other resources that can help you turn the tide against PTSD.

Icons Used in This Book

One handy device that *For Dummies* books use is the icon — a symbol in the margin that lets you quickly spot the types of information that interest you. In this book, I use the following icons:

This icon highlights an important bit of information that you won't want to forget.

The Tip icon marks practical advice that can be part of your action plan for defeating PTSD.

The Warning icon alerts you to be careful about a possible hazard or to seek professional help in handling a particular problem.

This icon lets you know that a piece of information is interesting but not necessary to read if you're pressed for time and want to zero in on the facts you need to jump-start your healing from PTSD.

This icon points you to inspiring, enlightening, or just plain interesting stories about real patients — mine and other doctors' — and the insights these survivors have to offer. Where I include stories about patients of mine, know that these people are real. However, I've changed their names and other identifying details to make sure I protect their privacy.

Where to Go from Here

Depending on who you are — a person with PTSD, friend, or family member — some parts of this book will be more important to you than others. That's why you don't need to start on page 1 and read straight through. Instead, you can use the Table of Contents or index to find the topics that interest you the most. For example, if the facts and figures about PTSD don't interest you, feel free to cut to the chase and start with Part II, where you can find info on effective treatments.

As you read this book, feel free to skip from section to section and read it in any order. I do recommend reading Chapters 2 and 3 if you're seeking a basic understanding of what PTSD is. And I suggest reading Part II for information on treatments if you're saying, "I'm ready to get better — how do I start?" If you're helping a child who has PTSD, or pitching in to aid a PTSD-affected friend in need, Part V is an excellent place to dive in.

Wherever you start, you're making an excellent move — because the advice and strategies in this book can help you take back control of your life (or effectively support someone you love in doing so) and make your future a better and brighter one. I wish you the very best of luck in achieving that goal!

Chapter 1

The Invisible Epidemic of PTSD

*Y*ou jump out of your skin if you hear a police siren or a car backfiring. You wake up screaming after terrible nightmares. You feel cut off from your life and the people around you, and you're angry or sad all the time. Worst of all, you experience moments of sheer terror when your mind pulls you out of the present and drags you into a horrifying time in your past.

If you suffer from symptoms like these, you probably feel very much alone — but in reality, you aren't. Instead, you're likely one of millions of people around the world who suffer from a disorder called *post-traumatic stress disorder (PTSD)*.

If so, you're facing a problem as old as humankind. The difference between the past and now, as you discover in this book, is that for today's PTSD sufferers, *effective help* for this pain is available. In the chapters that follow, I talk about the many ways to treat PTSD and explain why you can be very optimistic about your future.

As you begin your journey into a better tomorrow, it's a good idea to gain a little knowledge about the adversary you're facing. In this chapter, I take a quick look at what PTSD is, as well as why treating this disorder is crucial. I also offer an overview of the history of PTSD as a diagnosis and explain how people's understanding of this disorder has evolved over time. Next, I talk about the numbers of people (both adults and children) affected by PTSD, as well as the many types of traumatic experiences that can set PTSD in motion. In addition, I look at the toll PTSD takes not just on each individual sufferer but also on society as a whole.

The Diagnosis of PTSD: A Serious Matter That Requires Serious Intervention

PTSD is a major, life-altering disorder that strikes many people who survive traumatic experiences. I use the phrase *invisible epidemic* to describe this disorder because it affects millions of people of every age and in every walk of life, and many of them suffer alone and in silence. They feel scared, anxious, and isolated from the rest of the world — and they feel like no one can understand what they're going through.

To a casual observer, these people often seem to be doing just fine. But in reality, they're battling devastating symptoms that, if left untreated, make it difficult or impossible for them to hold down jobs, have meaningful relationships, or achieve their goals and dreams.

PTSD short-circuits people's lives by causing disabling symptoms that include a hyper-alert nervous system, numbness and detachment, and intrusive thoughts or flashbacks about the trauma (see Chapter 3 for an in-depth discussion of these problems). Living with these symptoms is a huge challenge, made even bigger by the fact that other problems such as depression or substance abuse often come along for the ride (another topic I cover in Chapter 3). People with complex PTSD, which stems from multiple traumas, may develop an even wider range of severe problems, including dangerous and self-destructive behaviors (see Chapter 2).

Getting treatment if you have PTSD is crucial because this disorder doesn't simply go away on its own. Unlike the normal, temporary stress symptoms that often occur after a life crisis, PTSD involves profound biochemical and psychological changes that cause the toxic memories of a trauma to remain strong instead of fading. (See Chapter 2 for more on the differences between normal stress responses and PTSD.) As a result, people with PTSD become trapped in their trauma, unable to process what happened and move on with their lives. In addition, untreated PTSD often leads to *secondary wounding* (a topic I cover in Chapter 8) because the problems caused by PTSD can lead to broken relationships, lost jobs, and other new traumas.

The good news — and it's very good news indeed — is that PTSD is highly treatable, and the vast majority of people with this disorder gain freedom from the disabling symptoms and get control of their lives again. In Chapters 8 through 10, I describe the wide range of treatments doctors and therapists now have to help adults with this disorder, and in Chapter 13, I look at interventions that can benefit children and teens. In addition, as I explain in Chapter 12, you can combine therapy with self-help steps that boost your healing power. So take heart: If you're in the depths of PTSD right now, the solutions are within your reach.

A Little Background on PTSD

PTSD is an age-old problem, but in a sense, it's also a new disorder because professionals are still learning about its causes, symptoms, and treatment.

As I explain in Chapter 2, PTSD can stem from any type of traumatic experience. However, much of the current knowledge about PTSD comes from one particular source — the military — for an obvious reason: War causes trauma on a massive scale. Throughout history, each successive war led to new names for the condition and new theories about its causes:

- During the American Civil War, doctors called combat-related trauma *soldier's heart*. (The name wasn't far off the mark because — as I discuss in Chapter 3 — PTSD can affect your heart as well as your thoughts, emotions, and behavior.)

- World War I doctors called it *shell shock*, thinking that it stemmed from changes in air pressure when artillery shells exploded.

- During World War II, doctors renamed combat trauma *battle fatigue* and made the terrible error (also made by many earlier generals) of blaming it on weakness or cowardice.

- By the beginning of the Korean War, psychiatrists began to recognize PTSD — then dubbed *gross stress reaction* — as a real disorder crying out for study.

PTSD made its way into the medical world as a legitimate disorder by finding a place in the *Diagnostic and Statistical Manual of Mental Disorders,* or *DSM* (the bible of modern American psychiatry) in 1980, following the Vietnam War. By this point, doctors recognized that civilians as well as soldiers could develop PTSD after a trauma. Even so, people who developed PTSD still found little sympathy, and the cruel myth that PTSD was a sign of weakness persisted. That myth finally died out (although not totally, as I explain in Chapter 17) toward the end of the 1900s, largely because soldiers from the Vietnam era and the first Gulf War fought hard to get the military — and the rest of the world — to take PTSD seriously.

Everyone dealing with PTSD, on either a personal or a professional basis, owes a big debt of gratitude to those wounded warriors who refused to sweep PTSD under the rug. Their persistence gave PTSD research a huge boost, and that research in turn opened doctors' eyes to the fact that millions of people — not just soldiers but also people who survived sexual assaults, natural disasters, illnesses, and other traumatic events — have a real medical problem and need real medical help.

The story behind PTSD: A problem as old as humanity

As I explain in Chapter 2, PTSD has a lot to do with biochemistry — that is, the chemicals that make your body tick. Because your ancestors had almost exactly the same biochemistry as you, it's no surprise that PTSD made its first appearance around the dawn of human history. In fact, the first person to describe it was an Egyptian doctor in 1900 BCE. But doctors didn't immediately figure out what *causes* PTSD. In fact, they came up with some pretty bizarre theories about it.

The oddest of these theories arose in the 1800s, when doctors studied people hurt in train wrecks (common events in those days). In addition to their physical injuries, many of these people reported having insomnia, nightmares, memory loss, and extreme fear of train travel — no doubt symptoms of PTSD stemming from the terrifying experiences they survived. The cause of these symptoms, the doctors said, was the incredibly fast speed of the newfangled trains of the era — which went about 30 miles an hour!

By the late 1800s, leading lights in psychiatry, including Sigmund Freud, began spotting the link between trauma and PTSD-like symptoms. Unfortunately, Freud set progress back again by changing his mind and deciding that these symptoms stemmed, at least in women, from sexual fantasies rather than real traumas. (For a genius, he could be pretty dim sometimes.) It took two World Wars, and several smaller ones, for experts to gain a true understanding of how PTSD affects people traumatized by war or other catastrophic events.

As a result, people who suffer from PTSD today are likely to get an accurate diagnosis and effective treatment instead of a cold shoulder and a brusque recommendation to "just get over it." (To increase your odds of success in diagnosis and treatment, see my advice in Chapters 5 and 6 on finding good professional help.) Better yet, treatments for PTSD grow more effective with each passing year. In fact, current research (see Chapter 4) hints that someday, doctors may be able to stop many cases of PTSD before they start.

Professionals still have far to go in fully understanding PTSD, but they're light years ahead of where they were just a few decades ago — thanks largely to generations of vets who finally won their battle against ignorance and stigma.

Stats on PTSD: The Numbers Game

It's easy to tell whether the man next to you in the checkout line has a head cold (all too easy, in fact!) or whether the neighbor you pass on the street has a broken leg. But PTSD is a silent problem whose sufferers usually hide in plain sight. Millions of people with PTSD don't even know that they have the disorder, and millions more keep their pain to themselves because they're afraid (for reasons I explain in Chapter 5) to seek help.

As a result, knowing the true scope of this tragedy is impossible. However, even the numbers that experts *do* know reveal a huge cost in human pain. According to the U.S. government's National Technical Information Service (www.ntis.gov), PTSD is "one of the most prevalent of all mental disorders, surpassed only by substance use disorders and depression as major public and mental health issues." Here's a quick look at the numbers of adults and children this disorder affects.

PTSD in adults

Once upon a time, experts thought that PTSD affected only soldiers. Now, however, it's clear that anyone — librarians, cab drivers, teachers, dentists — can fall prey to this life-altering disorder. All it takes to trigger PTSD is a trauma, and unfortunately, there are plenty of those to go around.

In fact, more than 70 percent of Americans suffer a traumatic event at some time in their lives. Of these trauma survivors, up to 20 percent develop PTSD. Put another way, approximately 13 million Americans — 5 percent of the population — suffers from PTSD at any given time.

Women develop PTSD at twice the rate of men, for reasons I talk about in Chapter 2. Studies suggest that rates of PTSD also are higher for people who are Hispanic or African American, possibly because people in these groups have a higher exposure to violence. For similar reasons, rates of PTSD are sky-high in refugees from countries torn by violence. For example, according to a 2005 study by Grant Marshall and colleagues in the *Journal of the American Medical Association,* more than 60 percent of a group of Cambodian refugees who resettled in the United States two decades ago exhibited PTSD symptoms.

PTSD in children and teens

No matter how hard they try, parents can't always shield their kids from trauma. Fires and earthquakes shatter the worlds of children as well as grownups, and so do car accidents, disease, and acts of terrorism. As a result, millions of kids and teens have a PTSD diagnosis, and millions more have undiagnosed PTSD symptoms. (See Chapter 3 for more on kids and PTSD.) Here are some statistics on the toll PTSD takes on youngsters:

- Of all children, 14 to 43 percent experience at least one traumatic event.
- Of these children, 3 to 15 percent of girls and 1 to 6 percent of boys exhibit PTSD.
- Of children who witness a school shooting, 75 percent develop PTSD.
- Among sexually abused kids, 60 percent develop PTSD, and so do more than 40 percent of physically abused kids.

Those numbers are hefty but don't tell the whole story because many children show few or no signs of PTSD after a trauma until years later, when they reach adulthood and grownup pressures cause symptoms to kick in. (For more on this condition, called *delayed PTSD,* see Chapter 2.)

Trauma Triggers: The Most Common Causes of PTSD

PTSD, as I explain in Chapter 2, stems from an experience that horrifies and overwhelms you. That experience can be anything from a hurricane to a terrorist attack to the very private moment of hearing a doctor say that you have a life-threatening disease. PTSD can begin after a tour of duty in a war zone, or it can strike after a freeway accident or sexual assault. What's more, the same event can cause PTSD in one person and leave another unscathed, for reasons I talk about in Chapter 2.

Although many types of catastrophes can cause PTSD, some life crises are far riskier than others. Figure 1-1 shows statistics on the events most likely to trigger PTSD. Several of these events score high on the PTSD scale in part because of their sheer magnitude. Others, although smaller in scale, make the list because of the depth of the pain they cause.

Figure 1-1:
The risk of developing PTSD after different types of trauma.

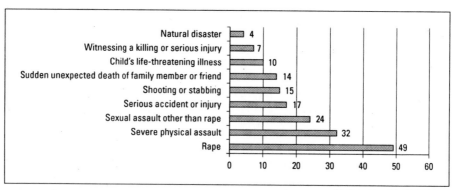

Graph courtesy of the PTSD Alliance

In this section, I look at several types of these trauma-provoking events and how they differ in their power to cause harm.

The ill winds (and fires, floods, tremors, and disease) that can lead to PTSD

For most of your life, Mother Nature is a kind friend. The sun smiles on you, the grass grows underfoot, and the river flows gently through your town. But Mother Nature has teeth and claws, and she can turn quickly from a kindly friend to a vicious foe. When that happens, your life can turn upside down in an instant.

Anyone who's watched a natural disaster unfold on TV — or worse, had to live through one of these calamities — can understand why these events leave a swath of PTSD in their wake. The biggest offenders, which can affect thousands of lives in a single day, include

- ✔ Hurricanes, tornadoes, and tsunamis
- ✔ Fires
- ✔ Earthquakes
- ✔ Floods

Natural disasters often trigger PTSD because they rain so many blows on their victims — lost homes, lost jobs, lost lives. Hurricane Katrina is a good example. Even after the winds and floodwaters subsided, many people remained without shelter, food, water, money, or medical aid for days. Thousands lost their jobs, and many lost loved ones. As a result, a single event turned into a series of traumas, and survivors suffered sky-high rates of PTSD. (One study by Lisa Mills, reported at the 2007 annual meeting of the Society for Academic Emergency Medicine, found that more than a third of Katrina survivors seen at a New Orleans emergency department had PTSD — a far higher toll than for most disasters.) Natural disasters also leave their scars on the rescue teams who lend a helping hand after catastrophe strikes, and many of these people experience secondary trauma (see Chapter 2) as a result of witnessing the suffering around them.

Mother Nature doesn't always strike with wind, water, fire, or earthquakes, however; often, she terrorizes people in quieter ways. One powerful risk for PTSD, often overlooked by doctors until recent years, is a serious illness such as cancer or AIDS.

People battling life-threatening illnesses (or watching a family member go through this experience) have very high rates of PTSD. In the *Journal of*

Clinical Oncology, a 2005 study by Anne Kazak and colleagues found that nearly 100 percent of parents of children being treated for cancer develop some degree of PTSD and that more than half of the fathers and three-quarters of the mothers of these children develop moderate-to-severe PTSD. PTSD often affects people for years or decades after a serious illness, even if the initial threat to the person's health passes.

The human acts that can cause PTSD

On September 11, 2001, the United States witnessed an act of human cruelty on a scale that shook the entire world. Other countries, too, have been rocked by episodes of genocide caused by wars or terrorism. Such dark moments in history are mercifully rare, but every single day, individual acts of violence — armed robberies, sexual assaults, and other violent attacks — derail the lives of thousands of people around the globe.

These acts, whether they affect thousands of people or a single life, put people at extreme risk for PTSD. As I explain in Chapter 2, intentional acts of violence or betrayal cut much deeper than traumas caused by the random acts of nature — especially when these acts happen in childhood or occur over and over.

The horrific scale of abuse in America

How big of a toll do domestic violence and other acts of partner abuse take on society? Here are some shocking numbers offered by the National Center for Posttraumatic Stress Disorder (www.ncptsd.va.gov):

✔ At least once in their lifetimes, 20 to 30 percent of American women are physically abused by a partner.

✔ Each year, 1.3 million women and more than 800,000 men are physically assaulted by an intimate partner.

✔ More than 200,000 women are raped by an intimate partner each year.

✔ Of those in same-sex relationships, 11 percent of women and 23 percent of men are raped, otherwise physically assaulted, and/or stalked by an intimate partner.

✔ More than 500,000 women and 185,000 men are stalked by an intimate partner each year.

✔ Of all women's emergency-room visits, 30 to 40 percent are for injuries due to domestic violence.

✔ Fifty percent of men who assault their female partners also assault their children.

✔ Each year, 3.3 million children witness acts of domestic violence.

The human-caused traumas that carry the highest risk for PTSD include

- Childhood sexual or physical abuse
- Rape and other forms of sexual assault
- Domestic violence
- Armed robberies and other nonsexual physical attacks
- Violent acts resulting in deaths that cause trauma in surviving relatives and loved ones
- Torture or acts of terror committed during war

Overall, according to the National Center for Posttraumatic Stress Disorder, the traumatic events most often associated with PTSD include the following:

- **For women:** Rape, sexual molestation, physical attack, being threatened with a weapon, or being abused as a child
- **For men:** Rape, combat experiences, or neglect or physical abuse in childhood

Violence also takes a huge toll on the courageous folks who put their lives on the line every day in the course of their jobs. As we count on police officers and soldiers to protect us from harm, we put these heroes directly in PTSD's line of fire. Police officers, for example, have rates of PTSD that may be four to six times higher than those of people in the general population, and for soldiers, the numbers are astronomical (see Chapter 2).

But although exposure to violence or abuse is a key cause of trauma, not all human-caused traumas involve violence, and not all of them are intentional. In fact, motor-vehicle accidents are the leading cause of PTSD in the general population. More than 6 million road accidents occur in the U.S. each year, causing around 3 million injuries and 40,000 deaths. Nearly one in ten people involved in a serious accident develops PTSD, and for kids, the rate of PTSD may be even higher. A 2000 study by Herb Schreier and colleagues, reported at the International Conference on Pediatric Trauma, evaluated kids injured in car crashes and other types of accidents; they found that 60 percent of the children reported PTSD symptoms a month after their traumas, and 40 percent still had symptoms six months afterward.

Other stressful events that occasionally cause PTSD

In the preceding two sections, I describe the catastrophes that frequently cause trauma. But as professionals discover more about PTSD, they're finding that many of life's events that people simply think of as tough breaks — the too-bad-but-you'll-get-over-it kinds of events — may lead to PTSD as well. Here are some recent findings:

✓ **People who live through events most experts consider to be upsetting but not traumatic have a high risk of PTSD.** In 2005, Saskia Mol and colleagues surveyed nearly 3,000 people to find out what stressful events they'd experienced and how many PTSD symptoms they had. The results surprised these scientists. They expected people who'd survived floods, hurricanes, wars, and near-death experiences to have an elevated rate of PTSD, which is just what they found; but they also reported in their article, which appeared in the *British Journal of Psychiatry,* that people who lived through events most experts consider as upsetting but not traumatic — for instance, a job loss or divorce — also had a high risk of PTSD.

✓ **A study of people chronically bullied on the job by bosses or co-workers found that many had PTSD symptoms.** Stig Berge Matthiesen and Ståle Einarsen, reporting in 2004 in the *British Journal of Guidance & Counselling,* said this finding isn't really surprising because "a traumatized person experiencing bullying at work may have a strong shattered experience of the world as not being a just place, with a strong anticipation of future misfortune to come." The same may be true for bullied children, a topic researchers are now studying.

Tolls of war

As professionals learn more about PTSD, trauma-scarred soldiers are finally starting to get the help and the respect they need. This change is a welcome one from past generations, when veterans often suffered in silence.

Because of that silence, many people think of war-related PTSD as a disease that appeared out of the blue during the Vietnam War. The truth, of course, is that combat-related PTSD occurs in every war. Here are some facts and figures about the toll of PTSD in past conflicts:

✓ A 2005 study of Korean War veterans in Australia reported that up to 33 percent of those soldiers met criteria for PTSD.

✓ During World War II, half a million soldiers developed battle fatigue (another name for PTSD). In 2004, as many as 25,000 World War II veterans still received disability compensation for symptoms related to PTSD.

✓ Britain recently issued pardons (a little late in the game) for about 300 soldiers executed during World War I on charges of cowardice. A review of these soldiers' records indicated that many of them actually had PTSD.

One lesson of these studies is that it doesn't take a hurricane, a war, or a near-death experience to trigger PTSD. The other lesson is that you shouldn't hesitate to seek help for PTSD symptoms, even if you don't think your life crises were major enough to affect you. Trauma is in the eye of the beholder, and a life problem that may look like no big deal to an outsider may actually be very damaging, depending on your life circumstances.

Adding It Up: The Costs of Untreated PTSD

Turn on the TV, and you hear public-service announcements about the perils of untreated diabetes, heart disease, or high blood pressure. You never see a commercial about the dangers of untreated PTSD, but you should. PTSD is a major public health crisis, affecting more people than diabetes or asthma. What's more, the cost of PTSD in dollars is staggering.

As experts begin to understand just how widespread PTSD is, they're also starting to realize the high price of this disorder — not just for each individual sufferer but also for society as a whole. Here are just a few of the ways that PTSD affects us all:

- ✔ **Lost lives:** Every year, society loses many of its best and brightest to the pain of untreated PTSD because the disorder significantly increases the risk of suicidal thoughts or behavior. The risk of suicide is especially high for people who develop both PTSD and depression, unless they receive effective treatment. (See Chapter 3 for info on the link between these two conditions.)

- ✔ **High medical costs:** People who don't get treatment for the fallout from trauma have higher rates of disability, more physical symptoms, more mental disorders, more medical diagnoses from doctors, and more risky health behaviors than other people. (See Chapter 3 for info on the health problems that PTSD causes.) The costs of untreated trauma-related alcohol and drug abuse alone are estimated to be $160 billion per year in the U.S. (Chapter 7 explains the substance abuse/PTSD link.)

- ✔ **Legal woes:** The out-of-control veteran on a shooting spree is a destructive Hollywood stereotype (see Chapter 17), but PTSD frequently does play a role in criminal behavior. PTSD can impair judgment, self-esteem, the ability to plan for the future, and the ability to control anger, putting people at increased risk for impulsive or destructive behavior. More than 60 percent of Vietnam combat vets with PTSD, for example, have a history of at least one arrest after returning from the war. Studies show that PTSD is a strong risk factor for both adult crime and juvenile delinquency and that it plays a powerful role in steering people into prostitution, drug dealing, and pathological gambling.

✔ **Poor work performance and, in turn, lost jobs:** PTSD can impair a person's concentration and productivity, create problems in getting along with co-workers, and trigger emotional outbursts on the job. All these factors, as well as the health problems associated with PTSD (see Chapter 3), can make it hard for people with PTSD to get and keep jobs, resulting in higher-than-normal rates of unemployment. In addition, people with PTSD often have difficulty making upward career moves and frequently stay stuck in a low-salary rut because of their symptoms. Experts estimate that the United States loses $3 billion each year due to work problems caused by PTSD.

✔ **Family troubles:** PTSD makes it hard to control emotions, empathize with other people, cope with financial matters, and handle the day-to-day pressures of relationships. It also ups the risk for substance abuse and other self-destructive behaviors. Because of this, the divorce rate for people with untreated PTSD is sky-high. In addition, children in families dealing with untreated PTSD have more learning and emotional problems than their peers. Rates of physical and verbal abuse are also high in families with a member suffering from PTSD. (For ways to cope if you're a family member of someone battling PTSD, see Chapter 13.)

That list is scary, but as you read it, don't be discouraged. Instead, focus on the word *untreated,* because that's the key. If you have PTSD and you get effective treatment, your risk for all these problems drops like a rock. (See Part III for info on medical treatments and Chapter 12 for self-help steps.)

Untreated PTSD almost always gets worse, putting you at ever-increasing risk for medical problems, broken relationships, and loss of quality of life. Conversely, *treated* PTSD almost always gets better (see Chapters 14 and 18 for some of the big and little changes you can expect). Recovery takes time and a lot of hard work (Chapter 11 details the therapy process), but it's well worth the effort. Just ask the millions of happy, healthy, creative, productive, joy-filled people who've left PTSD in their past.

If you're the friend or loved one of a person with PTSD, you can also take hope from another fact: Along with treatment, strong social support can play a powerful role in reducing the risks of the problems I outline in this section. (For details, see Chapters 13 and 16.) You can't shoulder the burden of aiding a person with PTSD all on your own — in fact, calling in the pros is essential — but your love and support can help give a trauma survivor the courage to break free from the chains of PTSD.

Chapter 2

Aftershocks: When the Past Won't Stay in the Past

"*W*e'll always have Paris," says Humphrey Bogart as he parts from Ingrid Bergman in *Casablanca*. It's a great movie line, and it says a lot about the amazing gift called memory. Like Bogey, you can keep your favorite places and people with you simply by pulling up your happy memories of them — even if they're miles away or long-gone. Without flipping open a scrapbook or putting in a CD, you can conjure up your newborn's first smile or first word, the ecstasy (or agony) of prom night, or even the aroma of Mom's freshly baked bread.

But memories have a dark side, too: They can make you feel devastated, furious, or humiliated (many of you just thought about prom night again, didn't you?), even decades after something bad happens. What's more, bad memories seem to stick more than happy ones — and that's especially true for terrible memories like the ones that can trigger PTSD. Minor crises such as a missed plane flight or a tiff with a friend may make you cringe when you recall them, but these memories don't change your life. Experience a terrible trauma, however, and the memories can torment you for months — or much longer — if you develop PTSD.

To understand why a single moment in time can change your life so dramatically, it helps to know just what a trauma is and how it can impact you both instantly and over the long run. In this chapter, I define what the term *trauma* means, explain why trauma is very different from stress, and describe how a trauma can turn a helpful tool — memory — into a destructive force. In addition, I look at the different forms of PTSD that can occur when a bad memory just won't let go, and I explain how triggers can set off the bad feelings in a snap.

Looking Closely at Trauma

Every case of PTSD starts in the same way: with a trauma. The word *trauma* comes from the Greek word for *wound,* and that's a good definition because trauma can wound the mind as well as the body. In this section, I look at what trauma is, dispel some of the confusion surrounding the term, and explain why a trauma is very different from a stressful event.

Defining trauma

Think of the word *trauma,* and you may conjure up a picture of a big, unusual event — a hurricane, an earthquake, the collapse of the World Trade Center towers. But traumas aren't rare at all, and most of them don't make the nightly news. In fact, nearly all people experience at least one major trauma in their lifetimes.

Here are the four elements that define a trauma:

✔ **It's an overwhelming event — large or small.** The level of distress an event causes, not the scale of the event, is what really counts. Anything from a life-threatening illness to a huge natural disaster can cause trauma.

✔ **It threatens life and limb — either your own or that of someone you love.** One exception is *secondary trauma,* which can affect police officers, paramedics, search-and-rescue teams, and other people who respond when a crisis occurs. At times, the sheer amount of human suffering these caring professionals see can make it hard for them to function. Thus, they can experience trauma even if their own lives, or the lives of people they love, aren't in danger.

✔ **It's unexpected.** Typically, a trauma — whether it's a car accident, an assault, or an act of nature — strikes when you're totally unprepared.

✔ **It's an event that causes fear, helplessness, or horror in the person involved.** A catastrophic event, in and of itself, doesn't always traumatize a person. If you feel like you have some control over what's happening, both physically and emotionally, then you may come through with few psychic scars. Again, the event itself doesn't constitute a trauma — it's how the event impacts *you.*

In short, a trauma is a dangerous, shocking event that shakes both your body and soul. It makes you fear for your life and your safety — or the lives and safety of the people you care about most — and it breaks down your psychological defenses and shatters your sense of security.

Differentiating between trauma and normal stressors

Every person has stressful moments, and those moments can be mighty intense. For instance, if you're pregnant, you lost your job yesterday, and the dentist says you need a root canal, it's a good bet that you feel stressed. However, that doesn't mean you've endured a traumatic event.

Here are three key questions that can help distinguish garden-variety stressors from a severe stress-inducing trauma:

- ✔ **What happened?** The day-to-day stuff causes minor stress: a job deadline, a fender-bender, or an argument with a partner. Bigger events, either good or bad — weddings, career changes, moves — can stress you out even more, but they're still part of the normal fabric of life. Trauma, on the other hand, knocks you totally off course, at least temporarily.

- ✔ **Did you feel in control?** If someone rear-ends you on the freeway, you get a rude shock — but after a few minutes, you pull out your cellphone and your insurance card and start putting things back in order. If an armed robber holds you at gunpoint, however, you have no control over whether you live or die. The first situation merely causes a brief uptick in your stress level; the second, however, can cause a long-term traumatic response.

- ✔ **Can you keep your feelings in their place?** If you're stressed by day-to-day problems, you can take a break from your anxiety by watching a funny movie or taking your kids to the beach. In the aftermath of a trauma, however, your feelings take over your life (at least temporarily). You can't simply tuck those bad feelings away and enjoy yourself.

Here's another way to look at the difference between stress and trauma: Stress is like a wrinkle in the rug of life, and you can step over it or straighten it out without changing course. But trauma pulls the rug right out from under you. Unlike simple stress, trauma changes your view of your life and yourself. It shatters your most basic assumptions about yourself and your world — "Life is good," "I'm safe," "People are kind," "I can trust others," "The future is likely to be good" — and replaces them with feelings like "The world is dangerous," "I can't win," "I can't trust other people," or "There's no hope."

Also, although stressors and their effects pass with time, the aftershocks of trauma continue to mount. In addition to the obvious first degree of damage done, trauma often causes secondary wounds — for example, financial crises after a natural disaster, broken relationships if a sexual assault leaves you unable to trust, sadness when good friends can't understand your trauma, or long-term injuries after an accident — that push you further into negative thoughts, negative actions, and a victim mentality.

Normal stress and trauma differ in another big way as well: One is often healthy, but the other is toxic. Ordinary stress, if it's not too severe or chronic, keeps you on your toes and challenges you to reach difficult goals. The severe stress that follows a trauma, on the other hand, can harm you both physically and mentally if you don't recover from its effects.

Understanding the Three Levels of Reactions to Trauma

When terrible things happen, you feel powerful emotions. These feelings aren't fun, but they're perfectly normal and healthy. In fact, *not* getting a big jolt from a traumatic experience is actually abnormal.

Mother Nature has a good reason for making you feel bad when a crisis strikes: She wants you to survive. The strong emotions you feel and the bad memories you form are her way of trying to tell you, "This is a bad thing — don't let it happen again!" (Of course, you can't always follow this advice, because most traumas are beyond your control — but try explaining *that* to Mother Nature.)

Although nearly everyone reacts powerfully when a trauma hits, these reactions fade quickly in some people and persist for a long time in others. In general, reactions to a negative event take three different forms: a normal stress reaction, acute stress, and PTSD. In the following sections, I explain each of these reactions.

The typical stress response

In a typical response to stress, you may experience physical reactions, such as a racing heart or trouble sleeping. And because being upset when something bad occurs is pro-survival, nearly everyone feels some or all of the following emotions when involved in a crisis (see Chapter 5 for an in-depth look at these reactions):

Mental Effects	Emotional Effects	Physical Effects	Relationship Effects
Difficulty concentrating	Anxiety	Increased "startle" response	Hostility
	Fear or terror		Withdrawal
Difficulty remembering some aspects of the trauma or of the time just before or after it occurred	Anger or irritability	Exhaustion	Lack of interest in sexual relations
	Shock	Insomnia	Poor work or school performance
	Grief	Headaches	
	A feeling of being "numb" or "detached"	Nausea and other digestive problems	Blame
Difficulty making decisions	Guilt	Rapid heartbeat	A desire to "nest" — that is, stay home and avoid contact with the outside world
Confusion	A feeling of helplessness	A "spacey" feeling	
Intrusive thoughts about what happened	Alienation	A loss of interest in, or pleasure from, usual activities	Overprotectiveness of family members involved in the trauma
	A feeling of vulnerability		
A sense of disorientation	A feeling of abandonment		

These feelings can be very powerful and may last for days, weeks, or even months, depending in part on the scale of the distressing event. The key factor that differentiates these typical stress responses from the other types of stress reaction is that they typically fade over time instead of staying the same or becoming worse.

Of course, not all post-trauma feelings are bad ones. You may also feel relieved, happy to be alive, and proud of how you handled yourself — as well as stronger for weathering the crisis. Most people feel a mixture of positive and negative feelings, and recognizing them as perfectly normal can really help.

Acute stress disorder

In many cases, people don't just adjust to the "new normal" in the days right after a trauma. As many as one-third of trauma survivors continue to experience very serious symptoms that significantly interfere with their lives instead of fading away in a few days or weeks.

According to the textbook definition, *acute stress disorder* starts within four weeks of a trauma, lasts between two days and a month (if symptoms last longer than that, the diagnosis is PTSD), and causes symptoms so severe that they interfere with a person's ability to handle normal, day-to-day activities. In real life, however, it's not so easy to draw a line on the calendar and say, "This is a typical response to trauma, and this isn't." Deciding whether a symptom is normal or a red flag for serious problems isn't easy, either.

One way doctors make that decision is by looking at how serious symptoms are. Typically, symptoms of acute stress disorder are much more severe than a normal stress reaction. Here's a list of the most common symptoms of acute stress disorder:

- *Dissociation,* in which you may experience changes in your sense of self, your sense of time, and/or your memory; these changes can include

  - Feeling spaced out or in a daze.

  - Feeling like the world around you is unreal. Your sense of time may speed up or slow down, familiar places may seem alien, and people or objects may seem like they don't really exist. Some people say they feel like they're watching a movie rather than living real life.

  - Unusual body sensations, as if you're looking at yourself from a distance or part of your body is split off from another part.

  - A numb feeling, as though your emotions are turned off.

  - Amnesia involving large parts of the trauma or its aftermath.

- Severe anxiety and hypervigilance — that is, an inability to let your guard down

- A strong desire to avoid people, places, or things associated with the trauma

- Flashbacks (see Chapter 3) and nightmares about the event

Giving stress a name: The behind-the-scenes battle over terminology

Pity the poor psychiatrists: They need to clearly define disorders that can't easily be captured on paper. To steal an old folk song lyric, this task is about as easy as trying to catch the wind.

Two good examples showing the difficulty of putting a name to a mental disorder involve acute stress disorder and PTSD. Acute stress disorder becomes PTSD if symptoms last more than a month. However, the *Diagnostic and Statistical Manual (DSM)* — the bible of psychiatry diagnoses — states that to have acute stress disorder, you need to have a symptom called dissociation (feeling disconnected from yourself), which isn't necessary for PTSD.

Why? Because when doctors wrote the definitions for these problems, they thought that dissociation in the early weeks after a trauma strongly predicted PTSD and thus helped to differentiate between normal stress that would fade and abnormal stress that wouldn't. Now, however, many studies fail to support this idea. As a result, some doctors don't think dissociation should be a criterion for acute stress disorder — and some don't think acute stress disorder should even be a diagnosis at all. (Instead, they think all severe post-traumatic stress reactions should fall under the umbrella of PTSD, with different categories for short-term and long-term symptoms.) So don't be surprised if the definitions I outline in this section are passé by the next time psychiatrists revise the *DSM.*

Because acute stress disorder is a risk factor for PTSD, you should tell your doctor if you have any of the symptoms listed. The doc can help you determine whether you're experiencing a normal stress reaction or a response that warrants therapy. But beware: Not all therapies for acute stress disorder are helpful. In Chapter 4, I explain what usually works and what doesn't.

Post-traumatic stress disorder

PTSD has a lot in common with a normal stress reaction; the big difference is that it's a much more powerful response, and it doesn't go away. PTSD also looks a lot like acute stress disorder — in fact, acute stress disorder becomes PTSD, diagnostically speaking, if symptoms last more than a month.

PTSD and acute stress disorder share three key symptoms: intrusive thoughts about the trauma, *hypervigilance* (always feeling like you're on red alert), and avoidance of places, people, or things that remind you of your trauma. One textbook difference between PTSD and acute stress disorder, however, is that the dissociative symptoms of acute stress, which I mention in the preceding section, don't need to be present for a diagnosis of PTSD, although they can be. (The reason for that is a little complicated — see the sidebar in this section on "Giving stress a name: The behind-the-scenes battle over terminology" if you're interested. Just think of PTSD as acute stress disorder that doesn't go away within a month or so after your symptoms begin, and don't worry too much about the details.)

Some general hallmarks of PTSD

If the symptoms you develop after a trauma don't start melting away within one month after they begin, then you may have PTSD. However, having symptoms after the one-month mark doesn't necessarily mean that your symptoms won't improve. Some people experience stress symptoms for several months and then recover completely; others do well at first and have problems later on.

That said, doctors do have some rules of thumb for identifying PTSD when it sets in. Here are two hallmarks of PTSD:

- ✔ **It seriously interferes with your life.** Typically, normal stress reactions are powerful, but they don't stop people from going to work or school, fixing dinner, or shopping for groceries. When PTSD kicks in hard, doing these everyday things can be a challenge.

- ✔ **It lasts a long time.** Doctors who go by the book don't diagnose PTSD until symptoms last at least a month.

The two primary types of PTSD: Simple and complex

Della begins showing symptoms of PTSD after she lives through a huge hurricane that destroys her house and car. Jenny, on the other hand, develops PTSD after suffering more than a decade of abuse at the hands of her stepfather.

Both of these women have the same diagnosis, but they may have very different symptoms and need very different types of therapy. That's because Della is likely to have simple PTSD, which typically stems from a single trauma. Jenny, however, is at risk of developing complex PTSD (sometimes called — how's this for psychiatric jargon? — *disorders of extreme stress, not otherwise specified,* or DESNOS for short). Here's how the two differ:

- ✔ **Simple PTSD:** This type of PTSD typically starts after a single event — for instance, a car accident, a physical attack, or a natural disaster. The symptoms of simple PTSD, which can be mild or serious, match the classic triad of symptoms that I describe in Chapter 3 (intrusive thoughts about the trauma, a nervous system that's always on high alert, and avoidance of reminders of the trauma). Simple PTSD responds well to basic treatments, and cognitive behavioral therapy (see Chapter 9) and related approaches can be quite effective in reducing its symptoms — often without the need for other intervention.

✔ **Complex PTSD:** Complex PTSD can occur when people suffer repeated traumas, particularly when these traumas occur at the hands of another person. It's especially likely to occur if these traumas occur in childhood and involve vicious acts by others (such as torture) or abuse by a close friend or family member. Here are some of the most common causes of complex PTSD:

- Childhood sexual or physical abuse or extreme neglect

- Urban violence — for example, growing up in a gang war zone and witnessing many shootings or other acts of violence

- Chronic abuse at the hands of a spouse or partner

- War-related traumas, including torture, the devastation of a person's community or country, or witnessing acts of genocide

These chronic psychic wounds can change people, both emotionally and physically, in ways that differ from the effects of a single trauma. That's why survivors with complex PTSD often have more symptoms and require a wider variety of interventions than other people with PTSD. It's also why treatments that work well for simple PTSD can sometimes be harmful for people with complex PTSD (see Chapters 8, 9, and 10 for more on treatments).

But take heart — complex PTSD, just like simple PTSD, is treatable. If you have this type of PTSD, finding the right path to healing may just take additional time and work.

A further category breakdown: PTSD types based on symptom duration

Earlier in the chapter, I mention that acute stress disorder lasts from two days to four weeks, at which point it's referred to as PTSD. But there's more: Doctors also divide PTSD into three further categories, based on the duration of the symptoms.

If this classification seems a little silly, it is. In real life, these tidy metrics don't really make sense. But scientists find them handy when they're doing research into PTSD, and these categories may affect your diagnosis or insurance coverage as well. Here's a breakdown of the three official timelines for PTSD:

✔ **Acute post-traumatic stress disorder:** A term used when the duration of symptoms is less than three months

✔ **Chronic post-traumatic stress disorder:** A term used when the duration of symptoms is more than three months

✔ **Delayed post-traumatic stress disorder:** A category describing cases of PTSD in which symptoms don't start until six months or longer after a trauma occurs (a fairly rare event, most often seen in combat vets and people abused as children)

In Chapter 3, I outline the symptoms of PTSD in depth.

Considering Factors That Influence a Person's Response to Trauma

Two vacationers, relaxing after a big day of sightseeing, decide to go out for a late-night snack. As they stroll from their hotel to a pizza joint around the corner, they run into an assailant who robs them at gunpoint.

Two years later, one of the vacationers returns to the same hotel and even pops into the same pizza place for dinner. Asked about the trauma, she shrugs off the incident, saying, "It was pretty scary, but at least nobody got hurt." But she's wrong: Her friend, who also survived the robbery, doesn't stay in hotels any more. He's afraid to travel, suffers terrible dreams about the trauma, and sometimes has flashbacks in which he feels like he's right back there on that dark street, with a gun in his face.

Why did one of these people but not the other develop PTSD symptoms? Forget the idea that it's because one person is stronger or braver than the other. In reality, the more we find out about PTSD, the more we discover that a wide range of factors — none of which has anything to do with being "weak" — can put a person at risk for this problem. In this section, I explain how biology, social supports, the type of trauma, and other factors play a key role in determining who recovers quickly and who develops PTSD.

Pre-trauma facts about you

You're not like anyone else — and that means your risk for PTSD is different from your neighbor's or your best friend's. In fact, a host of variables, from your gender and life history to your brain structure and genes, can affect your odds of developing PTSD. Here's a quick look at some of the factors that play a big role in whether you develop PTSD after a trauma occurs.

Your age

They say you're only as old as you feel, but age isn't just a state of mind with PTSD — it's also one factor that plays a role in whether you develop long-term problems after a trauma. Anyone, young or old, can develop PTSD. However, people in these two categories may be at higher risk:

- ✔ **Young children, especially if a trauma separates them from their families:** Kids often don't have the life experience to prepare them for a crisis or the thinking skills to understand what's happening, and the terror they feel — especially if Mom or Dad isn't there or isn't able to take charge — can be crushing. However, strong support from parents or other family members (either at the time of the crisis or later on) can buffer life's blows to a great degree.

> ✔ **Middle-agers:** This is a surprising high-risk category, but research consistently shows that the 40-to-60 age group is at increased risk for PTSD after a trauma. One possible reason: Because the sandwich generation is dealing with both kids and aging parents, they have more burdens to carry when a trauma strikes.

Seniors, on the other hand, often fare quite well when a crisis hits, especially if they're in good physical shape. A lifetime of surviving hard knocks apparently gives them the perspective they need to deal emotionally with traumas that can leave other people reeling.

Your life circumstances

A mix of different life circumstances can factor into your risk of developing lasting problems after a traumatic experience. Here's a sampling:

> ✔ **You have a lot of stress on your plate.** Here's one that pretty much goes without saying: If you have a huge pile of stress weighing you down already, a big life crisis can be the final straw — so the bigger your sack of troubles before a trauma, the greater your PTSD risk.

> ✔ **You're coping with a mental health disorder.** Not surprisingly, if you're dealing with psychiatric issues before a trauma happens — for instance, if you're depressed or have an anxiety disorder — a trauma is more likely to knock you for a loop.

> ✔ **You're a parent.** Being a mommy or daddy can add to your risk of having a long-term reaction to a trauma. That's probably because — as any parent knows — you worry more about your kids than yourself.

> ✔ **You aren't financially stable.** Money problems can make any crisis more traumatic because they add an extra layer of stress ("How can I afford new furniture now that ours is ruined?" "What'll we do about the doctor bills?"). If you're well-to-do, on the other hand, you have a lower PTSD risk. In large part, that's because a natural disaster doesn't affect you as much financially, and you can call on a lot of help to get your life back on track. Higher education also reduces your risk a bit.

> ✔ **You tend to see the glass as half-empty.** Several personality traits — for instance, a negative outlook on life or paranoia — appear to up your risk of getting PTSD; a sunny and optimistic personality may reduce your risk. Even the most Pollyanna-ish of people can develop PTSD, however, if a trauma is big enough or you have enough other risk factors.

In addition to the preceding personal situations, your ethnic group weighs in as well — different ethnic groups have differing risks for PTSD, possibly due to cultural or socioeconomic factors.

Your gender

Women are more than twice as likely as men to develop PTSD when a trauma involves a physical assault, whether it's a sexual assault or another form of violent attack. Many studies (although not all) also show that women react more strongly to other forms of trauma, such as natural disasters.

Why does gender cause such a big difference in a person's risk for PTSD? No one knows for sure, but here are some reasons scientists suggest:

- ✔ Women are physically smaller, so any crisis threatens their safety more — especially if it's a physical assault.

- ✔ Rape, one of the most terrible of traumas, affects far more women than men.

- ✔ Women often react even more strongly than men if a crisis involves their children.

- ✔ Xena the Warrior Princess aside, women tend to be less aggressive than men. Thus, when they experience a physical assault, they're less likely to be an active participant and are more likely to feel a lack of control over the situation.

- ✔ There's some evidence that the higher your rate of empathy for other people's suffering, the higher your risk of PTSD after a trauma — and although guys can be sensitive, too, women have a big edge when it comes to empathy.

- ✔ Women often have different symptoms than men. For instance, women may exhibit more stress — an easily-identified PTSD symptom — while men may turn to drugs or alcohol or may exhibit more anger. In addition, women often are more willing to own up to PTSD symptoms than men are. (Maybe it's the John Wayne macho prohibition against appearing weak that holds men back.) Thus, doctors probably find diagnosing PTSD in women to be easier.

Here's another odd gender-related tidbit, for what it's worth: If you're a woman, having a spouse in the house actually can increase your PTSD risk when a crisis happens, especially if your hubby is highly stressed. The reverse, however, isn't true: Men fare just as well if there's a better half in the picture.

Your genes

Genes appear to play a role in PTSD, but no single "PTSD gene" gets the blame when someone can't bounce back after a terrible life crisis. Instead, scientists speculate that a host of different genes — probably in different combinations in different folks — interact to increase or decrease the risk of PTSD, possibly by altering levels of brain chemicals associated with stress.

So far, experts don't have any hard data to pin down any specific genetic culprits. However, they have indirect evidence (based on studies of twins) that genes influence PTSD risk. Twin studies are neat because they allow scientists to compare identical twins (who share all their genes) to fraternal twins (who share half) and to non-twin siblings. By doing this, scientists can unravel the effects of genes and upbringing.

Most twin studies of PTSD rely on info from the Vietnam Era Twin Registry, and these investigations show a substantial effect of genes. One study of civilian male and female twins reported similar findings. In addition, studies show a strong influence of genes on PTSD-related problems such as alcoholism, drug dependence, panic disorder, and depression.

Your biochemistry

Best anyone can tell, PTSD stems from a normal stress reaction that just doesn't know when to quit. In other words, a person's internal stress switch gets stuck in the *on* position in PTSD because the normal mechanisms that flip this switch to *off* aren't working.

Just as with genes, scientists can't point a finger to any single chemical that goes haywire in the same way in every person with PTSD. However, some clues do point to abnormal levels of certain natural body chemicals as a risk factor for PTSD symptoms. For instance, researchers know that the fight or flight hormone, adrenaline (also called epinephrine), plays a key role (see Chapter 5 for a discussion of its effects and how new medical treatments may help to block them). So, most likely, does a hormone called cortisol (see the nearby sidebar "The cortisol connection"). Somewhere along the line, the feedback loops that control these and related chemicals go haywire, sending out too much or too little of them. Genes, life experiences, gender, and other factors add into the mix, increasing or lowering the risk that the chain of events kicked off by a trauma will end in PTSD.

Your brain structure

When researchers look at the brains of people with and without PTSD, they see some interesting differences. However, there's a big chicken-and-egg problem: Do these differences *increase your risk for PTSD,* or do they *result from PTSD?* It's a question experts can't answer for sure yet, although they have some clues.

One of the most consistent findings in people with PTSD is that many of them have a smaller-than-average *hippocampus.* The hippocampus (see Figure 2-1) is a little seahorse-shaped part of the brain. There's one on the left side of your brain and one on the right. This little brain region is a hard worker whose main job is to help you store new memories. Unfortunately, it's also highly susceptible to stress.

But here's the question: Does the stress of a trauma and its aftermath cause the hippocampus to shrink in people with PTSD, or is it the other way around? That is, are people with small hippocampi (that's the plural) more prone to develop PTSD after a trauma? Or — another possibility — could a mix of both scenarios occur?

Here are some studies that come down on different sides of this issue:

✔ A few years ago, a twin study looked at two groups of men. The first group included Vietnam vets who developed PTSD and their non-vet twins who didn't have PTSD. In the second group were vets who *didn't* develop PTSD and their non-vet twins (who also didn't have PTSD).

The study found that the military vets with PTSD had smaller hippocampi than the vets without PTSD (no surprise there). But here's the kicker: *their non-combat twins also had smaller hippocampi* than either the non-PTSD military vets or their twins. So this study clearly pointed to a small hippocampus as a risk factor for PTSD.

✔ On the flip side, many studies show that chronic elevation of cortisol, a stress-related hormone (see the preceding section), can damage brain cells and lead to a smaller hippocampus. These studies point the finger at the trauma itself and the resulting stress as the causes of hippocampal shrinkage.

To complicate the picture even more, some studies show differences in the size or function of other brain areas in people with PTSD. One key region that may be different in people with PTSD is the *amygdala* (see Figure 2-1), which alerts you to "watch out!" if something scary happens.

The short story is that in some but not all people with PTSD, experts see significant differences in brain structure or function. But until they sort out the chicken-and-egg question, no one will really know what it all means. They can say, however, that the symptoms of PTSD mesh in several ways with abnormalities in these brain areas. For instance, many people with PTSD have memory problems that can go hand-in-hand with impaired hippocampal function, and abnormalities in either the structure or function of the amygdala can trigger abnormal fear or anger responses.

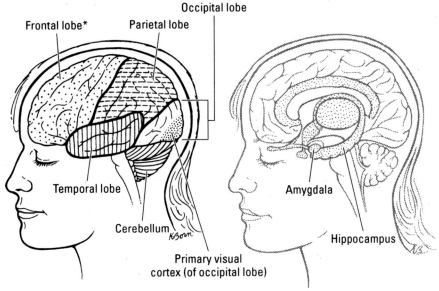

Occipital lobe

Frontal lobe*   Parietal lobe

Temporal lobe

Cerebellum

Amygdala

Hippocampus

Primary visual
cortex (of occipital lobe)

Figure 2-1:
The hippo-
campus and
amygdala,
two regions
of the brain
associated
with PTSD.

*All lobes of the brain are paired structures.

The type of trauma you experience

Traumatic events come in all shapes and sizes, from traffic accidents to tornadoes. Some pass quickly; others last for hours or keep recurring. Mother
Nature gets the blame for many, but human predators cause an enormous
amount of suffering as well.

Each trauma is one-of-a-kind, and some events have more potential to do
long-term psychic damage than others. Here are some of the key factors that
influence how traumatic a trauma is in terms of causing PTSD symptoms:

- ✔ **The severity of your trauma:** A trauma that ends quickly, with no lasting
  physical injuries to anyone, usually doesn't pack as much PTSD punch
  as one that causes injuries or deaths — especially when these terrible
  events involve loved ones.

  Traumas that cause long-term physical pain also up the odds for PTSD,
  as do life crises that cause serious financial problems — for instance, a
  flood that washes away a person's house, an earthquake that destroys a
  family business, or a hurricane that devastates an entire community.
  Traumas that separate a child from Mommy or Daddy can also raise the
  odds of long-term reactions.

✔ **The cause of your trauma:** If Mother Nature shattered the calm of your life in the form of a hurricane or an earthquake, that's bad enough. What's worse, however, is a trauma caused by another human being, such as a sexual assault or an armed robbery. Worse yet is an attack by someone you love and trust (for instance, a sexual assault by a parent or a trusted friend), especially if this betrayal occurs when you're very young.

✔ **The surprise factor:** Traumas that strike with no warning are riskier than the ones that offer at least a little heads-up. For instance, if TV newscasters warn you for days that a hurricane's coming, the actual event may shock you far less than a trauma that catches you totally off-guard. However, if an expected catastrophe hits much harder than you anticipate, the shock can be overwhelming — as when Hurricane Katrina struck New Orleans.

✔ **The degree to which the trauma violated your personal boundaries:** Your body belongs to you and you alone, and you should feel safe in your own skin. If a sexual assailant or armed robber attacks you, the shock of this breach to your personal boundaries can increase the odds of developing serious PTSD symptoms. That's why rape is one of the leading causes of serious PTSD symptoms.

✔ **The number of traumas you've suffered:** If you already survived one trauma, you may be at greater risk for PTSD when a second one occurs — even if the second trauma is entirely unrelated. The worst-case scenario occurs when people suffer repeated traumas for weeks, months, or years (for instance, if they live with an abusive spouse or suffer years of abuse as a child). This repeated trauma can set a person up for complex PTSD, which can cause more-severe symptoms than simple PTSD (see the earlier section "The two primary types of PTSD: Simple and complex").

On the other hand, getting through a natural disaster can sometimes make you better-prepared if another, similar crisis strikes. (And interestingly, veterans with PTSD actually reported having fewer symptoms in the aftermath of September 11. Nobody's sure why, but one guess is that the sense of patriotism and togetherness reduced their sense of isolation. That's in line with evidence that increased social support can reduce PTSD symptoms.)

✔ **The chance that the trauma will reoccur:** After September 11, people close to Ground Zero battled two emotional stressors: the aftereffects of the World Trade Center collapse and the fear that terrorists may be planning another attack. The massive initial trauma created a huge risk for PTSD, and being on red alert for weeks afterward magnified that risk.

Similarly, people victimized by stalkers or abusive spouses, or fighting in an ongoing war, can't simply relax and recover from a first trauma because they know the next one may be waiting in the wings. Their chronic hypervigilance ups the odds of symptoms setting in for the long run.

The strong link between war and PTSD

Combat is the perfect storm of risk factors for PTSD, so it's no surprise that nearly 10 percent of combat soldiers returning from current battle zones have at least some PTSD symptoms. War is a mix of primal fear, physical and emotional stress, guilt at taking lives even if the cause is just, and anger or grief when comrades die. It's intense, it often involves multiple traumas, and there's no chance to say, "Okay, I've had enough — I'm outta here." Add in often-primitive living conditions, the tender age of many combatants, and their worries about returning to "the world" — especially a world that rarely gives combat veterans their due — and it's easy to see why PTSD injures more soldiers than combat itself.

A few features of combat trauma, however, actually reduce the risk of PTSD or increase the odds of getting early diagnosis and treatment. Among these protective factors are the following:

- Soldiers in battle are in it together and can offer each other powerful moral support.

- Soldiers in today's volunteer military may feel more committed to their job and the cause they're fighting for than soldiers back in the days of the draft.

- Doctors look harder for signs of PTSD in veterans than in civilians, so getting a diagnosis is sometimes easier if you're a vet.

By the way, one misconception about PTSD in vets is that it happens only to people who directly experience combat. However, people in non-combat roles can experience severe trauma as well. Doctors and nurses in field hospitals, for instance, can be overwhelmed by the terrible injuries they see and the grief of losing many of their young patients — along with the guilt they feel over not being able to save every life. (Intellectually, they know that's not possible, but the mind doesn't always listen to facts.)

Not all people traumatized by war wear uniforms, of course. Armed conflicts also create an epidemic of PTSD among people uprooted from their homes, injured or terrified by bombings, and threatened with starvation or financial ruin. More than most other traumas, war turns entire communities upside down, leaving people with desperate needs and nowhere to turn for help, so you can easily see why the wounds of war don't always heal when peace arrives.

After the trauma: The influence of others

Whatever problems you face, from minor setbacks to major life crises, good buddies and loving family members can help you cope. That's especially true when an overwhelming trauma strikes and you need all the help you can get.

Studies show that strong support from friends and family, both before and after a trauma, can lower your odds of developing PTSD. That makes sense because your loved ones can offer moral support, healing humor, a sympathetic sounding board, and a lot of practical help — from dealing with insurers to keeping your groceries stocked or watching your kids.

Of course, that doesn't mean you'll get PTSD if you don't have a lot of connections. It does mean, however, that you should tally up your human resources after a trauma — whether it's a church group, your co-workers, or close friends and family — and see who you can call on for aid and assistance.

The opposite side of this coin, of course, is that an abusive or unsupportive family can up your risk for PTSD. (That's why your best bet is to avoid toxic people as much as possible, especially if your life is in chaos after a trauma — see Chapter 7 for details.) It appears, too, that wonderful parents can also have kids at higher-than-normal risk for PTSD if the parents themselves suffered a terrible event. For example, children of Holocaust survivors have an increased risk of PTSD, possibly because hearing their parents' stories stripped these children of their sense of security very early in life.

On a larger scale, how well you fare after a trauma also depends on how your community and your society treat you. If your neighbors (or your country) can grasp the magnitude of the suffering you experienced, express their gratitude if your trauma occurred in the line of duty, and support you as you recover, then the odds are strongly in your favor. If not, however, your risk of PTSD can climb steeply.

Other points to remember about risk factors

At this point, you may feel worried if you have several of the PTSD risk factors I list. If so, make sure you remember three things:

✔ **Risk factors aren't destiny.** If you don't have PTSD now, the odds are against your developing the disorder if you experience a major life crisis — even if you have quite a few of the risk factors I outline in this chapter. And if you *do* have PTSD, none of these factors will prevent you from progressing on your path to healing.

✔ **Many risk factors aren't cast in stone.** For example, one of the most powerful risk factors is lack of social support — and that's a factor you can change. If you live alone or your friends and family aren't supportive, you can make new connections through support groups, recreation centers, church groups, or even online communities. Granted, making friends when you're overcoming PTSD isn't always easy, but the benefits can be well worth the effort.

✔ **Research findings about risk factors are actually good news for you because this information may lead to new treatments or even cures.** For instance, identifying some people's wacky cortisol reactions to stress is helping doctors develop new drugs to rein these reactions in. As they say, every cloud has a silver lining — and the lining here is that insights into the roots of problems can jumpstart the process of solving them.

The wounds of war

During the Vietnam War, half a million soldiers — many of them kids still in their teens — faced unmentionable terrors in faraway jungles and then returned to a torn nation where their former friends spat on them and called them "baby killers." The horrors of the war and its aftermath left many of these young soldiers trapped by PTSD for years — or even for the rest of their lives.

One study showed just how destructive society's failure to support these veterans was. Collecting info from nearly 250 Vietnam vets being treated for PTSD, the study's authors found that homecoming stress outranked combat exposure, childhood and non-combat traumas, and other stressful life events as the strongest predictor of PTSD symptoms.

The toxic fallout of these soldiers' traumas included high rates of shame, negative relationships with other people, social withdrawal, and resentment — symptoms that stemmed both from the horrors they saw at war and the terrible injustice done to them when they came home deserving a welcome and got a cold shoulder instead.

The Role That Triggers Play

PTSD plays a lot of tricks with your memory. It can make you forget parts of your trauma (see Chapter 3 for info on the amnesia that can accompany PTSD). It can cause *time skew,* in which the chronological order of events during a trauma gets mixed up in a person's mind (many kids with PTSD experience time skew — see Chapter 3). It can also mess with your short-term memory, making it hard to remember to pick up the dry cleaning or take the dog for a walk (see Chapter 12 for ways to deal with this problem.) But the worst game PTSD plays with your memory is to keep dredging up bad memories and throwing them in your face instead of filing them away in a mental folder marked "over and done with."

Often, traumatic memories lie dormant for days, weeks, or even months, only to resurface when a trigger occurs. This trigger, which can be anything tied to the original trauma, can set off a cascade of physical and emotional reactions that make the trauma survivor experience the horror of the event all over again. This situation is called *traumatic coupling* — in the survivor's mind, the trigger is so powerfully connected to the original trauma that it cues the same response the trauma caused.

Sometimes, spotting a trigger is easy. For instance, survivors of car accidents often feel their hearts pound and their anxiety levels soar if they see pictures of crashes on the news. Other times, figuring out what's setting off symptoms takes some detective work. (For example, one teen realized that the smell of chlorine awakened memories of her assault, which happened in the restroom at a public swimming pool.)

Here are some of the most common types of triggers:

- **Sensory triggers:** Sensory memories are very potent, and they can bring back a flood of other memories. For a person with PTSD, triggers may include

  - Sounds such as fireworks, sirens, a car backfiring, thunder, or a person screaming in a movie

  - Sights such as a dented car fender, a fallen tree, light shining at a certain angle, a billboard resembling one at the trauma scene, or a photo of someone who looks like the perp who assaulted the trauma survivor

  - Tastes such as a food that a war vet once ate in-country or a spice that reminds a survivor of the dinner she ate just before the trauma occurred

  - Odors such as the aroma of the aftershave worn by an attacker or a whiff of freshly mowed grass that brings back memories of being attacked in the park

  - Sensations involving touch, such as a turtleneck that revives memories of being choked or a watchband that brings back a feeling of being restrained; some women recovering from a sexual trauma discover that an infant's contact during breastfeeding is a trigger

- **Actions:** For instance, running a sprint in a phys ed class may trigger memories of trying to escape from an attacker.

- **Physically painful experiences:** Experiences such as dental procedures or the sight of blood can trigger bad memories.

- **Dates:** Anniversaries of the trauma — or important dates, such as a wedding anniversary associated with someone the survivor lost in the traumatic event — can trigger PTSD.

- **Stresses or emotions associated with the trauma:** For instance, if a person experienced extreme terror during a bank hold-up, any event that causes fear — such as a near-miss on the freeway — can trigger a flashback. If a trauma destroyed a person's home or car, later financial stressors, even mild ones, can trigger feelings of helplessness and fear.

- **Legal proceedings following the trauma:** Legal proceedings can be triggers especially if the survivor needs to testify against an assailant.

- **Sexual intercourse or intimate touching (kissing, hugging):** Such contact may trigger PTSD if the trauma involved sexual or physical assault.

- **Milestones (such as reaching the teen years or heading off to college):** Because these events bring on a flurry of emotions, they're big culprits when it comes to dredging up memories. The onset of puberty can also be a trigger if a trauma involved sexual abuse.

These triggers stir up deeply disturbing emotions, which is why people with PTSD go out of their way to avoid them. However, triggers have a big upside: They're the key your therapist can use to unlock the door to your trauma and help you face it head-on and overcome it. In fact, confronting these triggers in the safety of the therapeutic setting is almost always the first step in healing from PTSD (see Chapters 8 and 10 for more info).

Chapter 3

Spotting the Clues: Signs and Symptoms of PTSD

In This Chapter

▶ Understanding the three core symptoms of PTSD

▶ Knowing the medical problems that often accompany PTSD

▶ Figuring out why PTSD symptoms are different for kids

*T*alk to a dozen people with PTSD, and you hear a dozen different stories about what it's like. Here's a sample:

> *I don't date anymore. Just thinking about getting close to someone romantically makes me feel sick.*

> *When I see a news story about a shooting, I feel my heart in my throat. It's like I'm right in the middle of the robbery again.*

> *I feel so cut off from everyone. My kids say, "You just don't care." And you know what? Sometimes they're right.*

These stories don't sound at all alike — but dig deeper, and you start to see common threads in each person's life. Doctors can weave these threads into a description that helps them spot PTSD, even though each person with this problem has a one-of-a-kind story.

Before looking closely at the actual symptoms, though, a doctor who suspects PTSD considers three general areas, all of which I cover in more detail in Chapter 2:

✔ **Whether a particular event (or series of events) kicked off the patient's symptoms:** PTSD always follows a trauma.

✔ **How long the symptoms have lasted:** The duration of the symptoms helps indicate whether the symptoms point to a normal stress reaction, an acute stress reaction, or PTSD.

✔ **The severity of the patient's symptoms:** PTSD isn't just a nuisance; it's a major problem that affects every aspect of life.

After weighing these factors, doctors look for specific clusters of symptoms that spell PTSD. In this chapter, I look at these symptoms as well as additional symptoms — both mental and physical — that aren't part of the core diagnosis but often come along for the ride. I also discuss how symptoms of PTSD can look very different in children and teens than they do in adults.

The Traumatized Person's Reality: Three Core Symptoms

Every medical disorder has its own signature, a pattern of symptoms that allows doctors to make a diagnosis and plan a treatment approach. In the case of PTSD, doctors look for three specific symptoms, which I explore in the following sections. *Every* person with PTSD displays these three core symptoms in some form:

- ✔ Intrusive thoughts
- ✔ Avoidance
- ✔ Hyperarousal

Recurring, intrusive thoughts

Normally, you can easily brush aside an unpleasant thought. If you have PTSD, however, thoughts and emotions force their way into your mind, leaving you completely at their mercy.

The intrusive thoughts that occur in PTSD almost always cause a strong surge of emotion — anger, fear, humiliation, helplessness. When you're asleep, they can show up as nightmares. In the daytime, they pull you away from present time, sometimes making you behave in ways that don't make sense to the people around you. The best-known type of these intrusions — although not everyone with PTSD experiences it — is a flashback.

A *flashback* is a memory from your trauma that intrudes into the here-and-now, making you feel like you're right back in the past. Flashbacks typically contain random bits and pieces of information — a sound, an odor, the color of a bystander's umbrella — rather than full-fledged memories. That's one reason it's hard to make sense of these blasts from the past or gain control over them without a therapist's help in understanding them and putting them in context.

Flashbacks usually involve sights and sounds (as when a soldier sees and hears the sounds of a long-ago battle) — but they can also include smells, tastes, or sensations of touch. Sometimes a flashback just won't go away. Here are some examples:

- Sheree, who survived a bad car accident years before, is sitting in rush-hour traffic when she suddenly finds it impossible to shake the thought "I need to escape right now, before something terrible happens." She has to force herself to stay in her car, when all she wants to do is run.

- Damon, a Vietnam vet, is setting a trap for a backyard gopher when he feels an overwhelming wave of fear and nausea. The trigger: the animal's hole in the ground, which caused Damon to flash back to his days as a "tunnel rat" assigned to crawl into booby-trapped tunnels containing enemy weapons caches.

Not all intrusive thoughts involve sensory flashbacks, however. Often, people with PTSD have other types of negative thoughts — for instance, "Other people are out to get me" or "Nothing goes right for me" — that stem from the trauma.

If you have PTSD, other people may mistakenly believe that a flashback or other intrusive thought is "all in your head." What they don't understand is that in reality, your whole body — not just your mind — gets in on the game. For instance, if you have a frightening flashback, your heart usually beats faster and your palms often sweat. That's because you're not just thinking about the past; you're reliving it.

Avoidance and numbing

After a trauma, you desperately want your terrible feelings to go away — but when PTSD strikes, unpleasant emotions don't just pack their bags and leave. In fact, they often grow even stronger over time, causing you intense distress. In order to cope, your mind tries to block or avoid these bad feelings with the intention of protecting you from the hurt. These mind games may lead you to change your behavior in different ways, such as the following methods:

- You may avoid going to the scene of your trauma or to places that resemble it.

- You may avoid activities involved in the trauma. For instance, if your trauma occurred in a restaurant, you may stop dining out.

- You may block out key parts of the trauma. (This blocking is called *psychogenic amnesia*.)

A time-machine trip for one

It was the busiest day of the holiday shopping season, and Lily had her hands full at the sales counter. Suddenly, a man stepped in front of her and demanded, "Where's the digital camera in your ad? I made a special trip to get it, and you'd better have it."

The threatening tone of his voice — just like the tone of the man who assaulted her — caused Lily to flash back to the night of her assault. Suddenly, she wasn't standing in a department store. She was in her bedroom, with a stranger in a ski mask in front of her.

Panicking, Lily shoved the startled customer in the chest, knocking him into the woman behind him. She turned and ran blindly toward the exit,

her heart pounding. After a few steps, the flashback faded and she realized what had happened. Behind her, she heard the angry man say, "I ought to sue this store" — and she wondered whether she'd still have a job at the end of the day.

Lily's actions made perfectly good sense, given the vision she saw in front of her — but they didn't make any sense to the camera-seeking customer or the boss who wound up giving him a huge discount in the hopes of forestalling a lawsuit. Like Lily, many people with PTSD experience flashbacks that can cause behavior that looks odd, rude, or even crazy to people who aren't along for the trip-back-in-time.

✔ You may resist taking legal action in a case involving the perpetrator of your trauma for fear that your feelings will resurface.

✔ You may avoid watching television or movies for fear of seeing scenes that remind you of your trauma.

✔ You may find it hard to fall asleep because you worry that nightmares will dredge up the fears you're trying to suppress. (And then, when you're awake, all you want to do is sleep as a means of escape from the thoughts that plague you. It's a real Catch-22!)

A related problem that occurs in PTSD is *emotional anesthesia,* a different trick your mind uses to help you avoid pain. It works to some degree — but it also makes feeling the emotions you *want* to feel more difficult. For example, people who viewed themselves as outgoing, fun, warm, and loving before a trauma often say that they now have trouble feeling an emotional attachment to others or reacting in a normal way to life events. Here are some results of this emotional distancing:

✔ **It hurts relationships.** You may find connecting with friends and family to be difficult, or you may find sexual relations and intimacy unpleasant or simply boring. If you have children or a partner, they can mistake your emotional numbness for a lack of caring.

✔ **It steals your joy in life.** You may lose interest in hobbies and recreational activities that you once enjoyed deeply. In addition, you may think, "What's the point?" when it comes to celebrating a special occasion or looking your best.

Emotional anesthesia can also make it harder for you to conjure up the emotions or enthusiasm you need to envision your future. As a result, you may find yourself thinking, "Who cares what happens next year? I might not even be here." The fancy term for this kind of thinking is *foreshortening,* which means that you have difficulty planning ahead and picturing where you'll be in years to come. Here are some signs of foreshortening:

✔ **Short-circuited goals:** You may abandon your long-term career plans and instead settle for something that pays the day-to-day bills. Also, you may focus on short-term romantic attachments instead of cultivating meaningful relationships.

✔ **Loss of interest in your health:** If you can't picture yourself being around in 15 or 20 years, you may eat poorly, stop exercising, resume smoking, or develop alcohol or substance abuse issues.

Hyperarousal and (possibly) panic attacks

When Germaine hears a car backfire, he starts shaking. Kim nearly jumps out of her skin if the dog barks suddenly. Jack's kids think he's an ogre because he can't tolerate their shrieks of joy when they're roughhousing.

All three of these PTSD sufferers show signs of hyperarousal, a hallmark of PTSD. Their nervous systems stay on red alert all the time, and they can't let their guard down and relax. This situation causes a range of problems that affect their relations with other people and their general well-being, such as

✔ Chronic irritability

✔ Quickness to anger

✔ A feeling that if they just relax and let go, something terrible may happen

✔ Difficulty sleeping or even resting

✔ Exhaustion stemming from nervous-system overload

✔ Heart palpitations, sweaty palms, and other types of reactions triggered by a fight-or-flight reaction when a trigger occurs (see Chapter 2 for a discussion of triggers)

The brain's equation: Less feeling = less pain

Scare an opossum half to death, and it rolls over and plays dead. The same is true for a bird caught in a cat's mouth or a mouse trapped by a hawk — and something very similar can also happen to you if you experience a trauma.

When a big scare first happens, your nervous system sends you the message "Run away!" or in some cases, "Fight!" If you can't do either, it offers a third option: "Freeze." As a result, your muscles feel stiff or slack and your body feels numb. Time seems to slow down, and a strange calmness descends on you. Your brain, expecting the worst, is trying to cushion the end it thinks is coming.

If you survive your terrible scare, this reaction usually fades away. However, in PTSD, elements of this freezing response hang on, and they can lead to a numb, surreal, wrapped-in-cotton feeling.

Hyperarousal often leads to *panic attacks,* which cause any, some, or all of the following symptoms:

- ✔ Lightheadedness, as if you may faint
- ✔ A feeling that the outside world is spinning
- ✔ A rapid, irregular heartbeat
- ✔ Shallow breathing
- ✔ Tingling fingers
- ✔ Flushed skin
- ✔ Nausea
- ✔ A feeling as if you're choking or suffocating
- ✔ An urgent and intense need to run away
- ✔ A powerful urge to scream
- ✔ A fear that you're dying or going crazy

Panic attacks can strike at any time, even when things are going along smoothly. They can lead to a vicious cycle, making a person with PTSD fearful of going to any location where a panic attack occurred. In severe cases, this can even lead to agoraphobia — a fear of leaving the house at all. (For info on how therapists can treat the panic attacks that may accompany PTSD, see Chapter 8.)

The Result of Long-Term Trauma: Symptoms of Complex PTSD

If you're a survivor of multiple traumas, such as prolonged sexual or physical abuse or torture, you may have a condition called *complex PTSD* (see Chapter 2 for more on the causes of this disorder). If so, you may experience a number of symptoms that differ from the pattern of simple PTSD stemming from a single trauma.

If you have complex PTSD, realize that one reason you have these symptoms is that *many of them helped you survive.* They may seem frightening or crazy, but during your trauma, these symptoms made perfectly good sense. (For instance, dissociation — feeling detached from your body — can make the experience of childhood sexual abuse easier to survive emotionally.) The trouble is that these symptoms are still hanging around when you need them to go away.

Getting the symptoms of complex PTSD under control is a tougher assignment than managing simple PTSD because complex PTSD reaches deeper into the core of who you are, what you believe, how you feel about yourself and your body, and how you relate to others. Here are some of the problems that often occur in complex PTSD, although not all of them occur in every case:

- **Wild mood swings and out-of-control emotions:** Complex PTSD can leave you confused about your emotions and unable to regulate them. For example, if you were sexually abused as a child, you may react to a loving partner by swinging from seductiveness to shame to violent anger. Extreme depression, anxiety, and suicidal thoughts and behavior are also common.

  People with complex PTSD often exhibit out-of-control behavior as well, including shoplifting, having one-night stands with strangers, gambling away large amounts of money, spending wildly, or participating regularly in dangerous behaviors such as speeding.

- **Dissociation:** When you experience this serious form of emotional numbing, you actually feel detached from your body or yourself, as if your life were happening to someone else. Dissociation is also a common feature in acute stress disorder (see Chapter 2 for more info) and can occur in simple PTSD, but it's more common in complex PTSD. It's your mind's way of saying, "It's okay. This is happening to someone else, not me." But dissociation comes with a severe penalty: It makes you feel like a shadow of a person rather than a real human being.

Going out and beating agoraphobia

Paula Deen, a famous chef with her own TV show, started her cooking career in an unusual way: She made sandwiches in her home and then sent her sons out to sell them. That's because she developed agoraphobia after a series of traumas, including being held at gunpoint during a bank robbery.

Her story is a good example of how agoraphobia can trap a person — and it also offers hope to anyone in the same situation. That's because this charming, vivacious woman eventually overcame her fears and managed to leave her house. But that's not all: She also managed to remarry, build a hugely successful career, and introduce thousands of people to the joys of cheese grits and collard greens.

I can't guarantee the same result for anyone with agoraphobia — especially the part about becoming a famous chef! — but her experience certainly proves that beating agoraphobia and rediscovering the joys of the great, wide world is possible.

✔ **Disturbances in how you feel about yourself and your body:** Complex PTSD often involves multiple assaults on your body or your dignity, and these can leave you with powerful feelings of shame, guilt, helplessness, or self-disgust. These feelings sometimes result in eating disorders, overeating, or self-injury such as cutting or burning yourself.

✔ **Distorted feelings about the person who perpetrated your trauma:** One common result of complex PTSD is *Stockholm syndrome,* in which you identify emotionally with the person who traumatized you and defend the person's actions. For example, you may stay with a spouse who abuses you, justify his actions, and protect him from arrest, even if you can safely escape the situation. (The name of this syndrome stems from a bank robbery in Stockholm, Sweden, in 1973, during which the hostages — held for days under terrifying circumstances — became emotionally attached to their captors.)

✔ **Alterations in your feelings toward other people:** If you have complex PTSD, you may be distrustful, afraid to let other people in your life, extremely jealous, or overly needy.

✔ **Loss of meaning in your life:** Complex PTSD can leave you feeling deep despair and hopelessness and make it hard for you to have faith in people or the goodness of life.

To triumph over complex PTSD, you need the help of a dedicated treatment team that can address each of your symptoms effectively. You also need to have courage and faith, because although progress will happen, seeing major progress can take time.

Body Language: Aches and Pains That May Accompany PTSD

Sometimes the first person who spots PTSD is a specialist who's looking for an entirely different medical problem, such as a heart condition or a digestive disturbance. That's because the chemical changes that are part and parcel of PTSD can affect many areas of the body, causing a wide range of symptoms. Certain medical problems, too, have a strong association with PTSD.

The most common physical symptoms of PTSD stem from hyperarousal or panic attacks (see "Hyperarousal and [possibly] panic attacks," earlier in this chapter, for more on these topics). These symptoms can include fast heartbeat, hyperventilation (rapid, shallow breathing that can make you feel faint or panicky), sweating, trembling, and lightheadedness.

In addition to isolated symptoms, certain diseases and disorders are often linked to PTSD. If you're wondering why, the answer is *we don't know*. Doctors who treat PTSD have a lot of chicken-or-egg questions, and this is one of them. PTSD seems to increase the risk of some medical problems, such as cardiovascular disease; but in some cases, a preexisting disease possibly ups the odds that person will develop PTSD or worsens symptoms when they occur. (For example, sleep apnea — which causes breathing problems during sleep — may increase your risk of panic attacks, nightmares, and insomnia if you have PTSD.)

The following medical problems aren't universal in PTSD, and they're not part of the basic diagnosis, but they do go hand-in-hand with PTSD fairly frequently:

- Cardiovascular problems, such as high blood pressure; PTSD is also linked to an increased risk for heart attacks.

- Chronic pain, such as that occurring in fibromyalgia (muscle pain) or headaches. Interestingly, however, many people with PTSD exhibit a *reduced* sense of pain.

- Stomach pain, irritable bowel syndrome, heartburn, or chronic diarrhea or constipation.

- Autoimmune disorders such as arthritis, asthma, or skin problems. These disorders occur when the body mistakes its own tissues for an invader and starts fighting its own cells.

- Obesity. According to a 2006 study by a PTSD center at a VA hospital, "Overweight and obesity among our male veterans with PTSD strikingly exceeded national findings."

- Pregnancy complications. One study hinted that women with PTSD may have more problems in pregnancy, such as miscarriage, severe nausea, or preterm contractions.

Double trouble: Why PTSD and other medical disorders often go together

Scientists are exploring the reasons PTSD raises the odds of several medical disorders. Here are some of their theories:

✔ PTSD alters levels of stress-related chemicals and other brain messenger chemicals. This change can set off a cascade of additional changes downstream, affecting multiple organs and possibly altering immune system function.

✔ Abnormal elevations of stress hormones may simply wear down the cardiovascular system over time.

✔ Because people with PTSD have trouble coping with the present and often find the future hard to plan for, they can easily fall into unhealthy habits such as overeating, smoking, and lack of exercise — and these in turn can lead to health issues.

✔ The same chemicals that affect the brain often affect the digestive system in very powerful ways. (That's why the digestive system is dubbed the "second brain.") Thus, the chemical changes that upset your mind can also play havoc with your digestion.

Psychological Disorders That Sometimes Hitch a Ride with PTSD

Rates of coexisting psychiatric problems are high in people with PTSD. The reverse is true, too: Rates of PTSD are very high in people with mental disorders. Neither of these facts is really surprising, because PTSD and other mental disorders interweave in the following ways:

✔ If you have a mental disorder, you're more vulnerable to being hurt or exploited because making rational decisions and protecting yourself is sometimes difficult. This makes you an easy target for a trauma and, in turn, for PTSD.

✔ Some mental disorders can impair brain function in ways that may make it harder for you to logically process the memories of a trauma, heightening the risk for PTSD.

✔ PTSD can trigger mental disorders such as depression or eating disorders in people who didn't have these problems before their trauma occurred.

✔ PTSD, like any major life problem, can also worsen symptoms of a preexisting mental disorder.

Different psychological problems often require different treatments, so identifying each problem on your plate — even if all your issues stem from PTSD — can help you and your medical team to come up with the most effective way of tackling each issue.

The good news is that treating either problem — PTSD or the coexisting mental disorder — nearly always leads to improvements in the other problem. For example, getting your PTSD-linked nightmares under control can ease your depression, and treating your depression, in turn, can give you the energy and positive attitude you need to succeed in your therapy for PTSD. The bottom line: Just as your problems go hand-in-hand, so do their solutions.

In the following sections, I discuss some of the most common psychological issues that can crop up in people with PTSD.

Depression

As many as 50 percent of people with PTSD have enough symptoms to warrant a second diagnosis of depression. We don't know why these two disorders often co-occur, but here are two logical explanations:

- ✔ PTSD can change the biochemistry and even the structure of the brain in ways that may also promote depression (see Chapter 2).
- ✔ PTSD makes life rough and plays havoc with careers and relationships. Sad life events, in turn, up the risk for depression.

Teasing out the symptoms of PTSD and depression can be tricky for doctors, but differentiating between the two may result in more effective treatment. Symptoms of depression include the following:

- ✔ Apathy
- ✔ Inability to concentrate
- ✔ A sense of hopelessness
- ✔ Insomnia or oversleeping
- ✔ A lack of interest in other people or activities
- ✔ Profound sadness
- ✔ Suicidal thoughts or actions
- ✔ Feelings of worthlessness

If you do receive a diagnosis of depression, *Depression For Dummies* (Wiley) can help you to understand your symptoms and the treatments your doctor may recommend. In some cases, these treatments are the same as those for PTSD. In others, they may differ; for instance, doctors are more likely to recommend medications when a patient has significant depression as well as PTSD.

Anxiety disorders

The symptoms of anxiety disorders resemble the symptoms of PTSD (which, after all, is a form of anxiety disorder itself). However, if your symptoms of anxiety are severe enough, fall into a specific category, or existed before your trauma, you may get an additional diagnosis of anxiety disorder. Here are some of the possible diagnoses you may receive:

✔ **Agoraphobia:** If you're afraid to go more than a short distance from your home or can't face leaving your home at all, your doctor will probably decide on agoraphobia as a secondary diagnosis (see more about this topic earlier in this chapter in "Hyperarousal and [possibly] panic attacks").

✔ **Generalized anxiety:** Your doctor may use this diagnosis if you have many disabling worries about a wide range of topics.

✔ **Obsessive-compulsive disorder (OCD):** Symptoms such as rituals and constant checking (for instance, going back to the kitchen six times to make sure you turned off the stove) may call for a diagnosis of OCD. Other symptoms of OCD include an obsession with germs, a compulsive need to touch or count objects, and intrusive negative thoughts.

✔ **Panic disorder:** If you frequently experience disabling panic attacks in which you feel like you're dying or losing your mind, your doctor may give you this diagnosis.

✔ **Social phobia:** An extreme fear of being around other people can warrant this diagnosis.

Some doctors may view problems such as social phobia or agoraphobia as part of your PTSD; others may see them as separate but related issues. Don't worry if the members of your medical team disagree on this score, because it probably won't affect your treatment — the therapy for anxiety disorders is much like that for PTSD. Recognizing severe symptoms of anxiety can aid in your treatment because it can guide your doctor to take even more precautions to create a safe space for you before therapy begins.

Alcohol and/or drug abuse

Rates of alcohol dependence and drug use are sky-high in PTSD. That's not surprising, because the disorder causes a mountain of anxiety, pain, and heartache. When you feel bad, you need relief — and it's easy to fall prey to a temporary form of numbing that causes far more problems down the road.

PTSD can lead to substance abuse problems in people who never struggled with drugs or alcohol, or it can worsen problems that already existed before a trauma. Violent traumas put survivors at especially high risk for developing dependency on alcohol or drugs. The highest-risk groups include veterans, survivors of childhood abuse, and men and women who are victims of rape or physical assault. In contrast, only about 10 percent of people traumatized by natural disasters develop substance abuse problems.

Here are some statistics that shed a little light on the link between PTSD and substance abuse issues:

- ✔ Thirty to 60 percent of people seeking treatment for substance abuse problems also have PTSD.

- ✔ People with severe PTSD symptoms are at greater risk for substance abuse problems than people with mild PTSD symptoms, indicating that drugs and alcohol are used as self-medication.

- ✔ Between 60 and 80 percent of Vietnam vets seeking treatment for PTSD also have alcohol problems.

To understand why millions of people with PTSD fall into the drug or alcohol trap, consider the most prevalent reasons:

- ✔ Drugs and alcohol can temporarily numb the terrible feelings of anxiety, fear, helplessness, hopelessness, loneliness, or anger that overwhelm the person with PTSD.

- ✔ In social situations, drinking or drug use can allow a person to relax and fit in — something that's very difficult when PTSD makes connecting with others a real challenge.

- ✔ Many people with PTSD use alcohol, street drugs, or an excess of prescription drugs in an effort to combat insomnia or keep nightmares at bay.

- ✔ Drinking or drugs can temporarily soothe the pain of injuries that can't completely heal — a common problem for people who suffered a physically painful trauma.

These are powerful reasons to reach for a pill or a bottle of Scotch, so it's not hard to see why so many strong and brave people — soldiers, firefighters, police officers, doctors, paramedics, and millions of other trauma survivors — fall into the snare of substance abuse. It's an easy mistake to make when you're desperate to ease overwhelming suffering.

In Chapter 7, I talk more about the link between PTSD and alcohol or drug issues. For now, the take-home message is that substance abuse — far from being a sign of shame or weakness — is a very common symptom of the medical disorder we call PTSD.

Borderline personality disorder

Borderline personality disorder, or BPD, is a fairly common diagnosis for people with complex PTSD. It's also very controversial because many practitioners believe the symptoms of BPD stem from chronic trauma in a high percentage of cases and should fall under the diagnosis of complex PTSD. Patients may receive a diagnosis of BPD from their doctors if they have five or more of the following symptoms:

- Desperate efforts to avoid real or imaginary abandonment (for example, many stalkers are diagnosed with BPD)
- Intense but unstable relationships, cycling between idealizing and devaluing the other person
- A disturbed self-image or sense of self; many people diagnosed with BPD are chameleon-like, assuming the personality traits they think other people desire them to have
- Impulsive behaviors (for instance, compulsive spending, promiscuous sex, substance abuse, reckless driving, or binge eating)
- Recurring episodes of suicidal behavior, gestures, or threats or self-injurious behavior
- Extreme mood swings
- Chronic feelings of emptiness
- Inappropriate, extreme anger or difficulty controlling anger
- Episodes of paranoia (the feeling that other people are plotting against you) or dissociation (see more on this symptom in "The Result of Long-Term Trauma: Symptoms of Complex PTSD," earlier in this chapter)

As you can see if you read the section on complex PTSD in this chapter, the symptoms of PTSD and BPD overlap quite a bit. Thus, this diagnosis is a judgment call on the part of a doctor or therapist. If you do receive a diagnosis of

BPD, your therapist may suggest a form of therapy called dialectical behavior therapy (which is different from the other treatments I discuss in Chapters 8 and 10 because it combines elements from a variety of psychological therapies). He or she may also suggest medications that can reduce some of your symptoms. However, because dialectical behavior therapy and medication may also play a role in treating complex PTSD, don't assume that your doctor thinks you have BPD just because he or she recommends these approaches.

Self-injury

Some people with PTSD develop a behavior called *self-injury* or *self-mutilation*. Typically, they make superficial cuts, burns, or needle sticks on their arms or other parts of their body. Family members sometimes mistake this act for suicidal behavior, but experts say it's a very different kind of cry for help — a statement saying, "I want to live."

People with PTSD are more likely to injure themselves intentionally if they have these risk factors:

✔ They're female.

✔ They suffered prolonged, severe physical or sexual abuse in childhood.

✔ They have eating disorders or substance abuse problems.

If you engage in self-injury, you may feel very ashamed and alone. However, you should know that self-injury isn't crazy or bad behavior. Rather, it's the only escape route a mind in pain can see at the time — it's your way of dealing with pain when you can't find any other way to cope. Here are some of the reasons people with PTSD engage in self-injury:

✔ **It says, "You're real — and you're alive."** People who feel unreal and disconnected from the world (see the earlier section titled "Avoidance and numbing") can be desperate for any sign that they truly exist, and pain can serve that purpose.

✔ **It helps them forget the bigger pain that won't go away.** The pain caused by self-injury acts as a counterirritant that briefly distracts a person's mind from the greater pain of terrible memories.

✔ **It can create a sense of control.** Intentionally injuring yourself can make you feel like you're in charge of one part of your life at a time when you feel powerless in other areas.

✔ **It creates an artificial emotional high.** Injuring your body releases feel-good chemicals called *endorphins.* These chemicals can help to dampen emotional pain as well. In addition, they help ease tension and anxiety.

- ✔ **It's a way of punishing the "guilty" — even though it actually punishes the innocent.** People who suffered abuse as children may unconsciously feel that they're bad people who deserve to be punished.

- ✔ **It's a way of denying the body.** To a person who lived through years of abuse as a child, the body can seem like an enemy: a source of pain, humiliation, fear, and helplessness. Cutting the body can be a way to deny its existence.

- ✔ **It's an S.O.S.** One legacy of child abuse is secrecy. But terrible secrets insist on battling their way to the surface — and if a person can't talk about her wounds, her mind may use cutting as another way to say, "I need help."

- ✔ **It offers an excuse to receive love.** A person abused as a child didn't get the love and nurturing he needed. He may cut himself in order to provide an excuse to love and nurture himself.

- ✔ **It can serve as a trigger for dissociation.** Earlier, I explain a symptom called dissociation, in which a person mentally disconnects from part of the body or mind. Often, people use self-injury as a way of triggering dissociation so they can temporarily escape from their problems.

Don't let misplaced guilt or shame stop you from seeking help if you develop self-injurious behaviors. Understand that the relief that self-injury brings is fleeting and that the price is terrible. Self-injury is a false solution because it only *adds* to shame and secrecy, increasing the toxic legacy of child abuse or other traumas. If you have this problem, overcome the urge to hide it and instead tell your doctor — therapy can offer you far more effective tools to overcome the pain caused by your trauma.

Eating disorders

Eating disorders have many roots — some genetic, some cultural, and some emotional — and PTSD is one possible trigger. The research is actually a little murky on this topic, with some studies showing a significant connection between PTSD and eating disorders and others showing only a weak link. Overall, however, traumas — especially sexually linked ones — appear to up the risk of developing an eating disorder, particularly if you're female.

The eating disorder that's linked most strongly to PTSD is *bulimia nervosa.* People with this disorder binge on food and then vomit, exercise excessively, or use laxatives to avoid gaining weight. Doctors also see a high rate of compulsive overeating in patients with PTSD. *Anorexia nervosa,* a serious food disorder in which people literally starve themselves, has weaker ties to PTSD.

The idea that a trauma can lead to bulimia or compulsive overeating (and perhaps to anorexia) may seem strange, but the link actually makes sense. Here's why:

- ✓ **Overeating and eating disorders can offer distraction from problems you don't want to face.** When you're focused on food (either eating it or avoiding it), you don't have as much time to worry about other things — such as past traumas, present fears, or worries about the future. Thus, overeating or eating disorders can make major problems fade into the background, at least temporarily — although they do so at a great price.

- ✓ **Overeating or eating disorders can be a way of distancing other people.** People victimized by a trauma involving sexual assault or abuse may want to reduce the risk that they'll suffer similar pain again. One way is to attempt to make themselves appear less attractive by gaining or losing large amounts of weight. The message they're unconsciously sending: "Don't notice me as a sexual being, and maybe you won't hurt me."

- ✓ **Eating disorders create a false sense of control.** A person who's controlling her weight through binging, purging, or starving herself feels like she's totally in charge of one aspect of her life. She may use this behavior to restore the sense of control and security she lost when crisis struck.

A Whole Different Ballgame: PTSD Symptoms in Children and Teens

In some ways, kids are just little people, and teens are just younger versions of adults. In other ways, however, the under-20 crowd is very different from their elders. (If you don't believe it, just look at their taste in clothes and music!) When it comes to diagnosing PTSD, some of the adult rules apply to children and teens, and some don't.

Here's what's the *same* for both kids and adults (see Chapter 2 for full explanations):

- ✓ PTSD stems from a specific trauma or series of traumas.
- ✓ Symptoms must last for a month in order to get a diagnosis of PTSD.

The *symptoms* that children and teens with PTSD show, however, aren't always the same as those that adults exhibit. In this section, I describe extra clues that savvy doctors look for in the younger set. Note that any child may show a handful of these symptoms at one time or another — so don't be overly concerned if your child exhibits several if she's generally happy and healthy.

When grief crosses the line into trauma

When you lose someone you love, the pain can seem unbearable at first. But that ache, hard as it is to endure, is part of the natural healing process. As a wise patient of mine once said, "Tears are the vehicle that grief uses to transport someone who is dead and gone from your life into your heart, where they live on forever."

Not everyone, however, is able to experience this form of healing. In some cases, a person remains trapped in grief — a condition that doctors call *traumatic grief*. This condition is closely related to both PTSD and depression, and the same treatments that are effective for these disorders (see Part III) can often help.

Holly Prigerson, a leading expert on traumatic grief, lists these warning signs of traumatic grief:

- Preoccupation with the lost loved one

- Physical pain in the same area where the person who died was afflicted — for example, chest pain in a person grieving for someone who died of a heart attack

- Intense upset at memories of the person

- Avoidance of reminders of the death

- Refusal to accept the death or a sense of disbelief about it

- A feeling that life is empty

- Longing for the lost person

- Hallucinating that you hear or see the person who died

- Being drawn to places and things associated with the person

- Anger or bitterness about the death

- A feeling that it's unfair to go on after the loved one's death

- A feeling of being stunned or dazed

- Envy of other people's relationships with their loved ones

- Difficulty trusting others

- Chronic loneliness

- Lack of concern for other people

Many of these symptoms are part of the normal grieving process, but if they don't improve or go away in several months, seeking professional guidance is smart. The advice that I offer in Chapter 16 to friends and family members of PTSD sufferers can also be helpful for families trying to help a person who's experiencing traumatic grief.

Warning signs in very young children

Spotting PTSD in a toddler or kindergartener is tricky because little kids don't think or act like grown-ups. Thus, letting their symptoms slip under the radar screen is easy. Here are some signs that can indicate PTSD in toddlers or kindergarteners (with a caution that these ages are approximate and that symptoms of different age groups overlap):

✔ **Fears and worries:** Often, these concerns seem unrelated to the trauma. For instance, a toddler may develop a fear of monsters and talk about them obsessively because he can't come up with a coherent picture of the person or event that actually threatened him.

✔ **Intense separation anxiety:** Separation anxiety is a normal behavior that sets in when children realize that parents can leave them. If a child develops PTSD, this fear of separation can become very intense — to the point that children shriek with terror if a parent leaves to go to work.

✔ **Irrational self-blame:** Young kids think the world revolves around them, so they may believe that something they did or thought caused the trauma. In the world of child development experts, this belief is called *magical thinking* — a child's belief that his thoughts or desires, or actions totally unrelated to an event, made the event occur. (Of course, you do the same thing every time you wear your lucky socks during playoffs season!)

Here's an example of magical thinking: A child who's traumatized by a parent's car crash may believe that he caused the accident by wishing that Mommy would quit pestering him the day before. Kids don't usually tell you when they have beliefs like these, so uncovering them may take a little sensitive dialogue.

✔ **Mood changes:** A toddler with PTSD may appear withdrawn, irritable, or even aggressive.

✔ **An overactive startle response:** Kids who once loved noise and commotion may cry, scream, or even experience a complete meltdown at a loud or sudden sound or an unexpected occurrence. These reactions can be even more extreme if they involve sights or sounds related to the trauma — for instance, the sound of a school bell if the crisis happened at school.

✔ **Post-traumatic play:** A child with PTSD may repeat certain elements of a trauma when playing with toys, blocks, or dolls — for instance, by crashing his toy cars together — or may draw pictures that show parts of the trauma.

✔ **Preoccupations:** Often, preoccupations can involve objects that seem unrelated to the event — for instance, a particular toy or character on TV.

✔ **Setbacks:** Traumatized tots can lose previously learned skills, such as language, toilet training, or dressing.

✔ **Sleep problems:** Any change can trigger sleep problems in a tot, so it's no surprise that a traumatic change can keep a young child from falling asleep at night or napping during the day.

✔ **Stomachaches or headaches:** These symptoms are common in kids traumatized by a life crisis, but make sure your pediatrician rules out other medical causes before assuming that these symptoms stem from PTSD.

Clues that can point to PTSD in elementary-school children

Like younger children, kids at the elementary-school stage may develop sleep problems or nightmares as part of their PTSD. In addition, they may display mood swings, anger, or aggression. They can also act "babyish," have stomachaches or headaches, or act out their trauma in play or art projects.

Here are some additional signs of PTSD in elementary-school-age children. Not all of these show on the surface, so listen for clues in your child's conversations or actions:

- **Fears about safety:** One common sign of PTSD in kids this age is an obsessive concern with safety or a constant fear of death.

- **Guilt:** Children traumatized by an event can think that it was somehow their fault. This mindset is a somewhat more mature version of the "magical thinking" of toddlers (see the preceding section).

- **Loss of interest in friends and activities:** A traumatized child may shut herself in her room after school each day and watch TV or play video games instead of hanging out with her buddies or talking on the phone.

- **Omen formation:** Children with PTSD sometimes believe they failed to spot warning signs of an impending trauma and that they need to be on alert so they can prevent a repeat of the event. For instance, a child who survived a hurricane may panic and say, "We need to go away!" when a small storm rolls in.

- **School problems:** Kids may let their grades slip, act out in class, or even refuse to go to school.

- **Time skew:** Kids with PTSD can seem very mixed-up about when a trauma occurred or about the order of events during the trauma. This idea is similar to the amnesia experienced by many adults with PTSD.

Red flags for PTSD in teens

PTSD in teens often reveals itself as acting-out behavior. That's a big problem because teens can express their inner pain in more dangerous ways than younger kids (especially if they're old enough to drive, date, or drink) and they don't have the self-control of adults. The following behaviors can be warning signs of PTSD in adolescents:

- Aggression
- Impulsive behavior

Bad kids — or bad trauma?

The police arrested Angela two days after her 14th birthday for shoplifting a dress from a mall store. They let her go home with her foster parents after giving her a slap on the wrist, but two months later, she got busted again — this time for stealing a classmate's purse. When a police officer asked her why she committed these acts, she simply replied, "Why not?" Her uncaring manner shocked the officer, who figured her for a bad apple.

But Angela, like many of the "bad" kids you read about in the papers, isn't bad at all; instead, she's deeply traumatized. She's living with a foster family because her father sexually abused her for years, and her behavior is a way of acting out the pain of her PTSD.

Therapists see a lot of children like Angela, and with time and hard work, they can often get these kids back on the road to a happier, healthier life. But the job is easier when everyone involved — parents or foster parents, schools, and the legal system — has compassion for the terror that lies behind the I-don't-care attitude of the abused child who turns troublemaker.

✔ Increased sexual behavior

✔ Rebellion

✔ Risk-taking, such as fast driving

Even if your teen is quiet after a trauma, however, don't assume that all's well. Teens with PTSD can also show their distress in more subtle ways. Here are the most common:

✔ Changes in friendships — for instance, dropping a lifelong friend or hooking up with a bad crowd

✔ Problems with grades or school work

✔ An increased interest in violence-related activities (for instance, violent video games or extreme sports)

✔ Depression or withdrawal

✔ An obsession with getting revenge on a person they blame for the trauma

✔ Sleep problems and nightmares

Because teens are drama queens even when life is going smoothly, sorting out PTSD symptoms from normal adolescent behavior isn't always easy. One key is to look for behaviors that are big changes from the way a teen acted before a trauma occurred. For instance, if a once-happy 14-year-old suddenly

gets heavy into Goth and starts skipping school, or if an outgoing teen quits the soccer team and starts hiding out in his room, that's a big red flag.

Signs of PTSD that abused kids and teens may exhibit

In Chapter 4, I talk about the betrayal effect that occurs when a trauma happens at the hands of someone a child loves and looks to for protection. Because this betrayal shakes a child to her core, the effects of sexual or physical abuse are much more profound for a child than the effects of other traumas. As a result, abused kids can display some very severe and frightening symptoms. These include

- ✔ Stealing
- ✔ Promiscuity or prostitution
- ✔ Running away
- ✔ Violence
- ✔ Self-injury (see additional info earlier in this chapter)
- ✔ Use of hard drugs such as heroin or cocaine, or heavy use of alcohol
- ✔ Severe depression or suicidal behavior

If you're dealing with a child or teen who suffered abuse somewhere along the line, recognizing the traumatic roots of violent, illegal, antisocial, or dangerous behaviors is very important. By addressing these problems through therapy when they first appear, you maximize the chances of turning a young life around before it's too late.

Chapter 4

First Response: Preventive Treatments for PTSD

*I*f you step on a nail, a tetanus shot can keep you safe, and if a cut puts you at risk for infection, an antibiotic can stop nasty germs in their tracks. But right now, doctors don't have any magic potions to prevent you from getting PTSD when trauma strikes. What doctors and therapists do have, however, are some tools they think may lower your risk of developing PTSD after a life crisis.

If you've experienced a trauma, you may have questions about one or more of these preventive measures. For example, if your trauma occurred just a few weeks ago, you may be asking whether any of these therapies can really lower your risk of developing PTSD in the long run. On the other hand, if you tried one of these approaches and still developed PTSD, you may wonder why these therapies failed. Was it your fault? Your treatment team's fault? Or the fact that these therapies have limits and don't work in every situation? (The quick answers are *no, no,* and *yes* — but more on that later.)

In the following pages, I give you the scoop on the medical and psychological interventions that doctors and therapists use right after a trauma occurs and info on how well each one works. Remember, though, that although these preventive measures can help a great deal, they don't come with any guarantees. If they make you feel better, excellent! If you already tried some or all of them and they didn't work, don't despair. In Part III, I describe a wide range of other therapies that can empower you to get your life back on track after a trauma derails it.

Be aware that nobody has all the answers about the best ways to prevent PTSD or about the odds of succeeding in this effort. After a trauma, you get a lot of advice — from doctors, friends, and relatives — about what you should do. But in many ways, the best expert on this topic is you. In this chapter, I offer you tools that can help you heal in the first few weeks after a life crisis. Which ones you choose depends on how serious your symptoms are, on how much support you have, and ultimately, on what you feel deep down is right for you.

Immediate Treatments Intended to Reduce PTSD Risk

When a trauma occurs, doctors and therapists have two forms of instant treatment up their sleeves. One is a common blood pressure drug that's gaining new interest as a PTSD therapy, and the other is what's called *crisis intervention.*

Do either of these therapies work? The answer is a little complicated because one therapy is very new and the other — although it's been around for many years — isn't really well studied. In the following sections, I look at both of these treatments and what doctors know (and don't know) about them.

Propranolol, the magical pill?

Imagine a magic bullet for preventing PTSD — a little pill you pop for a few days after a life crisis to protect yourself from any long-term psychological harm. Does it sound too good to be true? Maybe it is . . . but maybe it isn't.

New studies suggest that *propranolol* (Inderal) — the same pill that millions of people take for high blood pressure — can prevent some trauma survivors from developing PTSD if doctors first give it within a few hours after a traumatic event. (Researchers don't yet know if it can help prevent PTSD if it's given later than that.) The drug is still under study, but some doctors are already prescribing it as a preventive measure. The following sections explain what people know so far about this drug's effects and the pros and cons of using it.

How propranolol works

The memory-blocking effects of propranolol, which may take the long-term sting out of trauma in some cases, make a lot of sense in terms of brain chemistry. When you live through an event that causes fear and helplessness, your body immediately cranks out huge amounts of *adrenaline* — the fight-or-flight hormone. High adrenaline levels dramatically boost your ability to remember things, so scary stuff gets etched in deeper than run-of-the-mill events.

Propranolol, however, may short-circuit this process. Like a driver stealing someone else's parking place, propranolol sits on the spots on nerve cells where adrenaline usually goes (see Figure 4-1). When this happens, adrenaline can't do its job. As a result, bad memories still form, but they don't carry as much of an emotional punch.

The scientific scoop: Exciting but unproven

The propranolol story starts with Roger Pitman, a doctor at Harvard. In 2002, Pitman published the results of tests of this drug on a group of 22 people who survived car accidents or other life-threatening events. When these patients arrived at the emergency room at a Boston hospital, doctors gave eight of them the drug within the first six hours after their crises. To enable a comparison, the doctors gave fake pills to 14 patients after their crises.

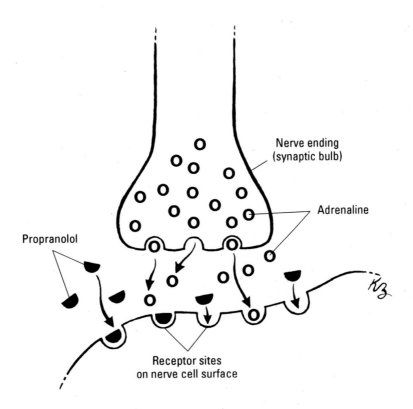

Figure 4-1:
Propranolol
occupies
the receptor
sites where
adrenaline
usually
attaches on
nerve cells.

Nerve ending
(synaptic bulb)

Adrenaline

Propranolol

Receptor sites
on nerve cell surface

Three months later, Pitman tested all 22 patients for PTSD symptoms. When the patients listened to their own audiotapes describing their crises, not a single person who took propranolol showed physical signs of anxiety. In contrast, 8 of the 14 people who got the fake pills showed strong signs of anxiety, including pounding hearts and sweaty palms.

A French study, which tested propranolol immediately after a trauma on patients at high risk for PTSD, also reported positive results. The study found that nearly all patients developed some PTSD symptoms after two months — but symptoms were only half as severe in the treated group. Only one of 11 propranolol-treated patients had symptoms severe enough to warrant a diagnosis of PTSD, but three of eight patients who didn't take propranolol received PTSD diagnoses.

More studies of propranolol's effects on PTSD are in the works, and time will tell whether these initial findings hold true for larger groups of patients. The early findings about propranolol are exciting, but they're just that — early. And medicine is full of promises that don't pan out, especially with miracle drugs. Propranolol is a promising treatment, but it doesn't help everyone — and when it does help, it often reduces symptoms instead of preventing them altogether. Because there's little research on this drug's PTSD-fighting effects so far, doctors still don't know who it can help, how much it can help, and whether its effects will last. They also don't know how long trauma survivors need to take the drug or whether there's a limited window of opportunity for the drug's effects to take hold.

If you received treatment with propranolol right after a trauma and you still developed PTSD, the drug quite possibly didn't work for you. It's also possible, however, that you have less-severe symptoms as a result of the treatment — there's no good way to know. Either way, the treatment likely didn't do you any harm, so it was probably well worth a try.

(Right now, you may be wondering whether propranolol can also alter PTSD symptoms if you take it months or years after a trauma occurs. If so, see Chapter 9 for the latest findings, which are preliminary but encouraging.)

Crisis intervention: Helpful or harmful?

After an earthquake, terrorist attack, school shooting, or similar crisis, experts rush to the scene to offer counseling to the survivors. These experts, often affiliated with government agencies or community mental health services, frequently start offering their services within hours of a terrible event. Their goal: to stop PTSD before it can get a toehold. It's a noble idea — but surprisingly, it may not work. In fact, some studies hint that crisis intervention (also called *critical incident stress management* or *psychological first aid*) can create problems where none exist.

How crisis intervention works

Crisis intervention professionals typically offer their services within the first two or three days after a crisis occurs, but in some cases (particularly after natural disasters), sessions may take place a few weeks after the event. If you undergo crisis intervention, you usually attend what's called a *debriefing* (probably as part of a group of survivors). At this single session, which typically lasts three or four hours, counselors ask participants to discuss

- ✔ What happened during the trauma
- ✔ How they felt and what they thought during the traumatic event
- ✔ What the worst part of the event was
- ✔ Any stress reactions they feel (at which point the professionals offer advice on coping techniques)

Afterward, the counselors describe the symptoms you can expect to experience as a trauma survivor. They finish up by offering to refer you for extra help if you have serious symptoms.

Big questions, few answers

Crisis intervention sounds like a very helpful strategy, which is why it's so popular. But when scientists set out to show that crisis intervention helps people, some studies showed just the opposite: It can actually make people experience *more* problems, not fewer (for possible reasons, see the following section). Among the findings:

- ✔ One team of researchers offered crisis intervention to a group of burn patients. A little more than a year later, these patients had higher levels of depression, anxiety, and PTSD than a group who didn't receive treatment.
- ✔ A similar study, this time with accident victims, found that three years after their traumas, people who received crisis intervention had more PTSD and psychiatric symptoms, and more fear of traveling, than those who didn't participate.

Other researchers, however, say that getting quick help after a trauma is a very good thing. These scientists say that the negative studies didn't use the right methods or study the right groups. In addition, they say that crisis intervention needs to be part of a larger treatment package — which wasn't the case in the thumbs-down studies — and that it works best if it's used with emergency workers who treat crisis victims rather than with the frontline trauma victims themselves.

What's the bottom line? Researchers don't have solid answers yet. What they can say for sure is that this therapy doesn't help everyone — so don't be surprised (and certainly don't blame yourself) if it doesn't prevent you from developing PTSD.

A Good Track Record for the First Few Weeks: Early CBT

If a trauma shakes your world, you may recover from the blow in a few days or weeks. If not, your doctor may diagnose you with acute stress disorder (see Chapter 2) and recommend a short course of therapy.

The leading therapy for acute stress disorder is a short form of the *cognitive behavioral therapy* (CBT) used to treat PTSD (see Chapter 9 for a full description of CBT). Unlike crisis intervention, which has mixed results (see the preceding section), early CBT is a treatment with some strong scientific support. Your doctor may recommend this approach if your symptoms are so serious that they interfere with your work, relationships, or daily activities. If so, scientific studies suggest that it's good advice to follow. Typically, this shortened version of CBT takes only four or five sessions.

Early CBT and crisis intervention have common features; for instance, they both provide info about the symptoms that trauma causes and about coping strategies you can use. So why does early CBT seem to work so much better than the crisis intervention that's also popular for trauma survivors? In short, CBT has two big advantages:

- ✔ Instead of asking you to describe your terrible experience a single time — which can send your feelings of distress into hyperdrive without letting you work through them — CBT lets you work through your trauma in a step-by-step approach called *graded exposure.*

- ✔ CBT helps you take control over the negative thoughts that can trap you in a cycle of trauma. (To do so, therapists use a technique called *cognitive restructuring,* which I also cover in Chapter 9). Crisis intervention typically doesn't address this aspect of post-trauma stress.

The only catch to signing on for a few sessions of early CBT is that you may not need them. Most people who experience acute stress disorder get over their symptoms on their own and don't need therapy. However, if your symptoms are keeping you from enjoying your life and functioning at work or at home, a few CBT sessions will probably do you good. And there's no evidence, at least so far, that it can cause problems.

Self-Help Strategies: Simple, Safe, and Often Successful

When you survive a traumatic event, your doctors do everything they can to help you recover — but you can do plenty for yourself as well. If you have minor symptoms such as sleep problems and trouble getting thoughts about the trauma out of your mind, you may try self-help approaches to chase away the clouds. In many cases, these steps, combined with time and patience, can help you heal completely after a trauma.

That's *not* to say, however, that you can prevent PTSD all by yourself. Many factors play into who gets PTSD and who doesn't, so don't feel like you failed if these steps don't prevent long-term problems. (That's a little like feeling guilty if washing your hands doesn't stop you from getting a cold!) And don't wait too long to seek professional help if you find that self-help techniques don't do the trick — generally, I advise that a person see a doctor if symptoms don't start to fade within a month. In Chapter 5, I guide you through a self-evaluation so you can decide for yourself whether you should talk with your doctor; I also discuss the most common fears and excuses people have about seeking a professional evaluation, so rest assured that if you feel this way, you're not alone.

That said, tapping into your own healing powers after you experience a trauma is an excellent idea. The following sections tell you how.

Getting help to meet your most basic needs

Traumas often strike on many fronts at the same time. Here's an illustration: Bob, who survives a huge hurricane, loses his home and car on the day the hurricane hits. He also loses his job because the catastrophe puts his store out of business. He suffers a serious injury during the hurricane, and his family barely escapes alive. Nobody can find his cat or his dog.

Telling Bob to simply relax, get support from his friends, and take care of himself — even though that's all good advice — is unrealistic. He needs time to get over his psychological scars, but he also needs practical, common-sense help — and a lot of it. The faster he can get a roof over his head, a car in his driveway, a check in his mailbox, and help for his medical problems, the better his odds of healing without long-term emotional scars.

Don't make the mistake of being too proud to reach out for help. The more quickly you meet your needs for food, clothing, housing, and medical care, the better you'll fare both mentally and physically in the long run. Depending on the type of crisis you survived, here are some agencies or individuals who can help:

- ✔ Charitable agencies such as the Red Cross (www.redcross.org) or Salvation Army (www.salvationarmyusa.org)
- ✔ Government agencies

- ✔ Your insurance company
- ✔ Your place of worship
- ✔ The Legal Aid Society
- ✔ Your employer
- ✔ Hospital social workers
- ✔ Friends and neighbors
- ✔ Animal shelters and humane societies

If possible, find a friend or family member — preferably someone not exposed to the trauma — to help you. This person can handle paperwork, phone calls, and other tasks that can otherwise overwhelm you.

Educating yourself

Mental, physical, and emotional symptoms are less scary if you know that they're normal reactions to a traumatic event — and the less scared you are after a trauma, the less likely you are to develop PTSD. Understanding the effects of a trauma can also help you to judge whether you're getting better on your own or you need to seek professional help.

Of course, by reading this book, you're already educating yourself about the aftereffects of a life crisis and how to handle them. Here are some other good ideas:

- ✔ Talk to your doctor about what you can expect in the days or weeks after a trauma.
- ✔ Visit the National Center for Posttraumatic Stress Disorder's information page at www.ncptsd.va.gov/ncmain/information.

Finding ways to relax

Stop for a moment and think about how your body feels right now. Are your muscles tight and tense? Is your jaw clenched? Does your neck feel stiff or sore?

After a catastrophe, you may subconsciously tense up, almost as if you expect another blow to fall. That tension can keep you awake at night, cause headaches and stomachaches, and lead you to breathe rapidly and shallowly — which in turn can trigger panic attacks. To chase away the tension, actively seek out ways to relax. The following sections explain some techniques.

Progressive relaxation

Progressive relaxation entails tensing and relaxing different muscle groups in order to release the muscle tension that occurs when you're stressed. You can do this technique lying in bed or sitting in a comfortable chair. Follow each of the following steps and then repeat them once or twice. As you do this activity, be careful not to tense your feet, back, or neck too tightly. If you have back or neck problems, check with your doctor before using this technique.

1. **Sit or lie with your feet slightly apart, your arms a little way away from your sides, your palms facing up, and your eyes closed.**

2. **Breathe in and out in a relaxed way, slowing your breathing as you do, while you count slowly and silently to 20.**

   Each count should last about one second.

3. **Tense the muscles of your feet and toes, counting to 5 as you do, and then relax them while counting to 20.**

4. **Follow the same steps with one muscle group at a time, in this order: calves, thighs, stomach, chest, fists (clench them tightly and then relax), biceps, upper arms and shoulders, neck (very gently), and face.**

Visualization

When practicing *visualization,* you close your eyes and picture yourself in a safe, beautiful, and relaxing place. Here's an example:

- ✔ Picture yourself lying on a soft blanket in a sunny glade, surrounded by a quiet forest where the only sounds are birds chirping and a brook babbling.

- ✔ Involve several of your senses: Feel the warmth of the sun on your face, hear the water running over the stones of the brook, and smell the piney scent of the trees and the fresh aroma of the grass beneath you.

- ✔ Imagine looking up at the clouds drifting slowly by and the birds flying in the distance.

- ✔ When you feel calm and relaxed, let yourself come back gently to the real world, take a few deep breaths, and stretch.

If your mind wanders during this exercise, don't worry. Just gently return your attention to the scene you're visualizing.

Other methods for promoting relaxation

Different people find different activities relaxing — and what soothes one person's soul may leave another person wound up like a top — so finding the right relaxation tools may take a little trial and error. Here's a list of relaxation techniques that you may find helpful:

- ✔ **Yoga:** Many people find this form of exercise calming and relaxing, but some people with PTSD have a very negative reaction to it. If you give yoga a try, listen to your body and continue with it only if it makes you feel better — not worse.

- ✔ **Meditation:** One form of meditation that many people find highly effective is mindfulness meditation, which several major U.S. hospitals now use to help patients with stress disorders, panic attacks, or physical pain. (See Chapter 12 for more info.) This form of meditation helps you focus on being present rather than being distracted by past memories or worries about the future.

   A good book that explains mindfulness meditation and describes how to use this method is *Calming Your Anxious Mind: How Mindfulness and Compassion Can Free You from Anxiety, Fear, and Panic,* by Jeffrey Brantley, MD.

- ✔ **Simple hobbies:** Taking your mind off the trauma and focusing on positive activities can foster healing. Spend time on a hobby that absorbs your attention, whether it's painting, gardening, building furniture, or playing the piano.

- ✔ **A personalized relaxation tape:** One good trick is to make your own tape describing a relaxing image (for instance, "I'm lying on the beach, listening to the gentle waves . . .") and listen to it during your sessions. The sound of your own voice gently walking you through your pleasant scene can be very calming.

If these do-it-yourself techniques don't take away the tension, talk to your family doctor about going to a therapist for a few sessions of relaxation therapy (see Chapter 10 for more on this). In this approach, a therapist walks you through various relaxation techniques and helps you find the ones that work best for you.

Getting plenty of rest

It's tempting, especially if you're an emergency responder who faces crises for a living, to suck it up, say you're fine, and keep going. But you're *not* fine right after a trauma, and your mind and body need time to cope with the shock you just suffered. Take time off from work if you can, especially if your work brings you into contact with stressful events. In the following sections, I explain some measures that can help you rest.

Easing anxiety so you can sleep

After a trauma, you need as much sleep as possible so your mind can get some rest. That's easier said than done because dozing peacefully in the aftermath of a trauma is hard, and acute stress can lead to terrifying nightmares. However, some very basic steps can help you rest more easily:

✔ If you live alone, having a close friend or family member stay with you for a few days sometimes helps. This company can make you feel safer (especially at night, when fears tend to take over), and you also get a sympathetic sounding board for when you feel like talking about what happened.

  Man's best furry friend can help in a time of crisis, too. One woman I know had the smart idea of borrowing her parents' dog to keep her company after she experienced a life crisis. She says, "Having a warm, comforting, familiar body to sleep next to, coupled with the distraction of someone else to care for, really helped me when I needed it most."

✔ Avoid watching violent TV shows, reading books with scenes of violence, or watching the nightly news before you go to bed. Instead, read something restful or watch something light and fun such as cooking shows or sports. Letting the TV lull you to sleep can be helpful, but use the snooze feature if you have one so you won't be rudely awakened by a loud or frightening show or commercial.

✔ Avoid caffeine or alcohol before bedtime.

✔ Leave a light (or all of them) on if doing so makes you feel safer.

✔ Play a tape of nature sounds or soft music, or use a fan or white-noise generator to block sounds that can wake you in the night.

✔ Use relaxation techniques (see that section earlier in this chapter) before bedtime.

✔ If your trauma occurred inside your home, consider changing the furniture arrangement, getting new rugs or bedding, or even repainting. The more you change the room's appearance, the less likely it'll be to trigger bad memories. Sleeping elsewhere, or installing a security system, may also make you feel more secure.

Avoid using sleep medications — either prescription or non-prescription — unless your doctor strongly feels that they're right for you. These drugs can cause their own problems, which are sometimes serious (see Chapter 9). One possible alternative is the over-the-counter sleep aid melatonin, a natural hormone that helps some people but not others. If you decide to try melatonin, check with your doctor first to make sure it's safe for you.

Dealing with nightmares

Dealing with the aftermath of a trauma is tough enough when you're awake, but it's even worse when you can't get a good night's sleep. Nightmares are a common aftereffect of a terrifying experience, and these bad dreams can interrupt your sleep and make you fearful of sacking out when the sun goes down. Here are some tricks that can calm your troubled nights:

✔ **Try consciously rewriting your nightmares in your mind so they have happy endings.** For instance, if you have recurring nightmares about being threatened by a faceless attacker, picture the attacker turning into a funny bug and visualize yourself squashing it. If you can get this picture firmly in mind, you may alter the course of your nightmare if it recurs.

Don't fall back asleep intentionally with the hopes of changing the nightmare's ending — chances are good that you'll just keep re-experiencing the same awful ending or other just-as-bad alternate endings. Rewrite the dream while you're awake, and if you begin to fall back to sleep, focus intently on the happy ending as you drift into Dreamland.

✔ **Remind yourself that nightmares, like dreams, are just a tool your brain uses to help you sort out events and file away memories.** If you think of a terrifying dream as part of your brain's filing system, you can take away some of its punch.

✔ **Ask your doctor whether he or she thinks you'll benefit from a brief intervention called *imagery rehearsal therapy*.** This therapy often reduces the frequency of nightmares in trauma survivors. In IRT, a therapist guides you through the steps of writing down your nightmares, changing their endings to more positive ones, and rehearsing your rewritten dream scenarios so they can displace the bad endings when your dream reoccurs (see Chapter 11 for more info).

Eating healthy foods and exercising

A life crisis throws everything out of whack in your life, and that includes eating. Getting back on track with meals is a big key to feeling better because your body needs nutrients to counter the effects of stress — especially B vitamins and vitamin C, which stress can deplete.

As soon as you can, get back to your typical eating schedule. Do your best to choose healthy foods, and try to eat at least a little at each mealtime even if you're not hungry. Avoid heavy doses of caffeine or alcohol, and if you live on fast food, take a good vitamin/mineral supplement, at least for a few months. Also, consider taking supplements of omega-3 fatty acids. (You can find these at most grocery stores and any health-food store.) Initial studies suggest that these nutrients may help to lower stress.

In addition to eating right, you can help yourself heal by adding exercise to your get-well plan. A good workout can release built-up stress and relax tense muscles, and it also produces natural feel-good chemicals called endorphins that can lift your mood. Lifting weights, pushing against exercise machines, or running or biking at a fast pace can help work out the anger that often follows in the wake of a trauma.

Some people become more anxious — not less — if they do aerobic exercises such as running or kickboxing. Pay attention to how you feel after an exercise session, and pick the routines that calm you rather than stress you out.

Taking charge to gain a sense of control

After you survive a trauma, take steps that make you feel like you're more in control of your life. The actions you choose can depend on the type of trauma you suffered, but here are some examples:

- ✔ Start a journal to work out your feelings.

- ✔ Take positive steps to increase your safety. Avoid the urge to crawl into a hole and never leave the house, but do sensible things. For instance, install better deadbolts and/or a home security system, buy pepper spray, increase your homeowner's insurance, or buy home-repair tools, flashlights, and first aid kits so you'll be better prepared in the event of a sequel.

- ✔ After you put a very big distance between yourself and the trauma — a long enough time that you're over the worst of the shock — consider taking a first-aid course, a self-defense class, or any other type of class that can make you feel more capable of handling a future emergency. (However, wait on these activities until you're quite sure they won't trigger stressful memories.)

- ✔ Donate to a charity that helps people in times of crisis — or if the idea appeals to you, volunteer to help other survivors. The old saying is true: Lighting a candle in the darkness can have a powerful healing effect.

Talking it out

Having your horror heard helps heal your hurt, so share your feelings with friends and family members you trust. When you share with a good listener, you feel less alone. When you feel less alone, awful feelings become, well, less awful. Getting panicky feelings off your chest and into a caring person's ear can help you go back to just feeling frightened; getting angry feelings off your chest can help you get back to just feeling frustrated.

If you're lucky, your friends and family will listen to you without rushing to tell you that everything will be fine (which people often say because you're starting to make them nervous). If they do try to reassure you that all's well when you know it's not, look elsewhere for a sympathetic ear — perhaps to a therapist or a support group (see info on support groups in the next section and info on finding a therapist in Chapter 6).

When you talk with friends or family, you don't need to relive every detail of the trauma you survived or dredge up the memories that scare you. Instead, talk about the parts of the event you're comfortable remembering. For example, it may be easier at first to offer a description of how the event unfolded than to talk about your feelings when it happened — or it may be easier to talk about the before-and-after parts of the trauma than to describe the scariest moments. If you're unable to talk about your trauma even weeks after it occurs, consider seeing a therapist who can help you work through what happened.

Attending a support group (if it helps)

Sometimes, even the people closest to you can't understand what you're going through. That's why support groups, which bring together people who share a similar problem, can be powerful healing tools. In a support group meeting, you're less likely to get blank looks when you talk about your post-trauma problems and are more likely to hear, "I know just what you mean" and "I feel exactly the same way." But although these groups can offer understanding and support, they're not for everyone. In the sections that follow, I talk about the pros and cons of support groups and where to find one if you want to explore this option.

Deciding whether a support group is right for you

Throw 10 or 12 strangers in a room together for a meeting, and you never know what'll happen. The outcome depends on the people themselves — and that's as true for support groups as it is for board meetings (or cocktail parties, for that matter).

Some people gain hope, help, moral support, and new friendships by attending support groups; others find them a waste of time or even a trigger for anxiety. And some people visit three or four support groups before they find one that clicks for them. Here's a look at the advantages and drawbacks of these groups to help you decide whether this option is right for you.

On the pro side:

> ✔ You meet other people in the same boat and realize that you're not alone. Also, discovering that many other wonderful, strong people have the same feelings as you can help you get rid of the destructive idea that you're "abnormal" or "weak."

✔ You can share your feelings in a safe environment. Other group members can offer support and security while also nudging you to work through your feelings.

✔ Often, interacting with people who suffered a similar trauma gives you a chance to meet both people who are newly traumatized and those who are moving through and getting over it. This range can show you that people do make it through.

✔ Sharing with others can help you stay out of your head, which is a good idea because your imagination can really scare the heck out of you.

On the downside:

✔ Sometimes, support group meetings trigger anxiety or flashbacks. This can leave you worse off, not better, if you haven't received therapy and don't have the tools to deal with these reactions.

✔ If you have severe symptoms, support groups (unless you augment them with professional help) probably aren't the right approach for you. That's because you need the more structured setting of therapy to work through serious PTSD symptoms in a controlled way.

Finding your niche: The search for the right group

If you think a support group can benefit you and you're willing to shop around to find the right one, you can locate support groups through the following sources:

✔ **Your family doctor (or your therapist if you have one):** These professionals can be a big help in steering you toward groups that meet your specific needs.

✔ **The Internet:** Just type in "support groups" and a description of the type of trauma you survived. (For example, a search of "support groups" and "air disasters" leads you to ACCESS, the AirCraft Casualty Emotional Support Services, which helps people whose loved ones died or suffered injuries in an air disaster.) Often, adding the name of your town or state helps to narrow your choices.

✔ **Your local hospital:** Some hospitals offer their own programs, and others can help you locate resources in the community. Your best bet is to talk to the community relations or social services department.

✔ **Clearinghouses:** Call or search online for support group *clearinghouses,* which are nonprofit groups that help you link up with the right group for you. (If you go to www.mentalhealth.org and click on "Resources" and "Mental Health Services Locator," you can find a state-by-state listing of various groups.)

✔ **Your local newspaper:** Many newspapers publish calendars of support group meetings.

- ✔ **United Way (www.unitedway.org) and similar organizations:** These organizations can provide referrals to agencies that offer the type of group you're seeking.

- ✔ **Your place of worship, particularly if it offers referrals to pastoral (religious) counseling services:** A pastoral counselor is in an excellent position to direct you toward community resources, including support groups.

- ✔ **Community clinics in your area:** Some of these clinics offer support-group services themselves, and others can give you appropriate referrals.

If you can't find a local group, try calling national groups and asking whether they know of groups in your area. Also, see Chapter 7 for a list of national organizations that may be able to help you.

Part I
The Basics
of PTSD

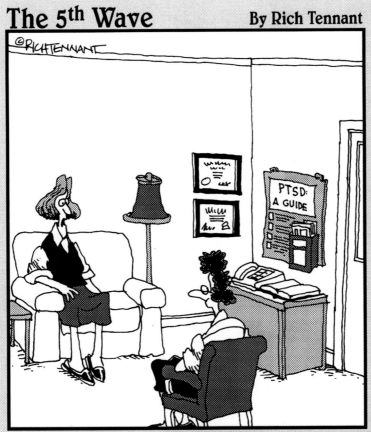

The 5th Wave   By Rich Tennant

"Of course I never get flashbacks of the 3rd item on a lost grocery list, or where I parked the car, or the names of my boss's children..."

In this part . . .

*H*aving some basic facts under your belt can be a big help if you're tackling PTSD. In this section, I look at the history of this disorder, the number of people it affects, and the big reasons getting help for PTSD is so important. Next, I talk about what doctors mean by *stress* and *trauma* and why some people are more vulnerable than others to PTSD. After that, I go through the signs and symptoms of PTSD, talk about other disorders that often are part of the package, and discuss why PTSD in kids and teens is different from the adult version. Finally, I talk about preventive treatments for PTSD and explain their benefits and limitations — and why you may still have PTSD even if you received one of those treatments.

Chapter 5

Getting Answers: Finding Out Whether You Have PTSD

*I*n my boyhood days, I once tried my hand at a paint-by-numbers kit. I still remember dabbing a blob of green here and a speck of black or red there and marveling as my little dabs gradually turned into a cow, a chicken, and eventually an entire farmyard.

Trying to decide whether you have PTSD is a little like watching a paint-by-numbers masterpiece unfold, because no single symptom or event can give you the whole picture. To find answers, you need to look at the pattern that emerges when you assemble your bits and pieces into a whole.

Of course, there's a huge difference between splattering paint on a piece of pasteboard and staring PTSD in the face — the latter is very serious business, and getting the right picture is vital to your future. In this chapter, I lend you a hand in that process by outlining the steps that can help you make an educated guess about whether you have PTSD. If your conclusion is *yes*, I offer advice on seeking professional help and tell you what to expect when you visit a doctor in search of answers.

A Quick Quiz: Identifying Your Symptoms

Feelings and behaviors don't always fit into tidy little boxes that you can label as *okay* or *not okay*. If you frequently blow up at co-workers, do you have PTSD, or is it just job stress? If you quit driving after an accident, is that a PTSD symptom or just common sense? Sometimes distinguishing a symptom from an everyday behavior is hard unless you look at the big picture.

An excellent place to start in this effort is by seeing how your symptom pattern stacks up against the official diagnosis of PTSD (see Chapter 3 for more on this). The following self-test, based on the clues doctors look for when they diagnose PTSD, can help you answer that question.

Answer *yes* or *no* to the scoring question at the end of each group of questions, writing your answers in the line to the left of the scoring question. *Note:* Don't score any questions except the scoring questions at the end of each section.

1. **Look back.**

   - Did you survive a traumatic event that threatened your life or threatened or killed another person?

   - If so, did that event make you feel terrified, horrified, and/or helpless?

   _____ **Scoring Question:** Did you answer *yes* to both questions?

2. **Spot intrusive symptoms.**

   - Do you have repeated, distressing recollections of the event?

   - Do you experience recurring nightmares about the event?

   - Do you sometimes feel like you're reliving the event? For instance, do you have flashbacks or hallucinations that make you feel like the event is happening again?

   - Do you feel mentally or physically distressed when something reminds you of the trauma?

   _____ **Scoring Question:** Did you answer *yes* to one or more questions?

3. **Identify avoidant symptoms.**

   - Do you try to avoid thoughts, feelings, or conversations about topics related to the trauma?

   - Do you try to avoid people, places, or activities that remind you of the trauma?

- Is your memory a complete blank when it comes to key parts of your trauma?

- Do you lack interest in day-to-day activities that you once considered important, interesting, or fun?

- Do you feel detached from other people?

- Is it hard for you to feel a normal range of emotions?

- Do you have difficulty picturing the future? For instance, is it hard for you to picture having kids, building a career, or living a long life?

_____ **Scoring Question:** Did you answer *yes* to three or more questions?

4. **Pinpoint symptoms of hyperarousal.**

- Do you have trouble falling asleep or staying asleep?

- Do you frequently feel irritable or have outbursts of anger?

- Is concentrating difficult?

- Are you always on guard and unable to relax?

- Do you startle easily? For instance, do you react much more strongly to noises or surprises than other people do?

_____ **Scoring Question:** Did you answer *yes* to at least two questions?

5. **Factor in how long and how strong.**

- Did your symptoms start more than one month ago? (No matter when the original trauma occurred — even if it was many years ago — answer this question based on your current symptoms.)

- Do your symptoms disturb you so much that they interfere with your work, your relationships, or other important parts of your life? (If you have trouble answering this question, see the next section in this chapter for help.)

_____ **Scoring Question:** Did you answer *yes* to both questions?

6. **Add up your score.**

Check your answers to the scoring questions at the end of each section. If you answered *yes* to every one of these questions — even if you didn't answer *yes* to all the questions in each numbered group — you likely have PTSD. Remember — the scoring questions are what count in your final analysis.

If you answered *no* to some of the scoring questions, you likely wouldn't get an official diagnosis of PTSD. However, pen-and-paper tests can't tell all, so if your symptoms worry you, talk to your doctor.

A note about timing: If your symptoms started at least six months after a trauma, you may have *delayed PTSD*. If less than one month has passed since your trauma but your symptoms indicate PTSD, you may have *acute stress disorder*. (See Chapter 2 for more about the timing of PTSD symptoms.)

Being 100 percent sure that you have PTSD takes more than a quick quiz, but your answers on the preceding self-test can allow you to make a pretty good guess — especially when you combine them with your gut instincts. You can get an even clearer picture if you take a long, honest look at just how much your symptoms interfere with the life you want to live.

A Reality Check: Assessing the Severity of Your Symptoms

Nobody's life is a bed of roses. All people have days when nothing goes right: They lose their jobs, break up with a lover, or do something foolish or hurtful.

If you have PTSD, however, these days happen far too often. What's more, you probably blame yourself when they do. But the truth is *it's not your fault.* That's because when your symptoms strike, you're not in the driver's seat — PTSD is. And PTSD symptoms can drive away friends and family, frighten the people you love, and hurt your chances at work (or even make keeping a job impossible).

However, spotting the damage PTSD is doing to your life can be hard when you're right in the middle of it. Now's the time to find some quiet time, during a period when you feel calm and relaxed, to analyze how your life is going and whether you're still in control of it. The sections that follow can offer some insight.

Are your symptoms affecting your relationships?

All relationships have rocky spots, but PTSD can throw giant boulders in the path of a marriage, friendship, or any other loving relationship. Here are some key signs that your symptoms may be driving you and your loved ones apart:

- Your emotional outbursts or extreme reactions to minor life events (for example, having a meltdown if a car alarm goes off or flying into a rage over a minor disagreement) worry, frighten, or alienate your friends and family.

✔ Your need to avoid certain things, places, or people that remind you of your trauma make it hard for you to be with your friends or participate in family activities.

✔ Your partner or family members worry about your lack of interest or negative attitude about your future.

✔ Your friends or partner say that you're distant, uncaring, or impossible to reach.

✔ You have extreme mood swings. For instance, you may be happy as a clam at breakfast and then upset or angry or weepy an hour later for no good reason.

✔ You're distrustful of people — even those who've earned your trust.

✔ You find excuses to avoid intimacy or sex with your partner.

✔ You avoid sexual relationships entirely or — conversely — seek out unsafe, temporary sexual partnerships.

✔ You avoid getting together with friends or family to the point that they ask, "What's wrong? Don't you like us anymore?" When you do accept an invitation to a get-together, you have trouble making small talk or being interested in the people you're with.

Are your symptoms affecting your work?

At some point, just about everybody says, "I hate my job," and everyone has occasional issues with a boss, co-worker, or client. But the work problems that stem from PTSD are a whole different ballgame because they can sabotage a job or even an entire career. If you have the following problems, then consider getting professional help:

✔ You have trouble keeping a job for more than a short time — or you find it impossible to work at all.

✔ You often have outbursts of anger or other emotional meltdowns on the job.

✔ You lose promotions or get bad reviews because your supervisors have trouble dealing with your symptoms. For instance, you may have trouble dealing with demanding customers, find it hard to concentrate on tasks, or miss too many days at work because you can't face the stress of a workday.

✔ You have trouble trusting co-workers or letting them develop relationships with you.

✔ You doubt abilities that you once felt confident about, and you don't feel positive about your professional future.

✔ You've lost interest in improving your job skills or getting ahead in your field.

Looking at legal protection: PTSD and the ADA

The Americans with Disabilities Act, or ADA, prevents employers from discriminating against workers with disabilities. But does that include you if you receive an official diagnosis of PTSD? The answer is a definite *maybe*.

The ADA doesn't spell out the medical conditions that qualify as disabilities. Thus, according to the Job Accommodation Network, "Some people with PTSD will have a disability under the ADA and some will not." Under the law, you're covered if you

✔ Have a long-term mental, physical, or emotional impairment that substantially limits your ability to perform a major life activity

✔ Have a record of having such a disability

✔ Are perceived as having such a disability, even if you don't (you don't need to figure out this brain-twister, because it doesn't apply if you have a PTSD diagnosis)

In real life, you may be covered if your PTSD causes significant symptoms that impair your ability to do a job without special help and if you can document this claim. If so, your employer may be required to make special accommodations for your PTSD. This could be anything from removing triggers from your work area (for instance, certain noises or aromas) to providing a driver if your PTSD prevents you from driving to a client's office.

Are your symptoms affecting your health?

Missing the connection between PTSD and physical aches and pains is easy, but the two often go hand-in-hand. If you have a number of the symptoms that follow and you find no other obvious explanation for them, a doctor can help you decide whether they're PTSD-related. If they are, therapy may help reduce their sting or eliminate them altogether:

✔ Heart palpitations

✔ Sleep problems

✔ Chronic exhaustion or fatigue

✔ Tension headaches

✔ Stomach pain, irritable bowel syndrome, or other digestive problems

✔ Chronic pain

Do your symptoms worry or frighten you or your loved ones?

If you have any of the symptoms that follow, you don't need to play the guessing game. It's time to seek help — no ifs, ands, or buts — because your life depends on it:

- ✔ Suicidal thoughts or impulses

- ✔ Alcohol or drug abuse

- ✔ Depression (see Chapter 3)

- ✔ Violent thoughts or actions

- ✔ Sexual behaviors that put you at risk for AIDS or other sexually transmitted diseases

- ✔ Eating disorders

- ✔ Reckless behavior, such as speeding or driving when you've had too much to drink

- ✔ Dissociation, in which you mentally disconnect from some aspects of your own identity (see Chapter 3)

- ✔ An unshakable feeling that your life is shattered and that you can never put the pieces back together again

- ✔ Feelings that you're worthless and don't deserve a good life

Adding it all up

After taking stock of your situation, you can assemble the facts you need to make some informed guesses. The self-test at the start of this chapter can help you spot patterns pointing to PTSD, and an honest look at your life can tell you whether your symptoms are standing between you and a happy life. Ask yourself how you feel after this self-analysis:

- ✔ **Relieved — you don't think you have PTSD.** If you didn't spot any big red flags, the preventive measures I describe in Chapter 4 may help you get any minor post-trauma symptoms under control.

- ✔ **Concerned — your answers make you realize that you have some serious problems.** If you're not sure your answers add up to PTSD but you spot some worrisome patterns, talk things over with a doctor who can help you make sense of your symptoms.

- ✔ **Scared — the PTSD symptoms and life problems sound like the story of your life.** If warning bells ring loudly when you take the quiz or analyze your life, then don't let worries or doubts get in the way of seeking professional help immediately.

If you picked either *concerned* or *scared,* I recommend taking action as soon as you can. The longer PTSD affects your life, the more secondary problems it can cause in the form of broken relationships, career problems, and missed opportunities. The following section tells you how to get help.

Facing Your Fears: Seeking Professional Help

If PTSD blocks the path to your happy future, getting a diagnosis is the first step to finding treatment and healing. Even so, the idea of sharing your fears and feelings with a doctor may make you wobbly in the knees. As a trauma survivor, you may feel that the world is unsafe and unpredictable. And if your trauma happened at the hands of another person, trusting a stranger with your deepest emotions can be tough.

In addition, just thinking about opening up to another person about your symptoms can reawaken powerful fears that you're struggling to keep under lock and key. What's more, you may worry about how people will react if you go public with your symptoms — will they think you're crazy or weak or possibly even dangerous? As a result, it's all too easy to sabotage your decision to see a doctor with excuses like these:

I'll get over it eventually, so I'll just wait.

I'm just too busy right now.

Everybody has problems. I'll learn to cope.

I have my friends and family to worry about. What would they think if I'm diagnosed with a "mental problem"?

If you keep catching yourself making these excuses — or scheduling appointments with your doctor and then canceling them — realize that fear, guilt, shame, and self-doubt are standing in the way of the future you want. When your heart is saying, "Go for it!" but your fears keep saying, "Whoa," the best way to move forward is to recognize and deal with the fears that hold you hostage. Here are the most common culprits:

✔ **Fear of what your friends and family will think:** If you're an overachiever — and people with PTSD often are — admitting that you're not superhuman can be tough. Like everyone else, you want your loved ones to think you're perfect (even though you're pretty sure that *they* aren't). But PTSD isn't a character flaw or a sign of weakness. It also has nothing to do with being "crazy." Wise friends and family members realize that — and if they don't, you can educate them. (Loaning them this book is a good start.)

✔ **Fear of telling your doctor about frightening or embarrassing symptoms or about drug or alcohol abuse:** Many people worry themselves silly about talking to their doctor, but the truth is that doctors are nearly impossible to shock. What's more, a good doctor knows that your behaviors and feelings are classic symptoms of a medical problem, not signs that you're weak or bad in some way. And the information you give your doctor is confidential, so you can safely tell the doc if you're using illicit substances.

✔ **Fear of giving up excuses:** Do your symptoms get you off the hook sometimes or buy you special privileges? For instance, do they make it easier for you to say *no* to family or work obligations or cause your family to walk on eggshells to avoid upsetting you? If so, you may secretly worry about having to shoulder more responsibility or accept some more emotional give-and-take as you begin to heal. Spotting this hidden agenda can help you overcome that fear.

✔ **Fear of giving up addictions:** Tackling a substance abuse problem is a very tough job, but you likely don't want to spend your entire life in thrall to alcohol or drugs (see Chapter 7 for more on this important topic). What's more, getting treatment for PTSD can give you a huge boost in finding the strength to conquer substance abuse problems.

✔ **Fear of losing control:** You probably go to great lengths to avoid situations that trigger your symptoms — and here I am, asking you to walk into the lion's den. But there's a big difference between being helpless and horrified when a trauma strikes and working through that trauma in a secure setting with the careful guidance of a therapist who'll protect you from harm. The techniques people use in therapy empower you to view the event from a position of strength — not a position of helplessness — and as a result, to gain power and control over it.

If you spot fears that are holding you back, banish negativity by focusing on what you'll gain when you heal — not what you may lose. True, getting a diagnosis can mean facing some scary parts of your life and tackling some tough issues. But confronting your problem can also mean opening the door to a future that's full of promise. It can mean less fear, more happiness, deeper relationships, greater career success, and — above all — the freedom to be the person you want to be. If you add up the pros and cons, taking action wins hands-down over a lifetime of *woulda, coulda, shoulda.*

What's more, you're likely to find that the simple act of admitting that you're scared or in pain takes a huge weight off your shoulders. Denying a bad feeling gives it more power, but acknowledging it instantly removes the heavy burden of trying to keep up a false front. And here's another tip: No matter how stoic you are, you're probably not fooling the people who know you best.

So decide that it's okay to say, "I feel bad," and take the next step toward feeling better. To help you gain more confidence to pick up the phone and make an appointment, the following sections explain how to prepare in advance and what to expect when you get to the doctor's office.

Preparing for Your Visit to the Doctor: What to Do, What to Bring

Just for a minute, pretend that you're a primary care doctor. You have six antsy patients in your waiting room, and you're already running an hour late — and in comes a patient with a problem that takes time, wisdom, and some serious detective work to diagnose. Such a situation can thwart even the best doctor's efforts to provide help.

Identifying strep throat or a sprained wrist is simple, but diagnosing PTSD is a different story — especially for a busy doctor who's not a specialist in this disorder. To decide whether your symptoms add up to a PTSD diagnosis — and to refer you to the right specialists if the answer is *yes* — your primary care doctor needs both plenty of time and a lot of facts. Here's how to be ready with both:

- ✔ **Give the doc a heads-up.** When you call to make an appointment, tell the receptionist that you need plenty of time and explain why. A doctor who's expecting a ten-minute appointment may not be ready to give you the attention you need. Also, make an appointment early in the day if you can. Doctors' offices tend to be less backed-up in the morning.

- ✔ **Write down every symptom you want to discuss with your doctor.** If you get emotional during your visit, remembering everything you want to say may be tough. (See the following section for info on the kind of information the doctor wants to know.)

- ✔ **Invite a friend along.** If you worry that you'll lose your cool when you talk with your doctor, consider bringing a trusted friend or family member along. Be sure to choose someone you can talk openly around so you won't need to edit what you tell the doctor.

- ✔ **Do your homework.** Assemble any paperwork that can give your doctor insight into your symptoms. For instance, bring medical records from the time of the trauma, lab tests from recent years, and any evaluations from professionals that may be useful.

- ✔ **Get your game face on.** Decide ahead of time to be polite but also assertive when you talk to your doctor. Sometimes if a doctor seems brusque or busy, you may feel like chickening out and leaving without asking your questions. But you need answers, so make sure you get them.

- ✔ **Be a good guest.** Be nice and respectful to the people in the doctor's front office. If the staff seems rushed, cut them some slack — you never know what traumas they're dealing with themselves! Thank them for their assistance.

    Thanking your doctor as well doesn't hurt. Many doctors feel that they care about others more than others care about them, so expressing your appreciation is a nice way to let your doc know that you're grateful for the extra time you're requesting.

If you start with a family doctor, expect to get a referral to a second doctor (most likely a psychiatrist or a psychologist). Primary care doctors usually send patients with PTSD to physicians who have extra training in treating this problem instead of creating a treatment plan themselves.

Read up on the different treatments for PTSD (see Chapters 8, 9, and 10) before you go for your appointment. That way, if your doctor recommends a particular approach or asks you to choose between treatments, you'll have the background info you need to make the right decisions.

Getting a Diagnosis: What Your Doctor Will Do

Careful doctors don't rush a diagnosis, especially when it's a tricky one like PTSD, so be prepared for a long chat. Sorting out the symptoms of this disorder and ruling out other look-alikes that can masquerade as PTSD takes time. You can help in this process by being prepared and being ready to talk straightforwardly about your symptoms.

Doctors vary in their approach to PTSD, but the following sections go over what your doctor is likely to do at your appointment.

Questions, questions, questions!

There's no blood test or X-ray for PTSD, so your doctor needs your help in diagnosing this problem. The more you're willing to share, the easier it'll be to get to the heart of the matter. Here's what your doctor needs to know:

- The type of trauma you suffered
- When you started having symptoms and what they are
- How serious your symptoms are — for instance, whether they interfere with your personal life or work
- Whether you have related issues, such as a drug or alcohol problem or an eating disorder

Your doctor may ask for specifics, so be prepared. For instance, the doctor may ask you to describe how often you have flashbacks and what occurs when you do — or he may ask you to describe the intensity of your nightmares or how many nights per week you can't sleep. Bring some concise notes if you think it'll help you remember important points.

Also, expect a lot of questions designed to explore your feelings and behavior. These questions can be upsetting or embarrassing, but your doctor has good reasons for asking them. You may want to rehearse a little beforehand — for instance, by writing about your emotions in a journal or talking out loud to yourself about them — so you're ready to face these probing queries. Here are some typical example questions:

✔ Can you tell me what happens when you have flashbacks?

✔ Can you describe how you feel when you go back to the place where the trauma occurred?

✔ Did you suffer abuse as a child? If so, can you tell me who hurt you and how?

✔ What do you think caused the trauma? What do you think could be done to prevent a similar trauma?

✔ Do you feel like you were to blame for the trauma in any way?

✔ How is your life going? Are you doing okay at work? Are your relationships with other people healthy? Do you have issues with sex or intimacy?

✔ How much do you drink? Do you use any street drugs?

✔ Do you feel suicidal? Depressed? Angry? Do you feel any violent urges?

Respond honestly to each question, and rest assured that anything you tell your doctor will stay in the room. If you find it hard to talk about some topics, a caring doctor understands — but do your best to hang in there, and don't be embarrassed if the tears flow during your conversation. (There's a good reason every doctor's office has a box of tissues.)

More-detailed questions

Typically, the second step in making a diagnosis of PTSD involves still more Q&A, this time based on standardized checklists developed by experts on this disorder. These questions cover pretty much the same territory as the more informal questions your doctor asks, but doctors often like the confirmation of an official test result, and these results can be useful for your medical records. (Not all primary care doctors use these tests, however. Many decide, after hearing enough clues to strongly hint at PTSD, to save the formal tests for a specialist.)

If your doctor uses one of these tests, be prepared to answer a lot of questions, and be as patient as possible. These tests are pretty good at teasing out the symptoms of PTSD, and the results can help support your diagnosis so you can get insurance coverage and other services.

An unexpected culprit: When meds trigger PTSD

Be sure to tell your doctor about *every* drug you're taking, because even the safest medications can have side effects — and sometimes those side effects look like PTSD. Here's a case in point.

In the journal *Psychosomatics,* Roy Reeves and Vincent Liberto report on a Vietnam vet who went for decades without suffering PTSD symptoms despite a history of harrowing combat. At the age of 64, the man suffered an episode of chest tightness and his doctors discovered that he had high blood pressure and early heart disease. They prescribed metoprolol, a drug that's very helpful in lowering blood pressure.

The drug worked its magic on the man's blood pressure — but it also did a number on his mental state. Within a few weeks, he started to have violent nightmares about his days in Vietnam. The dreams disrupted his sleep, and he became irritable and had trouble concentrating. He started therapy for PTSD, but his symptoms worsened. He started avoiding things that reminded him of his time in combat, and he grew depressed and anxious.

Luckily, the man's doctors noticed that his symptoms started at the same time as his new medication, and they put two and two together. They switched him from metoprolol to a different drug, and after about ten days, his nightmares started to fade and his other symptoms improved.

The doctors say metoprolol can change REM sleep (the sleep stage in which most dreams occur), which may explain the man's terrible nightmares. Interestingly, this drug is related to another drug, propranolol, which is currently being tested as a treatment to *prevent* PTSD symptoms (see Chapter 4).

As this vet's case helps illustrate, a medication for *anything* — from back pain to high blood pressure to acne — can cause mental changes that are easy to mistake for PTSD. That's why your doctor needs the rundown on all your meds (including over-the-counter ones), as well as any herbal remedies or nutritional supplements you take.

A physical exam

If you think that PTSD is all in your head, think again — PTSD can affect you all over, from raising your blood pressure to upsetting your digestive system. That's why you need a top-to-toes checkup when you visit the doctor.

Your doc also wants to rule out medical conditions, some of them very common, which can mimic PTSD. Here are some of the biggest culprits:

- ✔ **Thyroid problems:** An underactive thyroid can make you feel depressed, and an overactive thyroid can cause severe symptoms of anxiety.

- ✔ **Mitral valve prolapse:** In this condition, a bulge in a heart valve allows blood to leak backward, causing symptoms ranging from heart palpitations to anxiety attacks.

✓ **Lupus or multiple sclerosis:** These autoimmune disorders (in which the body attacks its own cells) can alter both thinking and emotions.

✓ **Anemia caused by low levels of folic acid, vitamin B12, or iron:** Anemia can make you feel tired, moody, and depressed, and it can cause trouble concentrating and handling day-to-day activities.

✓ **Hypoglycemia (low blood sugar) or diabetes:** Alterations in blood sugar — either too high or too low — can cause a host of changes in your emotions and thinking, including spaciness, anger, confusion, and mood swings.

✓ **Meniere's syndrome (an inner-ear problem):** This problem can lead to anxiety and even to panic attacks.

✓ **Head injuries:** Head injuries can either mimic or complicate PTSD. These injuries can impair your thinking and memory and can cause emotional problems.

✓ **Hormone imbalances:** In women, mood swings, depression, and problems with memory or concentration sometimes occur just before or during menopause. In middle-aged or older men, low testosterone levels can lead to depression and fatigue.

✓ **Sleep apnea:** This problem, which is especially common in people with weight issues, can cause fatigue, confusion, hostility, and mood swings.

✓ **Medication reactions:** Disturbances of emotions and thinking are some of the most common side effects of drugs; see the sidebar titled "An unexpected culprit: When meds trigger PTSD" in this chapter.

Your doctor should give you a careful check-up to rule out these or other problems and to see whether PTSD is affecting your health. When the time for this exam arrives, be sure to tell your doc if you have issues that affect your ability to tolerate the level of closeness usually involved in an exam. For instance, let the doctor know if you have any of the following concerns:

✓ **A strong reaction to being touched:** Although some touching is necessary during a physical exam, a sensitive doctor can take care to respect your needs and keep hands-on evaluations to a minimum. If being touched by a person of your doctor's sex upsets you, see whether your doctor has a partner or physician assistant of the opposite sex — or make a separate appointment with a different doctor.

✓ **A strong reaction to any process or piece of equipment that triggers memories of your trauma:** These things can include tongue depressors, sedation, and certain positions or types of exams. You doctor may be able to avoid some tests or think of work-arounds that won't trigger your anxiety.

> ✔ **Fear of undressing in front of a stranger:** A sensitive doctor may find a way to limit the amount of undressing you need to do (for instance, by having you take off only one or two articles of clothing at a time) or minimize the time it takes to do the exam.
>
> ✔ **Fear of being trapped:** Tell your doctor if you feel more comfortable having a clear path to the door. Some survivors of assault feel panicky if a stranger — even a doctor — stands between them and an escape route.

If you find any part of your exam overwhelming, feel free to ask whether you can postpone some steps until your next visit. Talking about your symptoms and undergoing a physical exam on the same day can be overwhelming, and a sensitive doctor won't push you past your limits.

Taking the Next Step: What to Do If Your Doctor Says You Have PTSD

At some point, your doctor makes a diagnosis or refers you to a specialist. Reaching this point may take two or more visits, plus tests to rule out the mimicking disorders I talk about earlier in "Perform a physical exam."

If either your family doctor or a specialist says you have PTSD, now's the time for a heart-to-heart about what comes next. If you know what type of therapy you want (see Chapters 8, 9, and 10 for more info), ask for a referral that jibes with your wishes. If you don't know which approach is best for you, investigate each option your doctor recommends before selecting one. Also, if you have drug or alcohol issues, be sure your treatment plan addresses these problems.

After you decide on a course of action, see Chapter 6 for ideas on picking a therapist. You can also find tips on figuring out your insurance coverage or finding free or low-cost therapy if you don't have insurance.

Of course, you may not agree with your doctor's verdict. If you think the doc's full of beans, get a second opinion, because PTSD isn't always clear-cut and different doctors can come to different verdicts. Sadly, too, running into a doctor who's totally clueless about PTSD is possible. If that happens, don't give up — just find a better doctor.

If your doctor orders medical tests for you, be sure to get copies of the results, even if you need to pay a little for them. Keep them filed away because future doctors or your insurance company may need them.

Making the right moves if you're a veteran

If you're a military vet who can prove that you have combat-related PTSD, you're entitled to treatment at a Veteran's Affairs Hospital or Vet Center (see Chapter 6) and, in some cases, to financial compensation. First, however, you need to prove two things:

- **That you have PTSD**: To demonstrate that you have PTSD, you need a diagnosis from a medical professional (psychiatrist, psychologist, therapist, or social worker), preferably one with extensive experience in diagnosing PTSD. Many vets recommend getting your initial diagnosis from a private professional rather than starting with a VA doctor.

- **That your PTSD is linked to a stressful event that happened during your military service:** The Compensation and Pension Service of the Veterans Benefits Administration — not your doctor or therapist — makes this decision, based on information you provide.

The professional who initially diagnoses you needs to write an extensive report, offering information on your diagnosis, the link between your PTSD and your military service, and the connection between your PTSD and any other problems such as drug or alcohol abuse.

That's just step 1, because the Veterans Administration (VA) then schedules a second exam to confirm your diagnosis. This exam can include extensive interviews and a lot of paperwork.

Convincing the VA that your PTSD is service-related can be a challenge. This step is pretty cut-and-dried if you have a Purple Heart or other solid evidence of combat experience, but otherwise, the VA may balk. If you need assistance, call in the troops in the form of a Veterans Service Organization (VSO) that can hook you up with a Service Officer to help you. (This assistance is free, and many Service Officers are pros at navigating the murky waters of government bureaucracy.) To find a VSO that can help you, go to www1.va.gov/vso.

For more information on getting a diagnosis and proving that your diagnosis is combat-related, see the VA's Web site, www.va.gov, or the VA-sponsored National Center for Posttraumatic Stress Disorder at www.ncptsd.va.gov.

Chapter 6

Building Your Treatment Team

In This Chapter

▶ Assembling the right team to meet your needs

▶ Looking at the professionals who treat PTSD

▶ Getting referrals and recommendations

▶ Interviewing a prospective therapist

As you prepare to take on your PTSD, visualize the path that lies ahead of you. It's full of twists and turns and even some sheer cliffs to scale. You may get off to some false starts or even feel lost and frightened at times. But the farther you go, the less threatening and more rewarding your journey becomes. With each step, you draw closer to your goal: strength, happiness, a regained sense of connectedness, and healing.

That's not to say that the journey is short or simple. It isn't. That's why picking the best treatment team to guide you is so crucial. The people who help you face and fight PTSD are partners in the most difficult and important quest you'll ever undertake — the quest to get your life back — so take time to choose them carefully.

The task of picking a therapist can be frustrating, but don't let it slow you down. Just think of it as the next hurdle for you to catapult over on your road to healing — a much smaller challenge than the mountain you already conquered simply by saying, "I have PTSD." In this chapter, I help you tackle this job by describing the different types of therapists who treat PTSD and where to locate them. I also explain how to start off on the right foot by interviewing potential therapists before you decide which one is the best guide for the journey you're about to undertake.

Taking the Whole-Person Approach

If you're like many PTSD survivors, you're fighting more than one problem right now. Alcoholism, substance abuse, and mental disorders such as depression often go hand-in-hand with PTSD (see Chapters 3 and 8 for more information), and you can enhance your recovery by confronting and handling all these issues. As doctors are fond of saying, "If you have five nails in your shoe and remove only one, you'll still have a sore foot."

Often, therapists recommend that you first get treatment for any mental disorders and then address issues with alcohol or drugs before you start psychotherapy for PTSD. Another approach is to tackle the biggest problem first. For instance, if you're an at-risk drinker but not an alcoholic and you have severe PTSD symptoms, starting with your PTSD symptoms may make sense. Still another technique that's gaining favor is to tackle your problems as a whole (see Chapter 8).

No matter which approach proves to be right for you, your primary care doctor can offer help in assembling the team that best suits your needs. When you talk to your doctor, be honest about *all* your medical issues — even if doing so is difficult or embarrassing — so you and your doctor can develop a plan to treat all aspects of your condition. Trust me: Nothing impresses a doctor more than a patient with the courage to say, "I have a drinking problem (or a drug problem, or frightening mental symptoms) — and I need your help." The patients who give us heartburn are the ones who can't take this step.

As soon as your doctor has the full picture, he or she can find out what your insurance will cover and can give you referrals to each professional who should be part of your team.

If your recovery plan includes getting help for a mental disorder and/or addiction as well as PTSD, your treatment may include — in addition to the therapist treating your PTSD symptoms — some or all of these professionals:

- ✔ Counselors or therapists specially trained to treat alcoholism or drug addiction

- ✔ A physician, psychiatric nurse, or psychiatric nurse practitioner capable of prescribing medications needed to address your substance abuse issues or your particular mental disorder

- ✔ A social worker who can help you with issues related to your job, housing, or finances

When you start therapy, keep all the members of your team up-to-date about every treatment you're receiving. That way, they won't duplicate efforts or step on each other's toes.

Considering Your Options

Finding a therapist to treat your PTSD isn't as easy as picking a name from the phone book. No single therapy is best for every PTSD survivor, and many factors — including the type of trauma you suffered, your financial resources, and the other health issues you're addressing — play a big part in which therapist you choose.

Before you get started selecting the therapist who's right for you, you should know who's out there. In this section, I give you the lowdown on the different types of professionals who treat PTSD and the advantages and limitations of each. With this info in hand, you'll have a good idea about what each one can and can't do for you. When you're ready to begin your search, head to the section on picking the professional who best suits your needs.

Each type of professional has a different set of skills, but your therapist's title is less important than you'd think. What matters most is that you click with your therapist and that the person you choose is an expert with plenty of experience in the type of therapy you select.

Psychiatrists

A *psychiatrist* is a medical doctor (MD) with special training in treating disorders that affect thinking and behavior. Because psychiatrists are MDs, they can prescribe medications. This option can be a big help if you're battling additional problems such as depression or alcoholism, which may require drug treatments. A psychiatrist also can identify medical problems that can cause or worsen symptoms of anxiety or depression (see Chapter 7 for more on this).

A psychiatrist is by far the best choice if you have severe symptoms and especially if you have suicidal thoughts or violent impulses. This doctor is also the best option if you have any significant health problems.

Not all psychiatrists, however, practice psychotherapy, which is the core treatment for PTSD. Also, not all insurers cover PTSD treatment by a psychiatrist.

Clinical psychologists

Clinical psychologists are doctors but not MDs. Instead, they have doctoral degrees in clinical, research, or educational psychology. Typically, they list a PhD, PsyD, or EdD after their names. To be licensed, a clinical psychologist needs to have completed 6 or 7 years of graduate classes and clinical training.

Clinical psychologists are often highly trained in psychotherapy, and many have particular expertise in PTSD. Also, your insurer may require you to see a psychologist rather than a psychiatrist because it's less expensive.

On the other hand, except in New Mexico and Louisiana, clinical psychologists can't prescribe medications. Thus, they may not be the best choice if you have severe PTSD or additional problems such as depression or substance abuse. They also can't check for the medical disorders that can be invisible culprits in PTSD.

Clinical social workers

Clinical social workers (CSWs) earn their master's degrees or doctorates in social work. Licensed clinical social workers (LCSWs) are trained in psychotherapy, and they often treat PTSD. They can be an excellent option if you don't have severe PTSD and don't have complicating health or substance abuse issues.

Because licensed clinical social workers don't always receive as much upfront training as psychiatrists or clinical psychologists, you should look for an experienced LCSW who specializes in treating PTSD if you choose to go this route.

Psychiatric nurses and nurse practitioners

Psychiatric nursing is a relatively new specialty in nursing. *Advanced practice registered nurses* (APRNs) have master's degrees and can assess, diagnose, and treat problems such as PTSD. In most states, they can also prescribe medications. Although they have less training than psychiatrists, they offer some of the advantages of a medical doctor and can be more cost-effective.

Professional counselors and pastoral (religious) counselors

Among professional and pastoral counselors, you can find dedicated and brilliant therapists. The catch? Because *counselor* is a catch-all term, you may get a highly experienced therapist, or you may wind up with a complete amateur who does more harm than good.

If you're thinking of choosing a professional or pastoral counselor, ask what specific training the person has in treating PTSD. And because counseling is less intense than therapy, put this option low on your list if you have moderate or severe PTSD. It may be your best bet, however, if your PTSD symptoms are mild.

Marriage and family therapists

Marriage and family therapists look at problems such as PTSD in the context of a person's personal relationships. This setup can be an asset if you have a committed partner who's willing to commit to the healing process with you. However, a 1995 survey by *Consumer Reports* found that people in therapy rated marriage and family counselors as far less effective than psychiatrists, psychologists, and clinical social workers.

Marriage and family therapists typically have a master's degree or doctorate in psychology, psychiatry, social work, nursing, pastoral counseling, or education. But qualifications vary widely, so if you decide to go with a marriage or family therapist, be sure the person you pick is licensed and has experience in treating PTSD.

Non-psychiatrist MDs

Very few family doctors are experts on PTSD, so your primary care physician shouldn't play a big role in your day-to-day treatment. However, he or she can help a great deal by providing referrals and monitoring your progress. Your doctor can also help you address health habits — poor diet, smoking, and so on — that often accompany PTSD and can make recovery harder.

If you choose a therapist who's not an MD, seeing your family care provider before starting treatment is vital. Ask for a complete workup to identify any medical issues that can cause or worsen PTSD symptoms.

If you're seeing a clinical psychiatrist or social worker who can't prescribe medications, your therapist may be able to work hand-in-hand with your primary care physician if you need drug treatments.

Finding a Therapist

After you have an idea of what type of therapist to look for, you can begin your search. Of course, your insurance company has a big say in what type of treatment you receive, so talk with their reps before you start your search for a therapist.

Note: If you're a military veteran who qualifies for a diagnosis of PTSD, you can get free treatment through Veterans Affairs Medical Centers. (See the "Taking advantage of your veteran status" sidebar, later in this chapter.)

First things first: Consulting your insurance company (or other resources)

Before you start calling therapists' offices, you need to make a call to your insurance company. Different plans offer different types of coverage for PTSD treatment, so ask your insurer

- ✔ Whether the treatment you're seeking is covered by your plan
- ✔ If so, what percentage of the cost is covered
- ✔ Whether there's a limit to how many hours of treatment your insurance will cover or which type of therapist you can use

If you don't have insurance, you still have options. Here are some resources you can try:

- ✔ **Community clinics:** Such places often offer mental health care for free or for a reduced charge.
- ✔ **Your place of worship:** Some religious organizations can help you find free or low-cost pastoral (religiously oriented) counseling.
- ✔ **Self-help groups:** Many communities have free self-help groups led by a professional.
- ✔ **Government programs:** You may qualify for programs, such as Medicaid, that can help cover the costs of therapy.
- ✔ **Programs that compensate victims of crime:** Every state in the U.S. has one of these programs. To locate the program in your state, use the directory provided by the Office for Victims of Crime (a program of the U.S. Department of Justice) at `www.ojp.usdoj.gov/ovc/help/progdir.htm`.

If you need help exploring these options, these organizations can assist you:

- ✔ The National Mental Health Information Center (`mentalhealth.samhsa.gov/default.asp`) can provide referrals and assistance.
- ✔ The American Association of Pastoral Counselors (`www.aapc.org`) can refer you to religion-based counselors.
- ✔ The National Alliance for the Mentally Ill (`www.nami.org`) offers referrals and sponsors self-help groups and online communities where you can find support and advice.

If you're a college or university student, visit your campus clinic and ask what resources are available. If the clinic doesn't offer PTSD counseling, the staff may be able to steer you to free or low-cost community programs.

Networking your way to a good therapist

Finding a good therapist is much like finding any other good thing in life: The best way to begin is by asking the people you respect for recommendations. One good way to start is by asking your primary care doctor for a referral. If you prefer to have a variety of options, consider asking the following people whether they have any recommendations:

- ✔ Friends or relatives you trust
- ✔ A minister, priest, or rabbi
- ✔ The social services department at your local hospital
- ✔ A local support group for individuals with PTSD or anxiety disorders
- ✔ A university clinic (if you're a student)
- ✔ Your employer's human resources department

Note: If you decide to consult your work's HR department, do so cautiously if you prefer to keep your treatment confidential. If you have any doubts about your company's ethics when it comes to employees with medical issues, avoid this strategy. In a perfect world, getting treatment for PTSD wouldn't affect your job . . . but this isn't a perfect world.

Taking advantage of your veteran status

If you're a military veteran, the first step in getting help is to establish that you have PTSD and that your disability stems from your military service. For information on this process, see Chapter 5.

After you qualify for treatment, you're eligible for a wide range of free services. Veterans Affairs Medical Centers (VAs) offer outpatient, brief-treatment, and residential programs, including programs designed to treat both PTSD and substance abuse. They also offer special PTSD programs for women. The VA's treatment teams typically include psychiatrists, psychologists, social workers, counselors, and nurses.

In addition, more than 200 community-based Vet Centers, staffed by health care providers (many of them combat veterans), also offer what's called *readjustment counseling.* This service can include individual, group, and marriage and family counseling, as well as help in finding a job. In addition, these centers offer a safe haven where you can get moral support and practical advice from people who've walked in your boots. To find a Vet Center near you, visit www.vetcenter.va.gov.

If you need additional help in finding the right person, here are some excellent resources:

- ✔ The Association for Behavioral and Cognitive Therapies (www.aabt.org), a professional organization, offers a database of therapists trained in PTSD therapy.

- ✔ The Madison Institute of Medicine (www.miminc.org), a nonprofit organization, sponsors an online referral network that lists professionals with expertise in treating PTSD.

- ✔ The Anxiety Disorders Association of America (www.adaa.org) provides a referral network for both professionals and self-help groups.

- ✔ The Sidran Institute (www.sidran.org) offers referrals to qualified therapists.

If you have a friend, relative, or client who's a therapist, ask whether he or she can recommend a colleague. But remember these tips:

- ✔ As close as you may be to your business clients, always exercise the rule about not mixing your business and personal lives. It complicates issues a thousandfold if you use a therapist who's a client of your law firm or a customer of your plumbing service, so pick someone you won't see outside of the therapeutic relationship.

- ✔ Don't ask a relative or friend to be your therapist — it's unethical, and it doesn't work.

No matter who refers a candidate, do your own homework. Don't assume that anyone who claims to be a counselor or a therapist has any expertise in helping people with PTSD. In some states, those two terms can be used by just about anybody. Make sure the therapist you pick has good training — preferably a master's degree or doctorate — and at least a few years of experience in treating PTSD.

If your symptoms are severe or complicated by drug or alcohol abuse, be sure you're treated by a medical doctor (at least initially). If you're suicidal or in crisis, you may need emergency treatment or temporary hospitalization.

Making Sure You Meet Your Match

Picking a therapist isn't as easy as choosing a dentist. Your relationship with your therapist can be very intense, and you'll weather some major storms together. In a sense, you're putting your future in this person's hands. So take time to find someone you like and trust, and listen to your gut instincts. If you have good vibes on your first visit, you're likely to have a rewarding long-term relationship as well.

When you understand the terms of your insurance coverage and know what type of therapist you'd like and can afford, your best plan is to make a short list of three or four prospects and schedule an appointment to interview each one. If you have lots of choices, narrow your list to therapists close to your home. That way, following through on your commitment will be much easier.

Interviewing your prospects

Don't hesitate to ask your potential therapist lots of questions, because that's the best way to know whether you're a good match. A good therapist welcomes your questions if they're appropriate. (What's *not* appropriate? In general, questions about the therapist's personal life.) Here are some of the best questions to ask:

- ✔ **"What training do you have?"** Unless you're absolutely certain that a therapist is good enough to make up for the lack of a degree, choose someone with at least a master's degree in a field related to counseling or therapy. Also insist on someone who's licensed. A lack of licensing is a deal-breaker because it means you have no real assurance that the therapist is qualified. Also, if you pick a licensed professional, you'll be able to appeal to the licensing agency if problems arise.

- ✔ **"How much experience do you have?"** Good therapists have a gift for helping other people, but even the best get better through trial-and-error. If possible, pick someone with at least four or five years of experience in treating people with PTSD, because such therapists have a better grasp of what works and what doesn't.

- ✔ **"What approaches do you use?"** Different therapies work for different people, and you're the best judge of what's right for you. Review Chapters 8 and 10, which outline the most popular therapies for PTSD, and see whether your prospective therapist uses the approaches that make the most sense to you. (If not, ask why. A good therapist is glad to explain, and you may change your mind.)

- ✔ **"What's your feeling about using medications?"** There's no one-size-fits-all answer to this question, but it's helpful if you and your therapist have similar philosophies about the role and limitations of drug therapies in treating PTSD. Before you start interviewing therapists, reading Chapter 9 (on medications in PTSD treatment) is a good idea.

Be wary of any doctor who recommends drugs as a sole or primary treatment. The consensus of both medical and nonmedical professionals who treat PTSD is that psychotherapy is the most effective approach to treating PTSD.

✔ **"What's your philosophy about the therapist/client relationship?"** Look for a therapist who'll work with you as an active partner in the healing process. Your therapist should respect your opinions and concerns and recognize that when it comes to the causes and symptoms of your own PTSD, you're the expert.

At times during treatment, your therapist will ask you to do things that are alarming or unpleasant in order to help you face and overcome your fears. If you have a relationship of trust and mutual respect, going through these experiences as a team will be easier for you.

✔ **"Will you be sensitive to my cultural or religious beliefs?"** A therapist who doesn't understand cultural differences can misinterpret a client's remarks, miss signs of recovery or crisis, or make other major errors that impede recovery. One who's grossly insensitive to a client's religious or cultural beliefs can do even greater harm by sowing the seeds for additional trauma, doubt, and discord in a patient's life.

What your therapist's own beliefs are doesn't matter (and a good therapist probably won't tell you what they are) — but it matters a great deal that he or she can work within the framework of your culture or religion. Don't hesitate to ask whether your therapist has experience working with people from your culture or religious background or whether he or she has strong views about your religious beliefs that may interfere with your therapy.

✔ **"What's your session schedule like?"** Find out whether your prospective therapist can see you at times that suit your lifestyle. The better your schedules mesh, the more likely it is that you'll make it to all your appointments — and that's a big key to recovery.

✔ **"How much will my therapy cost?"** Patients often hesitate to ask this question, but they shouldn't. The time to handle money matters is now, before you commit to a therapist and a plan of action. A good therapist checks with your insurance, finds out what's covered, and gives you a ballpark figure of what your out-of-pocket costs will be. Also ask whether the therapist accepts direct payments from your insurer or if you need to pay upfront and be reimbursed by your insurance plan.

✔ **"How long is my therapy likely to last?"** A therapist who's seeing you for the first time typically can't tell you exactly how many sessions you'll need, because each patient is unique. However, you should be able to get an idea about whether your therapy will be short-term or long-term. The length depends, in large part, on the type of approach you select and the severity of your symptoms. If your insurance doesn't cover long-term therapy, a professional who insists on this type of approach may not be best for you.

✔ **"Can I reach you outside office hours?"** Therapists have their own lives, but they should be reachable (or have someone on call to forward messages) if you have a real emergency. Find out whether your potential therapist is willing to take calls outside of office hours in times of crisis.

Evaluating the candidates

After you interview all your candidates, analyze your feelings and the information each prospective therapist offered. Ask yourself the following:

- ✔ Which therapist has the best credentials and qualifications?
- ✔ Which one has the most experience in treating PTSD?
- ✔ Which one made you feel the most comfortable?
- ✔ Who seemed the most in tune with you?
- ✔ Whose approach to therapy seems best for you?
- ✔ Whose schedule and costs best suit your lifestyle and finances?

Your answers to these questions can steer you to the best therapist for you. (And don't feel bad about the runners-up. Therapists understand all about a concept called *goodness of fit,* which, translated into plain English, means, "I'm okay, and you're okay — but we may not be right for each other.")

As you make your decision, listen to your gut — even if your feelings don't seem fair to your candidate. For instance, if you were assaulted by a 6-foot-2 red-headed Yale grad, then a therapist who's a tall redhead from Yale probably isn't the best choice for you — even though he may be the best therapist in the world. Normally I advise people to overcome mindless prejudices, but now may not be the time.

After you make your choice, keep your momentum going by calling right away and booking the first convenient appointment time.

Working with Your Therapist

Finding a therapist you like and trust is crucial, but don't worry if your leading candidate doesn't score a perfect ten during your initial meeting. Therapists, like their clients, are human, and each has strong points and weaknesses. As long as you click on the important points (see the preceding section), don't sweat the details.

Also, remember that your relationship with your therapist, although it's important, isn't necessarily long-term. Give your therapist a fair chance — at least a few months — but if it isn't working at all (see Chapter 11 for more on this), feel free to look for someone new. And remember that each step you take in your therapy (even if it seems like a misstep at the time) is bringing you one step closer to healing. All that matters is that you keep walking!

Chapter 7

Setting the Stage for Recovery: The First Steps toward Healing

***

In This Chapter

▶ Making your environment safer

▶ Handling problem people who can sabotage your therapy

▶ Recognizing drug or alcohol abuse issues

▶ Addressing coexisting mental health problems

▶ Preparing to start therapy sessions

***

*P*icture this: You're a world-class swimmer aiming for a gold medal in the Olympics. The big day arrives, and you're crouched on the starting block waiting for the starter's pistol to go off — and suddenly you notice a 10-pound ball-and-chain attached to your ankle.

It's a silly image, but it illustrates a very serious point: Just like an Olympic swimmer, you're embarking on one of the most important jobs of your life. In fact, your mission is far more crucial than winning a medal because the therapy you're starting can get your entire life back on track. But therapy is hard work, and you'll have greater success if you're not saddled with physical, emotional, or mental health problems that can weigh you down.

In this chapter, I look at some of the biggest burdens that can get in the way of healing: a dangerous environment, unsupportive people, untreated drug or alcohol problems, and coexisting mental health problems that may complicate recovery. In addition to talking about how these problems affect you, I offer suggestions for taking control of them so you can head into therapy with more strength, energy, and resilience. In addition, I offer tips on identifying the right moment to start your therapy sessions and what you can expect when you meet with your therapist for the first time.

Making Sure You're Safe

To work toward healing in therapy, you need to start in a safe place — both inside and outside of the therapy room. Unfortunately, that's sometimes easier said than done. An inner-city resident who can't afford a safer neighborhood or a person who's being harassed by a stalker is in some degree of danger no matter what steps she takes to protect herself.

In many cases, however, you can make big or small changes to increase your safety. (For advice on getting your basic needs taken care of and regaining a sense of control in your life, please see Chapter 4.)

Seeing safety's role in helping you heal

The biggest reason for taking steps to ensure your safety, of course, is to protect your health and your life. In addition, each step you take to make your life safer can better prepare you for therapy and for healing from PTSD. That's because

- ✔ The safer your situation, the easier it is to keep your PTSD triggers under control.

- ✔ When you're living in an unsafe situation, your nervous system is stuck on red alert — and therapy works best if you're calm and as relaxed as possible.

- ✔ A dangerous life situation constantly distracts you from the work you need to do in order to heal.

- ✔ Dangerous situations set the stage for new traumas so that healing becomes harder and harder as time goes on.

One big danger that many people with PTSD face is ongoing abuse by a violent spouse, partner, or relative. In fact, domestic violence is a leading cause of severe PTSD, and ongoing abuse makes healing nearly impossible.

If you're trapped in an abusive relationship — whether it's psychological, sexual, or physical abuse — take any steps you can to get out of the situation. Otherwise, therapy can help only to a limited degree because you can't put a trauma in the past if it's still happening. Also, chronic, long-term trauma can lead to *complex PTSD* (see Chapter 3), a condition that's much harder to treat than PTSD stemming from an isolated event. And most important of all, your life and your future are at stake.

Finding help if you feel harassed or abused

Where can you find help if you have an abusive partner or if you're a senior citizen or child who's being abused by a family member? Going to the police is an obvious first choice, but sometimes battered partners, children, or seniors have reasons for hesitating to take this route. If you want to avoid that option, here are some other good places to seek help:

✔ Online resources such as

- **The National Domestic Violence Hotline (www.ndvh.org):** You can also reach this hotline at 1-800-799-7233 (1-800-799-SAFE).

- **Safe Horizon (www.safehorizon.org):** This site offers advice on how to leave an abusive relationship and provides a virtual tour of a domestic violence shelter to help you decide whether moving into a shelter is the right option for you.

  Note: If you're worried about your partner's discovering that you're using the Internet to find ways of getting out of an abusive situation, use your public library's computers instead — or consult someone who's savvy about computers to get info on how to delete the cyber trail you leave on your computer when you do Internet searches.

✔ Your local battered women's shelter (you can find these in your local phone directory, usually under a heading such as "Crisis Intervention" or "Domestic Violence Information")

✔ Your local Child Protective Services or Adult Protective Services agency

✔ A place of worship

✔ Your doctor

✔ A teacher or school counselor, if you're a minor

Another situation that can cause or complicate PTSD is long-term harassment by a stalker — often an ex-lover or ex-spouse. If this is happening to you and police can't catch the perpetrator (or they don't have enough evidence to arrest the person), here are some good resources that can help you protect yourself:

✔ **Safe Horizon:** This group (also a domestic violence resource) offers valuable info about steps you can take if you're being stalked. Visit www.safehorizon.org.

✔ **The Stalking Resource Center:** Check out this service, provided by the National Center for Victims of Crime, at www.ncvc.org/src.

If you can't get out of an abusive or threatening relationship before you begin therapy, your therapist can help you find ways to escape this situation. Bring this subject up *immediately* so your therapist knows the score right off the bat.

Ditching the Negative Nellies Who Can Sabotage Recovery

Sometimes, roadblocks to success in therapy don't stem from your own fears but from other people's failure to support or protect you. Worse yet, the people around you may actively put you in danger. If you're in either of these situations, now's the time to take stock of your relationships and see whether you need to make changes before you start therapy.

When you surround yourself with people who love and support you, weathering storms — and soaring when the skies are clear — is easier (see Chapter 13 for ways you can help these good people help you). Conversely, if you let stress-producing, energy-sapping people control your life, they can magnify your problems and stand in the way of your victories. That's why sidelining the emotional vampires is an excellent move as you prepare to start therapy.

If your Negative Nellies are absolutely unavoidable, don't panic. As soon as you're in treatment, your therapist can help you find ways to deal with problem people. But if you can get some of these jerks out of your life *before* therapy, you'll be ahead of the game when you start. In this section, I tell you how to spot the people who can sabotage your success, and I offer advice on getting them out of the picture so they can't harm you.

Spotting the people who can hamstring your healing

How can you spot the turkeys who may hold you back as you head into therapy? Some people, such as a spouse who hits you or threatens your life, are clearly bad news. However, most jerks trip you up in more subtle ways: a discouraging word here, a subtle chop to your self-esteem there. Added up over time, those digs have the power to sap your confidence, steer you away from positive goals, and weaken your resolve to heal. In the following sections, I explain how to tell these people apart from the supportive folks you want to keep in your life, and I describe the most common varieties of negative people you're likely to encounter.

Sorting out the good guys from the bad guys

The good people in your life come in lots of varieties: the true-blue friend, the lover who sticks by you through the rough spots, the boss who lets you take off early for therapy sessions without docking your pay, the parent who's always in your corner. Keeping these people close at hand when you begin the tough work of therapy is crucial.

Negative people, too, come in different varieties — and each one can interfere with your healing. If you can get at least some of these folks out of the picture prior to starting therapy, you'll be much better off.

In the following section, I describe some of the most common types of problem people to watch out for. Of course, as you read through this list, you may spot some behaviors that *you* (and everyone else you know) exhibit now and then. That's because nobody's Suzy Sunshine all the time.

So how can you tell the difference between a negative person who needs the boot and a good guy who deserves some slack when he's acting like a scamp? Here are some pointers:

- ✔ **Look for a pattern.** A negative person exhibits toxic behaviors chronically, day in and day out, to a degree that seriously affects your relationship with him.

- ✔ **Look for a reason.** The nicest person in the world can behave badly if he's dealing with a serious problem — for example, if he's undergoing chemotherapy or he just lost his job (or if he's battling PTSD!). A negative person, however, exhibits bad behaviors even when he doesn't have any major life problems that could justify his awful actions.

- ✔ **Look honestly at *your* role — if any — in causing the behavior.** For instance, if you have PTSD, your loved ones may develop a pattern of behaving called *codependency*. In other words, they develop a set of dysfunctional behaviors in response to *your* dysfunctional behaviors. They do this because it's the only way they can think of to survive in a stressful environment. (For more info on this situation, see Chapter 13.) Codependency *doesn't* mean that they're negative influences in your life. It just means they're stuck in the PTSD trap right along with you. So if any of the people you love exhibit codependent behaviors, don't cut them out of your life; instead, get them into therapy with you!

General personality types to watch out for

If you analyze your relationships carefully, you can get a good feel for who should stay and who should go. Here's my short list of people to show the door if possible (if not, the next section offers some suggestions for dealing with them):

- ✔ **Haters:** These people live in a constant state of anger and hostility. They turn every minor issue into a major confrontation, and they don't compromise — they just get madder and madder until they get their own way. You can't win with these people, because no matter how much you sacrifice your own needs to keep the peace, they'll be angry again an hour later.

  A hater can mess up your therapy by keeping you tied up in knots emotionally when you need to be calm and relaxed — and by forcing you to ignore your own needs and feelings in order to cater to hers.

- **Whiners:** A whiner is a low-level, annoying variant of the hater. (Think of the hater as an emotional sledgehammer and the whiner as a mosquito that drives you crazy.) No matter what you do, a whiner isn't happy with you, anyone else, or the world in general. The first sentence out of a whiner's mouth in the morning, and the last sentence at night, is generally a complaint.

  Because whiners are so negative, they drag you down, too. You don't need that when you're being buffeted by the strong feelings that therapy can trigger.

- **Weepers:** This type of person falls apart at the least whiff of a problem. If you're stuck with a weeper in your life, you spend much of your time walking on eggshells because you're terrified that a stray remark or minor disagreement will send the person spiraling into a scene worthy of a daytime soap actor. Just like haters, weepers get their own way all the time — but they do it by playing on your guilt, your sympathy, or your urge for peace and quiet.

  A weeper can sabotage your therapy by focusing all your attention on her drama-queen antics when you need to be focusing on helping yourself.

- **Esteem sappers:** Remember kryptonite — that green rock that makes Superman feel weak as a kitten when he gets close to it? If you think about it, you may realize that certain people affect you the same way. For example, if you say, "I lost 6 pounds!" the Human Kryptonite may say, "Wow, that's great. Another 20 pounds, and that double chin will start to go away."

  This kind of person makes you feel a little weaker, a little less competent, or a little more flawed after each encounter with him. That's especially harmful during therapy, when you need to recognize and build on your strengths, not magnify your weaknesses.

- **Bullies:** Not all bullies hang out at the playground. Many are adults who pick on co-workers, relatives, or even lovers. Bullies target people they think are weak and twist the knife in them every chance they get.

  Bullies are bad for your mental and physical health, especially when you're tackling the challenging task of therapy. They push all the wrong buttons, triggering your PTSD symptoms and sending your anxiety levels through the roof. A bullying boss, for example, can send you into a tailspin by constantly ridiculing or browbeating you in front of your colleagues.

- **Scapegoaters:** In these people's eyes, it's all your fault, all the time. If your girlfriend is a scapegoater, for example, she may constantly say things like, "You're the reason I don't go back to college. If you made more money, we wouldn't need to share the rent and I could afford school."

Scapegoaters get in the way of therapy because they constantly reinforce your own negative thoughts and feelings. When you're trying to offload toxic ideas such as "everything's my fault" or "I'm to blame for what happened in my trauma," a scapegoater is the last person you need in your life.

✔ **Narcissists:** To the narcissist, it's all about him. The whole world's a stage, and he's the only actor on it. Your role, in his eyes, is to sit in the audience and applaud.

A narcissist can be very dangerous when you're trying to heal from PTSD because therapy asks you to focus on your own thoughts and needs — and the narcissist doesn't like it when you turn your attention away from him. As a result, he may try to undermine your new feelings of confidence and happiness.

Saying goodbye to toxic people

If you spot destructive people in your life, don't let them continue to walk all over you — take action! (I call it doing a "jerkectomy.") The following sections mention some steps you can take to eliminate or reduce the influence these people have on you.

Disconnect if you can

If you don't have any hard-to-break ties to a toxic person, the best approach is often simply to walk away. To decide whether that's the best idea, look carefully at your relationship with the problem person and ask yourself the following:

✔ Do you really need this person in your life?

✔ If you have an emotional or sexual relationship with this person, would being alone really be worse than the problems the person creates?

If the answer to these questions is *no*, either say goodbye or do a gradual fade. Try to get the person out of your life before you start therapy — but if you can, do it in a cordial way with no hard feelings so he or she won't make trouble for you in the future.

Minimize contact if possible

If you're stuck with a problem person — for instance, if your dad's a hater, your boss is an esteem-sapper, or you're sharing your home with a whiny grandparent — think of ways to keep your contact with the person to a minimum. For instance,

A wake-up call

You don't need to suffer from PTSD to wake up and get rid of the toxic people in your life. Three years ago, someone I know very well had emergency, life-saving surgery. During his recovery, he had a chance to take a long, hard look at the stressors in his life — stressors that damaged his physical health and kept him from enjoying his life to the fullest.

The biggest stressors, he realized, were the toxic people in his life — the ones who always made excuses or blamed others for their problems, rarely kept promises, didn't learn from their mistakes, wouldn't cooperate, and were easy to upset and difficult to please.

In the days after his surgery, he vowed to not let any new people like these into his life. To this day, he's kept that promise — and he's healthier, happier, and more successful in every area of his life as a result.

I know this for a fact, because that someone was me!

✔ If Dad expects you over for dinner once a week, tell him you need to cut down to once a month.

✔ If your boss is the problem, see whether you can change your work hours, your assignments, or your physical location in the office in order to reduce your contact with him during the time you're in therapy.

✔ If you're living in the same house with a problem person and you're stuck with the status quo for now, see whether you can find ways to physically create some space between you. For instance, designate one room as your therapy room and declare it off-limits to other people for several hours of the day so you have a peaceful place to relax or do your therapy homework.

Ask your therapist for help

If negative people are really dragging you down and you're not in a position to cut them out of your life, talk with your therapist about this problem *before* you even start tackling your PTSD. She can offer powerful strategies for managing these people's toxic behaviors.

Facing Substance Abuse Issues

Jacob, a combat veteran, drinks to forget the faces of the friends in his platoon who didn't come home. Surani, a firefighter, downs a pint of vodka each night because alcohol numbs the emotions she feels when she remembers the horrors of 9/11. Mia was raped three years ago; she uses cocaine because it makes her mind feel less fuzzy on her bad days. Tad survived a terrible car accident; he smokes pot because it helps him sleep and keeps the nightmares at bay.

All these people have PTSD, and all of them are getting ready to take a huge positive step: the step into therapy and a healthier, happier life. To take that step successfully, they need to address not only their PTSD but also their substance abuse problems. The same is true for you if you're battling both PTSD and substance abuse and you're serious about getting your life back on track. In this section, I look at the reasons reliance on drugs or alcohol can complicate healing — and why you need to face down your substance abuse issues in order to heal.

Determining whether you're just using or abusing (it's trickier than it seems)

Stress and anxiety send your risk for substance abuse through the ceiling. In fact, people with anxiety disorders have double or even triple the normal risk for developing drug or alcohol problems at some point in their lives. And if you have PTSD — the mother of all anxiety problems — you're at even greater risk. (See Chapter 3 for more on the high rate of substance abuse problems in people with PTSD).

Owning up to a drug or alcohol problem takes great bravery. It's easier to fall into the trap of denial and use comforting strategies like the following to avoid facing your pain:

- ✔ **Minimizing:** In this strategy, you try to make light of a serious problem. For instance, you may say, "It's only two drinks a day," when each of your drinks contains 4 or 5 ounces of hard liquor.

- ✔ **Rationalizing:** In this strategy, you make excuses for your behavior instead of facing it. For example, you may say, "Hey, I'm a child of the sixties. We all used pot back then, so there's nothing wrong with smoking a little now." Or you may make excuses such as, "Of course I drink. It's because the kids drive me nuts."

Here's the hard truth: If you have a drug or alcohol problem, the only person you're actually fooling with excuses is yourself. And if you're making excuses in the first place, that's pretty strong evidence that you *do* have a problem.

If you're torn between saying, "I'm fine" and "I need help," the best favor you'll ever do for yourself is to overcome your fears and face your situation honestly. Here are some key questions that can help you decide whether you have a substance abuse problem; a *yes* answer to any one of them should tell you to seek help:

- Have you ever tried to cut back on your drinking or drug use?
- Have family members, friends, co-workers, or loved ones expressed concern about your drinking or drug use?
- Do you ever feel ashamed or guilty about your drinking or drug use?
- Have you ever had a drink in the morning to settle yourself down?
- Did your doctor ever express concern about your use of alcohol or drugs?
- Did you ever experience a memory loss or blackout when drinking or using drugs?

For more guidance in honestly evaluating your drinking or drug use, check out these Web sites:

- The U.S. government's Substance Abuse and Mental Health Services Administration offers an online self-test to help you decide whether you have an alcohol problem. The test is available at getfit.samhsa.gov/ Alcohol/tests/alcoholtest.aspx.
- A similar test is available from Alcoholscreening.org (www.alcohol screening.org), a service of Boston University's School of Public Health.
- Narcotics Anonymous offers a self-quiz that can give you insight into how drug use is affecting your life. Visit www.na.org/ips/ an/an-IP7.htm.

Reflecting on how a substance addiction worsens PTSD

The problem with substance use, of course, is that a pill or a drink solves your problems for only a few minutes or a few hours — and the price tag is steep, especially when you're dealing with something as devastating as a trauma and as life-shattering as PTSD. Here are the big downsides to the temporary relief that drugs or drinks offer when you're struggling with PTSD:

> ✔ The helplessness you feel as a result of your PTSD increases tenfold when you add the helplessness of drug or alcohol dependence or addiction.
>
> ✔ You experience new traumas and greater pain if drug use or an alcohol problem ruins your relationships, causes you to lose your job, creates legal troubles, or ruins your health.
>
> ✔ Your craving for drugs or alcohol and your behavior when you're intoxicated or high can lead you to harm your loved ones emotionally, financially, and sometimes physically. As addiction experts like to say, "People with substance abuse problems don't have families; they have hostages."
>
> ✔ An untreated drug or alcohol problem can prevent you from seeking effective treatments for your problems, limit the benefits that these treatments can offer, and greatly increase the risk of relapse after therapy ends.

The take-home message: Being smart or strong can't protect you from falling for the lure of drugs or alcohol when you're in pain. But if you're smart, you know that your future depends on escaping from this trap. And if you're strong, you overcome your denial and say those powerful words: "I have a problem, and I need help."

Opening up about substance abuse to foster therapy gains

If you have PTSD and you feel ashamed about a drug or alcohol problem, here's the most important advice I can give you: *Don't!* Having a substance abuse issue does *not* mean that you're weak or bad. Instead, it means that you're in so much pain that you turned to a desperate short-term solution in an effort to protect yourself.

As you prepare to enter therapy, you may be tempted to hide a problem with drugs or alcohol from your therapist (even if you admit this problem to yourself). However, resist the urge! A smart therapist will figure out what's going on, anyway — and more importantly, you'll only hurt yourself by failing to be upfront with the person trying to help you. What's more, your therapist will *not* think less of you for admitting your problem. Instead, he'll admire you for having the courage to face it head-on.

The best approach, no matter how reluctant you are, is the no-secrets strategy. Be prepared to acknowledge your substance abuse problems at the *very beginning* of your relationship with your therapist, and be ready to answer his questions about these issues:

What's in a name? Understanding the vocabulary of substance abuse problems

When people talk about drug or alcohol use, they bandy about terms that can be confusing. Here's a quick look at some of them:

✔ **Dependence:** If you become *dependent* on a drug or alcohol, quitting the drug causes significant physical or psychological effects — for instance, headaches, depression, or problems in thinking or concentration.

✔ **Tolerance:** If you develop a *tolerance* to a drug or to alcohol, you need more and more of it to achieve the same effect. For instance, if you need two drinks to make you relax at first and four or five drinks a couple of years later, your brain and body are developing a greater tolerance for alcohol. (That doesn't mean, however, that your body can *handle* alcohol or drugs more effectively. In fact, the longer you use drugs

or alcohol and the higher your intake, the more harmful the physical effects are.)

✔ **Addiction:** If you become *addicted* to a drug or alcohol, you exhibit three behaviors. The first is that you lose control over how often you use the substance. The second is that you ignore the consequences of your substance abuse. (For instance, you may continue to drink even if you lose your license for driving while intoxicated.) The third is that your life starts to revolve around getting and using drugs or alcohol.

If any of these terms describe your relationship with drugs or alcohol, now's the time to get help. The sooner you get that help, the higher your chances of kicking the habit are — although it's never too late to free yourself from the chains of a destructive habit.

✔ How longstanding your substance abuse problem is

✔ Whether you abuse one substance or several

✔ The severity of your problem

✔ What treatments, if any, you've undergone for your substance abuse problem and what effects (good or bad) those treatments had

✔ Whether the people you live with also have substance abuse problems, which can greatly complicate your efforts to heal

Addressing these issues upfront is crucial because it enables your therapist to make important decisions about your treatment. These decisions include

✔ Whether you'll benefit more from getting your substance abuse issues treated first or from tackling them at the same time as your PTSD (for a look at some therapies that treat both PTSD and substance abuse at the same time, see Chapter 8)

✔ Whether inpatient therapy may be more helpful than an outpatient program

✔ Which type of therapy will benefit you most and how intense it should be

✔ Whether medications should be part of your treatment plan

✔ What additional interventions — such as support groups — may help protect you against relapses

✔ Whether you and your therapist need to work on getting you into a safer environment where you'll have less contact with people involved in drug or alcohol abuse

In addition, a therapist who's fully informed about your drug or alcohol issues can coordinate with other pros if your treatment needs to be a team effort and can steer you to social and financial resources that can help you get the drug or alcohol monkey off your back. Kicking a destructive habit is a very tough but also very achievable mission, and a therapist's help can often make the difference between success and failure.

Addressing Any Coexisting Mental Disorders

In Chapter 3, I talk about the mental disorders that often occur along with PTSD. However, *any* mental disorder can coexist with PTSD. (As doctors like to say, "Having one problem doesn't prevent you from having another one.") A coexisting mental disorder may either predate your trauma or stem from it.

If you have a mental disorder in addition to your PTSD, you may feel very much alone — but you shouldn't. In reality, millions of Americans are living with one or more mental disorders. To show you just how many people are walking in your shoes, here are some stats from the National Institute of Mental Health:

✔ In any given year, approximately 26 percent of Americans 18 and older suffer from a diagnosable mental disorder. That's more than 57 million people.

✔ One in every 17 people suffers from a serious mental illness.

✔ Mental disorders are the leading cause of disability in the U.S. and Canada for people between the ages of 15 and 44.

✔ Nearly half of people with a mental disorder meet criteria for two or more mental disorders.

Tackling PTSD when you have another mental disorder is a challenge, but millions of people meet that challenge successfully — and you can, too! Here's one big key: getting your mental illness under as much control as possible before you head into the therapy room to address your PTSD. The fewer problems you have on your plate, the better you'll do in therapy for PTSD. Many mental disorders are chronic, but minimizing your symptoms as much as possible can maximize your therapy gains.

Talking to your current physician

To minimize symptoms of a mental illness before starting therapy for PTSD, make an appointment with the doctor who manages the treatment of your mental illness. At this appointment, tell your doctor that you're planning to start therapy for PTSD, and have a heart-to-heart talk about the following issues:

- ✔ Are the medications (if any) that you currently take to treat your coexisting mental disorder working well, and are any side effects as well-controlled as possible?

- ✔ Should you consider additional medical treatments to bring the symptoms of your disorder under greater control before starting therapy for PTSD?

- ✔ Is this a good point in your life to start therapy, or are there reasons for waiting a little while? For example, if your doctor recommends adding, dropping, or changing your medications, giving your new meds a few weeks to settle in before you start therapy may be a good idea. That way, you can handle any side effects that may otherwise interfere with addressing your PTSD.

During your appointment, be clear to your doctor that you're very open to the idea of her communicating with your new therapist. Both professionals will ask you to sign forms allowing them to exchange information, but they'll be even more likely to share their ideas if you give them the green light verbally.

Gathering the info your therapist needs

After your visit to the doctor, gather the materials your new therapist will need in order to be up-to-speed on your condition. If possible, get copies of the medical records describing your mental disorder and the treatments you've received. Here's some information you should have ready:

✔ Facts about any mental illnesses for which you've been treated, even if you're not having a problem with these conditions now

✔ The names and dosages of any medication you're taking

✔ How long you've been taking these medications

✔ Any side effects you're currently experiencing or have experienced in the past

✔ Other treatments you've undergone — including inpatient therapies, electroshock therapies, medications, or psychological therapies — and the results (good or bad) of these therapies

This information can help your therapist plan his own approach, allow him to watch for drug effects that may complicate the therapy picture, and aid him in coordinating with the rest of your medical team.

Also, if you suspect that you may have a mental disorder but you don't have an official diagnosis, plan to discuss this with your therapist at your first appointment. Together, you and your therapist can sort out the symptoms that PTSD can cause and those that may stem from additional disorders so you can tackle all your issues in the most effective way.

A Few Final Details: Getting Your Ducks in a Row

After you address any major life issues, your path is just about cleared for takeoff. Here are a few additional pieces to put in place so you're set for success when you start your therapy:

✔ **Finalize your plans.** Be sure you're happy with the therapist you selected and the approach he plans to use. (See Chapter 6 for info on selecting a therapist and Chapters 8, 9, and 10 for information about the different approaches used to treat PTSD.) Also, make sure you've addressed any questions about insurance coverage (see Chapter 6).

✔ **Line up your allies.** Tell trusted friends or relatives that you're starting therapy. These people can encourage you to stay the course and can offer practical help — for instance, by driving you to sessions or babysitting your kids when you're at the therapist's office.

✔ **Clear your schedule.** Now's the time to minimize your outside obligations so you'll have more time for your own needs. Keep up the activities you love, but say *no* to extra work hours or other commitments if they'll get in the way of your therapy.

✔ **Handle any logistical issues.** Make sure you have a reliable ride to and from your therapy sessions. If your car's a little hinky, get it fixed. Don't have a car? Get a bus pass and learn the route to your therapist's office. Also, make sure you have sitters lined up and have work responsibilities covered if you need to attend therapy during work hours.

These details are more important than you may think. That's because at some challenging points in therapy, you'll be tempted to use little issues like this — "Gee, it's raining, and my brakes aren't all that reliable" — to give yourself an out to avoid therapy sessions. The fewer excuses you have, the more likely you are to do the right thing!

The last and most important stage in preparing for therapy is to get your game face on. To strengthen your resolve as you start on this new journey, visualize the future you want — a future in which your hopes and dreams, not your fears and nightmares, steer your life. Therapy is the first and most important step into that future, so head into your first session with hope and confidence — as well as pride in yourself for having the courage to heal.

Getting Acquainted with Your Therapist

If you interviewed several therapists before picking one (see Chapter 6 for more on this), you and your therapist will already know a little about each other. If not, you'll be starting from scratch. Either way, here's what to expect.

Right off the bat, your therapist will want a broad overview of the trauma you survived, what symptoms bother you the most, and when your symptoms developed. In addition, the therapist will probably bring up the following topics early on in order to plan an approach that works just right for you:

✔ **Your goals for therapy:** The two of you will probably talk upfront about your expectations and what you can anticipate from your sessions.

✔ **Your ability to confront your trauma and your triggers:** Lots of approaches are in the therapy toolbox, so a good therapist can decide whether you can benefit more from a slow-and-steady approach or an all-at-once face-off with your demons. (More on these options later, in Chapter 8.)

✔ **Your pre-trauma history:** Sometimes the trauma you blame for your symptoms is only the tip of the iceberg, and facing it can bring earlier, buried traumas back to the surface. Thus, your therapist may ask you questions about things that happened years or even decades earlier.

✔ **Your readiness:** Your therapist will help you decide whether the time is right for you to start your sessions. For instance, if you're in the middle of a divorce and moving to a new home, the therapist may recommend that you wait a little while. Also, the therapist may decide that first tackling other problems, such as alcohol or substance abuse, makes sense. (But don't assume that this will happen; many therapists prefer to treat these issues at the same time as your PTSD.)

✔ **Your backup bench:** Strong support from the people close to you — a loving spouse or partner, caring relatives, good friends, an Alcoholics Anonymous sponsor if you have an issue with alcoholism — can be a huge help. Conversely, relatives or friends who don't back you up can impede your progress. It helps if your therapist has a clue upfront about allies as well as potential skunks at the garden party.

✔ **The ground rules you can expect:** Generally, a therapist uses the first session to outline the basics of your relationship. This info usually includes the following:

- How long your therapy will take (cognitive behavioral therapy, or CBT, is usually a short-term therapy, but short-term can mean anything from 1 to 12 months; your therapist can probably give you a guesstimate, if not a firm answer)

- How much work you'll need to do outside of your sessions

- What rights and responsibilities you have as a patient

You may also talk about mundane stuff, such as billing and scheduling, just so you can get those details out of the way and clear the path for the important work that lies ahead.

Part II
Getting a Diagnosis and Drafting a Plan

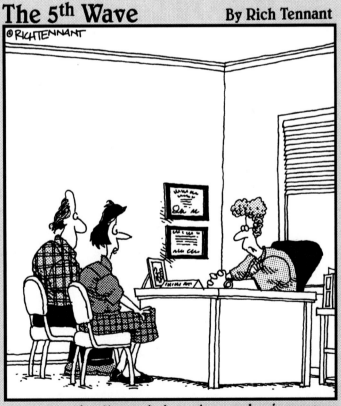

The 5th Wave   By Rich Tennant

"I realize the diagnosis is serious and raises many
questions, but let's try to address them in order.
We'll look at various treatment options, make a list
of the best clinics to consider, and then determine
what color ribbon you should be wearing."

In this part . . .

If you're reeling from the effects of a trauma and you think you may have PTSD — or if you already know you have PTSD and you're wondering what to do next — this part offers the advice you need. I start by providing a self-quiz to help you spot potential PTSD symptoms. Next, I tell you the steps to take if your answers point to PTSD, and I describe ways to maximize your chances of getting an accurate diagnosis from your doctor. If your physician does diagnose you with PTSD, I give advice here about finding a good therapist and creating the right environment to plant the seeds of healing.

Chapter 8

Putting PTSD in Its Place with Cognitive Behavioral Therapy (CBT)

*I*n an old sitcom episode, a character finds a pistol and decides to cash it in at a New York pawn shop. The clerk sees the gun and hits the alarm button, and this hapless fellow is arrested. Complications follow, but in the end, the character convinces the court that he's innocent. Before letting him go, however, the judge says, "It is against the law to sell a gun in New York. What will you do if you find another one?"

"Pawn it in New Jersey," replies our hero.

What's the point? That incorrect thoughts can steer you in wrong directions, which may be funny when you're talking about pawned firearms but not when you're talking about PTSD — a problem that creates patterns of thinking that lead to a vicious cycle of helplessness, anxiety, and self-destructive behavior.

To break that cycle, you need to replace it with a cycle of healing and resilience — and an excellent way to do that is a treatment called cognitive behavioral therapy (or CBT for short). CBT has a strong track record in treating PTSD, so it's an approach your doctor is likely to recommend. In this chapter, I look at what CBT is and how well it works as a treatment for PTSD. I also explain why CBT — although an excellent form of therapy — isn't the right treatment for everyone. In addition, I walk you through the steps of CBT and describe some of its many forms.

Understanding What CBT Is All About

CBT is a popular and effective treatment for a wide range of disorders. In particular, it's a powerful therapy for anxiety disorders, including PTSD. As you can guess from its name, this therapy addresses two issues:

- ✔ **Thinking (cognition):** The patterns of thinking that PTSD fosters can keep you trapped in the PTSD cycle. The *cognitive* part of CBT tackles these harmful thought patterns and helps you to break free of them.

- ✔ **Acting:** A trauma can lead you to act in ways that get in the way of healing. The *behavioral* part of CBT empowers you to spot and change these behaviors and to replace them with behaviors that work for you.

Because CBT deals with thinking and behavior, some people conclude that a trauma survivor's thoughts and behavior *caused* PTSD in the first place. Far from it! The trauma is the culprit, and the self-destructive thoughts and behaviors that result are *symptoms* — just like the runny nose and icky throat you get when a cold attacks you. In fact, doctors also use CBT to help people cope with chronic pain due to back injuries or diseases. You're in the same boat — your trauma simply caused a different type of pain.

In the sections that follow, I explain the basic principles that underlie CBT.

The foundation: Key principles that guide CBT

CBT is designed to produce results in a short time frame — usually a few months — so if the word *therapy* conjures up pictures of spending years on a couch talking to Sigmund Freud, you can chase those images away. CBT isn't the kind of therapy where you look at ink blots or talk about how your mom toilet-trained you. Instead, it's a practical approach that's based on the following principles:

- ✔ You're a strong, resilient person who can develop the tools you need to get a handle on your PTSD.

- ✔ The physical, biochemical, and emotional effects of your trauma created patterns of thoughts and behaviors that now interfere with your life.

- ✔ Just as you can train yourself to kick a soccer ball or play the piano better, you can change your life by challenging counterproductive cycles of thinking and behavior and replacing them with effective, self-affirming thoughts and behaviors.

> ✔ You're an active partner in therapy, and the ultimate goal is for you to leave with tools you can use to handle your PTSD independently.
>
> ✔ The more information you have about your trauma and how to treat your symptoms, the better you can heal. That's why CBT also includes education about how and why PTSD occurs.

CBT assumes that you're highly motivated and willing to invest in your recovery. It's hard work, and your therapist will expect you to do lots of homework outside of your sessions— for instance, practicing the healing thoughts and actions you discover in therapy or possibly keeping a journal about your progress and setbacks. That's because changing thoughts and behaviors, just like building muscles or learning to play a Beethoven sonata, takes practice. The good news is that the more effort you put in upfront, the more rewards you're likely to reap down the road.

The focus: Correcting destructive thought patterns

If you have PTSD, you suffered a terrible trauma that no one should ever experience. However, it's not the trauma itself but the thoughts, behaviors, and emotions that evolved from this crisis that keep you trapped. In the next sections, I describe how these negative cycles arise and how CBT can replace them with positive cycles of thinking and behaving that lead to healing.

Seeing healthy and unhealthy feedback loops in action

A simple thought can hold amazing power. The thought "I'm as good as you!" led Rosa Parks to refuse to sit in the back of a bus and jump-started the American Civil Rights movement. The thought "You are not hopeless!" led Annie Sullivan to give a young blind and deaf child, Helen Keller, the tools she needed to become a bestselling author and an inspiration to the world.

Unfortunately, destructive thoughts have an equally astonishing power to change lives. (Some patients and therapists like to call these *negative useless thoughts* — or NUTs for short!) That's why chasing these thoughts away is a key goal of CBT.

To understand how CBT works, think of your thoughts, feelings, and actions as interconnected loops: Jiggle one, and you set off a reaction that alters the others. Your thoughts affect how you feel and behave, and in turn, your feelings and behavior affect how you think. Normally, this creates a healthy feedback loop. Here's an example:

1. You think, "I'm good with a hammer and saw — I can tackle this broken gate."

2. Based on that thought, you get out your hammer and saw, and a few hours later, presto: Your old, broken gate looks good as new.

3. You feel proud and you think, "Hey, maybe next week I'll fix that attic ladder."

Feedback loops play a big part in PTSD too, but in this case, they create a vicious cycle. That's because your trauma generates self-destructive thoughts and behaviors that feed on each other, creating a downward spiral. Here's an example:

1. A man attacks Jane, beats her, and steals her purse as she leaves the mall at night. Because of this trauma, Jane develops certain thoughts and beliefs that change how she behaves. One thought, for instance, is "Going out of the house after dark is very dangerous."

2. As a result, Jane stops leaving her house at night. She makes so many excuses to stay home that her boyfriend, initially supportive after her trauma, finally leaves her, saying, "You're hopeless. You won't even go out to dinner. In fact, you won't go out the front door at night. That's just nuts."

3. Her fears and anxieties, and her boyfriend's reaction to them, make Jane think, "I'm going crazy. I can't even go to the mailbox after dark. There's something really wrong with me. I'm getting worse, not better."

4. To soothe herself when these thoughts upset her, Jane has a drink. It works at first: A shot of Scotch calms her for at least a half-hour and lets her read a book or watch TV in peace. That good feeling reinforces her urge to drink, so she starts having two drinks each night — then three and then four.

5. Jane's drinking eases her stress for a few hours, but it brings on a new wave of self-destructive thoughts: "I'm turning into a lush, just like my grandpa. I'm weak." It also makes her even more isolated: She now refuses to open her door to friends, for fear that they'll discover her secret drinking, and sometimes she won't answer the phone for fear that people will hear her slurring her words.

6. The more isolated Jane becomes as a result of these new behaviors, the worse she feels. And the worse she feels, the more she drinks.

Jane's story shows how a single counterproductive thought — in this case, that going outside after dark is dangerous — can start a chain of behaviors, thoughts, and emotions that break up relationships, alter lifestyles, and even lead to problems with drugs or alcohol.

Identifying the most common types of negative self-feedback

The list of negative thoughts that can stem from PTSD is virtually endless. However, these thoughts tend to fall into some common patterns. Here are some of the typical thoughts that trip up people with PTSD:

- **Overgeneralizing thoughts:** These types of thoughts occur when you mistake a single negative event (or person or thing) as part of a bigger pattern. For instance, if your trauma involved a traffic accident, you may generalize, "It's not safe to drive anywhere"; if your trauma involved a person who attacked you, you may think, "People are cruel."

  Your therapist can help you to spot the error of this thinking. For example, if you were assaulted during an evening walk, you may generalize that "Walking outside in the evening is dangerous." Your therapist can help you see that if you took a pleasant stroll around the block every evening for 20 years before a mugger attacked you one night, then you had more than 7,300 nice walks and only one time when a trauma occurred. Giving up your walks, on the tiny chance that a similar trauma will occur, makes no sense when viewed this way.

- **Always/never thoughts:** , These thoughts — such as "I always fail," "I never win," "My bosses always hate me," or "People never give me a fair shake" — are similar to overgeneralizing thoughts because they make you follow an extreme course. For instance, you may shun romantic relationships and break bonds with good friends if your always/never thoughts say, "I can never trust anyone again," or "I always get hurt by my friends."

  If your always/never thoughts involve people, your therapist may ask you to consider how many people you've known in your entire life and how many actually hurt you. Odds are, your *helped* list will be a whole longer than your *hurt* list.

- **One-side-of-the-equation thoughts:** In this kind of thinking, you look at only one limited (and negative) set of facts when making a decision instead of considering all the data. For instance, these thoughts may tell you, "If I avoid dating, I won't get hurt." True, maybe, at least in the short run. But do a loss-versus-benefits analysis, and you realize that in avoiding the small risk of being hurt by a boyfriend or girlfriend, you give up fun, sexual pleasure, the possibility of having a family down the road, and the long-term safety and comfort of having another person who cares about you deeply. Your therapist can help you see how changing this kind of toxic thinking can make you happier — and safer — in the long run.

✔ **Catastrophizing thoughts:** These thoughts take several forms. In one, you mentally transform small events into catastrophes. For example, you may think, "Oh great, a flat tire. That's a sure sign things are falling apart all over again." In another form, you constantly anticipate the terrible things that may happen to you. For instance, if a friend invites you to take a quick trip to the mountains, you don't think, "Hey, that'll be fun. I could use a break." Instead, you may immediately start thinking things like, "I'd better not leave. Someone could break into the house if I'm not here and take my stuff. And if they take my computer, they could get my personal data and rifle my bank account."

Catastrophizing can send you into a tailspin by making each minor puddle seem like a flood of misfortune or by making you afraid to have new experiences and trapping you in fear. In therapy, you can discover how to replace catastrophizing with positive thinking patterns that let you experience and enjoy life again.

I take a look at some more negative thinking patterns — and how a therapist can help you root them out — in "Step 3: Undoing false ideas," later in this chapter.

Setting sights on the goal: How CBT works

The goal of CBT is simple: to nip the negative thought cycle in the bud. It does this by

1. Identifying the toxic thoughts your trauma caused

2. Challenging these false and self-defeating thoughts, replacing them with thoughts that make sense, and turning your life in a positive direction

3. Spotting unproductive behaviors that stem from false thoughts and replacing them with behaviors that further your goals

Here's a good example of how this works:

Maxine, an avid nature lover, decides to take an early-morning hike. She starts at 7 a.m. because she wants to avoid the summer heat. Halfway up the mountain, she takes a little-used trail and falls, breaking her leg and cutting herself badly on a branch as she tumbles into a ravine. Maxine lies on the out-of-the-way path for two hours, terrified and in horrible pain, before another hiker finds her and calls for help.

Maxine develops symptoms of PTSD after this frightening event. She also develops a host of negative thoughts that alter her life, such as the following:

It's not safe to be in the mountains or even outdoors.

I always make stupid decisions — just like when I went hiking alone.

I'm just staying home from now on because it's safer.

If I try to have a good time, it'll probably go wrong and I'll wind up in trouble.

When Maxine's symptoms finally become overwhelming and she seeks therapy, her therapist helps her to identify these thoughts and replace them with more realistic and positive thoughts like these:

Being outdoors isn't perfectly safe, but the odds that something bad will happen are actually very small. If I take precautions, such as hiking with a friend and bringing a whistle or emergency flares along, I can make my favorite outdoor activities even safer.

I make thousands of decisions, and the vast majority of them are very smart and practical. Deciding to go on a hike alone early in the morning may not have been the best decision I ever made, but nobody makes perfect decisions all the time.

I could get hurt again if I go camping or hiking, but it's more likely that I'll have a great time and be healthier because of the exercise and fresh air. Staying shut up in the house won't make me much safer, and in the long run, it'll keep me from enjoying my life.

I don't need to focus on the bad things that could happen to me if I say yes to a fun activity. Instead, I can look forward to the good things that could happen.

As a result of her insights, Maxine gradually gets back into her favorite outdoor activities. She attends a hiking-safety class to make sure she's prepared for emergencies and hooks up with some hiking buddies — both practical responses to her traumatic experience. Maxine no longer feels terrified at the thought of being in the great outdoors. In fact, she now plans on heading up a hiking group for a local recreation center.

Figuring Out Whether CBT Is a Good Match for You

CBT is good medicine for PTSD. However, it's not for everyone. First off, you need to be very motivated, because CBT (as I mention earlier) is hard work. In addition, your therapist will look for these signs that CBT is the right approach for you:

✔ You're not living in a dangerous situation (for instance, with an abusive spouse).

✔ You're not currently suicidal or very violent.

✔ You don't have another psychiatric disorder than needs treatment first.

✔ If you have a substance-abuse problem, it's under enough control for you to participate successfully in CBT (or your CBT takes your substance use issues into account — see the upcoming section titled "Combined treatments for people with PTSD and substance abuse issues").

✔ Your health is good enough to allow you to cope with the temporary stress that CBT can cause.

If you don't meet all these criteria right now, your therapist may recommend handling other problems first so you can clear the way for CBT to work successfully — or he may suggest a different treatment approach.

The effectiveness of CBT

Overall, a CBT approach that includes directly confronting your trauma is highly effective according to studies. Here are some of the latest findings:

✔ Paula Schnurr asked 277 female veterans and 7 active-duty female personnel with PTSD to undergo either ten weeks of *prolonged-exposure therapy* (a type of CBT that involves mentally re-experiencing a trauma and working through it) or a different type of therapy that focused only on the women's current problems and avoided exposing them to their traumas. She reported in 2007 that women in the prolonged-exposure group were more than twice as likely to achieve a complete remission after therapy — as well as more likely to lose their PTSD diagnosis — as women in the other group.

✔ The Cochrane Collaboration, a group that reviews medical research to help professionals figure out what works and what doesn't, reported in 2005 that trauma-focused CBT and stress management

(which is typically a part of CBT) reduced PTSD more effectively than other standard psychological therapies.

✔ In 2007, Barbara Rothbaum compared the drug sertraline (Zoloft; see Chapter 9) alone to a combination of sertraline and CBT. The researchers found that patients who responded to sertraline got even better when they later underwent CBT, and those on the drug alone didn't continue to improve.

The National Center for Posttraumatic Stress Disorder notes that there are more published, well-designed studies on CBT (more than 30) than on any other PTSD treatment. And according to these studies, CBT is a highly effective treatment that produces marked reductions — generally 60 to 80 percent — in PTSD symptoms. It's especially effective in survivors of rape. Vets with combat-related PTSD show smaller benefits, but for this group as well, CBT produces better and longer-lasting treatment effects than other approaches.

When you look at the stats on CBT's usefulness (see the nearby sidebar, "The effectiveness of CBT"), remember that your mileage may vary. Different people respond differently to treatments, and what works like a charm for you may not work for the guy next door (and vice versa). That's why Chapter 10 describes many other treatments that can help you tackle PTSD if CBT isn't your best road to healing.

If your therapist does use CBT to treat your PTSD, remember that you may need other therapies as well. That's especially true if you have issues with alcohol or drugs or if you have complex PTSD (see Chapter 3).

The ABCs of CBT

CBT is a little like banana nut bread: It comes in different flavors, and every practitioner has a slightly different recipe for success. Thus, ten different therapists may go about CBT in ten slightly different ways, and therapists often mix and match approaches. Also, your therapist may switch from one approach to another, based on your responses. (For info on some relatives of CBT, see "Variations on a Theme: Offshoots of CBT," later in this chapter.)

However, just about every standard version of CBT follows a basic pattern, and in this section, I outline the typical elements of the CBT approach.

Step 1: Gaining the tools you need to feel safe in the moment

Right now, your trauma is like a painfully infected tooth: More than anything, you want to prevent anyone from touching it. But to win your battle with PTSD, you need to confront the problem and overcome it — because just like that bad tooth, it's not going away on its own.

Looking your trauma straight in the eye is a daunting prospect, so letting down your guard and digging down to the roots of your symptoms is tough. To take that big step, you need ironclad assurance that it's safe. Therapy works only if you can face your trauma, put the pieces of your experience together, and come to a new understanding — and that requires strong protection from the overwhelming emotions your memories can release.

Getting on the same page: Permission to heal

Todd's wife and two daughters counted on him, so he knew he needed therapy when he developed PTSD after the trauma of losing his son Jamie to an illness. But without consciously realizing it, he viewed therapy and healing as a form of betrayal — a way of forgetting his son. His mixed feelings came up in the first session with his therapist.

"Forgetting what happened to Jamie," he told his therapist, "makes it seem like he didn't really count. I don't ever want to feel that way."

The therapist reassured Todd that CBT *doesn't make a person forget.* Instead, it empowers an individual who's lost a loved one to comprehend, integrate, and deal with this loss in a positive way. That accomplishment, the therapist explained, would allow Todd to honor Jamie's life and what it meant to his family instead of remembering only his death.

When Todd realized that CBT could help him deal with his memories positively — not block them out of his life — he felt ready to tackle therapy. He made remarkable progress, and one year later, he sent his therapist an invitation to a 10K run — organized by Todd and named after his son — to raise money to combat the illness that took Jamie's life.

Like Todd, you may have some big questions about the goals of CBT. If so, don't feel embarrassed; after all, you're not a professional therapist. That's why talking openly with your therapist at the very beginning of your relationship is important. That way, you can get a feel for what will and won't happen over the course of your therapy — and what realistic goals you can have.

A good therapist offers you that protection by giving you the tools to put the brakes on when memories get too intense. With these tools always handy, you can confront the worst of your memories and know that you're safe and secure at all times. Sometimes, these tools are sufficient treatments in and of themselves (see Chapter 10), but more often, they're a first step in therapy. Typically, after giving you some basics about your PTSD and about CBT, your therapist will begin your treatment by focusing on these techniques.

One of the tools you use may be *stress inoculation training* (SIT). In SIT, you discover why certain situations cause stress, how stress affects you, and ways you can cope when a stressful situation arises; then you practice a specific set of stress-reducing skills in your therapy session, with your therapist helping by offering feedback. These skills vary depending on your needs, but a few of the most common are

✔ **Breathing techniques:** Controlling your breathing can short-circuit a stress response.

✔ **Thought stopping:** To train you in this skill, your therapist asks you to think about a distressing topic and then forcefully says, "Stop!" and asks you to immediately think about a pleasant topic — for instance, playing with your dog or baking cookies with your kids. As you practice, you gradually take over this "Stop!" response yourself so you can prevent distressing thoughts from spiraling out of control.

✔ **Positive self-talk:** All day long, people talk to themselves. Much of this talk is just random stuff such as, "Oops, I forgot to pick up the dry cleaning." But mixed in are some recurring themes, and the negative ones can cause big trouble if you don't root them out. People with PTSD, for instance, can say mean things to themselves — things they'd never say to a friend or loved one. (For instance, "I know I'm going to screw this up," or "I'm going to panic if I try this.") Your therapist can help you spot some of these messages upfront and replace them with validating messages.

This practice is much like the cognitive restructuring you do later in therapy (more on this in "Step 3: Undoing False Ideas," in this chapter), but practicing positive self-talk is more general and less specific to your trauma.

✔ **Muscle relaxation:** You can use techniques to ease the tension that builds up in your body in order to calm your mind.

✔ **Biofeedback:** You learn to spot your body's signals of tension so you can nip that tension in the bud. For example, as you watch a display of your heartbeat increasing or decreasing, you can actually figure out how to calm your racing heart.

You then practice these new skills in real life, and you and your therapist fine-tune them so you know they'll work when you call on them.

Your therapist also keeps you safe during therapy by deciding when you're ready to press ahead and when you need to take a breather. As an outside observer, he's capable of monitoring your emotions, behavior, and physical responses and ensuring that you don't push too hard or too soon.

Step 2: Confronting your trauma

To change the thoughts and behaviors that sprang from your trauma, you need to face what happened and how it damaged you. CBT allows you to safely confront your trauma in an environment where you're totally in control.

After you and your therapist know that you have the tools to face your fears (see the preceding section), you're ready to shed sunlight on the event that changed your life so dramatically.

Understanding the necessity of this step

In most cases, a therapist starts this process of confrontation by explaining *why* this face-to-face meeting with your foe is crucial. To give you a bit of a preview, here's why you must face your fears in order to be free of them:

- ✔ The initial event you experienced caused you to suffer terribly. Just thinking about this event causes you distress.

- ✔ Other seemingly innocuous objects or events — such as a parking lot where an assailant attacked you or the brand of shoes he was wearing — can cause you to feel distress, too, because your mind now connects them to the event.

- ✔ Avoiding memories and thoughts about the initial trauma or your triggers makes you temporarily feel better. Thus, you're rewarded (at least in the short run) for escaping your negative feelings. (In doctor talk, you're *reinforced* for avoiding your issues.) In the long run, however, this sets you up for far worse problems, because hidden wounds fester.

The best way to stop this downward spiral is to look your trauma — and the triggers that are linked to it — right in the face. When you do this repeatedly, a process called *habituation* occurs: The emotions attached to your memories start to fade, causing you less pain or anger or fear each time.

To understand habituation, think about those flying monkeys in the *Wizard of Oz*. The first time you saw them as a tyke, they probably scared the you-know-what out of you. But each time you watched the movie, you responded a little less — and eventually you could view the scene from a relaxed point of view and think about things like, "How did they get all those monkeys to fly?" A similar thing happens in exposure therapy, because each time you confront your fears, you take more of the sting out of them.

A related word you may hear from your therapist is *extinction*. Remember Pavlov's dog from high school science class? Pavlov rang a bell every time he fed the dog, and soon the dog started slobbering any time he heard the bell — even if no food was in sight. The food was the main event. The bell, because it became linked to the food, gained its own power. (The bell is called a *conditioned stimulus* because salivating at the sound of a bell is a learned response, not something that comes naturally.) But when Pavlov rang the bell time after time without offering any food, the dog eventually caught on and stopped drooling. That's called extinction.

Now, you're not a dog, and you don't slobber. (At least I hope not!) But extinction is a key idea to understand if you have PTSD. That's because your triggers, like Pavlov's bell, are conditioned stimuli. When you keep facing these triggers and nothing terrible happens, your mind finally sits up and takes notice: "Hey, this isn't really connected to the terrible thing that happened to me." When that happens, you break the spell that your trigger has on you — you stop responding to that bell — and you take a big step on the road to healing.

Renovating your mind at your own pace

Patients who hear the word *extinction* (the disappearance of a conditioned response) sometimes joke, "I may *become* extinct if you make me do this." Behind that joke lurks a very real and very big fear: A person who lives through a trauma feels, deep inside, that he couldn't have survived it — and that he can't survive *now* if he confronts that trauma head-on. So you can expect that your urge will be to run away rather than to stand your ground. Take heart, though: Your therapist starts you on this journey only when you're clearly ready to face and conquer your fears.

When you start therapy, you may worry that tearing down the barriers that hold in your emotions will cause your fears to flood in. But don't fear: A good therapist doesn't take away those walls. Instead — like a landscaper suggesting a picket fence instead of a barbed-wire fence — your therapist gives you options and lets you choose your own path.

For example, if you avoid driving, your therapist isn't going to say, "Bob! Get off your fanny right now and get into that car — or else!" Instead, she'll probably say something like this: "If you feel better not driving, using the bus is a fine solution. But if you decide at any point that it'd make your life better to be able to drive to work or to the store, here are some tools to help you feel safe when you get in your car. Go ahead and practice them, and then you'll be able to use them if you decide that you want to try driving again. At that point, we can take one step at a time and see how it goes."

In short, you can keep using your old defenses, or you can explore the new options your therapist offers without feeling like you have to commit to them — sort of a lease-to-buy option. At every point, you're the person in charge, so don't worry that your therapist will force you into a corner. She may encourage you strongly to take scary steps, but she won't push you past your limits. (If she does, find another therapist.)

Be prepared, however, because your PTSD is going to get worse before it gets better. To realize why, think of a splinter. Covering it with a bandage and pretending it doesn't exist is easier, but unless you pull it out, it'll keep hurting and possibly get infected. Removing the splinter hurts — sometimes a lot — but in the long run, it's the only way to heal. The same is true for tackling PTSD, so be ready for tears, anger, grief, guilt, shame, and even physical symptoms such as shaky hands or a racing heart. These reactions are a good thing, because they mean that you're getting to the root of your problem. And here's the good news: As you face and conquer each fear, you'll start to experience positive feelings of hope, relief, and joy. Most important of all, you'll experience the feeling of getting back in control of your life.

Getting to work: Spotting your triggers

When you and your therapist decide that you're completely ready, both of you can get to work. Your therapist may start by asking you to list the situations that trigger your flashbacks or bad memories and to describe how severe each one is. Therapists call this score *subjective units of distress,* or SUDs, and they typically use a rating system of 1–10 or 1–100, with the highest end of the spectrum being the most intense distress. Your therapist also asks you to describe how you react to a trigger. Table 8-1 shows one patient's list.

Table 8-1	Triggers Identified before Exposure Therapy	
Trigger	**Rating**	**How Do You React?**
Young men with long dirty-blond hair and the same build as the man who assaulted me	9	Sometimes I flash back to my attack, and I feel like I need to run away. Other times, I can block the impulse to run away, but I can feel my heart pounding and I'm filled with so much nervous energy that I can't stop moving.
The sight of the fast food restaurant where my trauma occurred	8	I can't eat at this restaurant anymore. One time I tried going through the drive-through and panicked and had to back out and drive away. Sometimes I hear commercials for this restaurant and I feel trapped, like I need to run somewhere.
The feel of a man's beard against my face	7	If my husband doesn't shave every day, I feel sick to my stomach when his whiskers touch my face.
The sound of rap music	3	I remember there was a rap song blaring from a car parked outside the restaurant when the man who assaulted me cornered me in the alley. Now, when I hear rap music, I feel scared and sick.
Movies or news stories about women being assaulted	10	I feel like I'm freaking out if I turn on the TV and hear something about a rape or an assault. My heart beats really fast, and I panic. If I was on my way out of the house, I can't make myself leave. Instead, I lock all the doors and stay home.

As you continue with your therapy, you may spot other triggers. If so, you and your therapist add them to this list.

Thinking about your triggers is hard, and so is confronting them (see the next section). When the going gets tough in therapy, patients often find themselves coming up with excuses to miss sessions. If this happens to you — and it's a good bet that it will — understand that it's very natural and normal. After all, it's human nature to stop doing what's unpleasant to you. So don't kick yourself. Instead, just do your best to remember the long-term gains you seek, and get back in the groove as quickly as possible. And don't worry about your therapist's thinking you're a failure if you ditch a session or two. She knows it's often a normal part of the process.

Facing your dragon by your therapist's side

When you're ready, the next step after identifying your triggers is for you and your therapist to take on your trauma together. Earlier, you described your experience to your therapist in a conversational way, probably touching only briefly on the most disturbing parts of it. Now, however, is the time to shed light on every dark corner of that experience. (This process is called *exposure therapy.*) Therapists approach this step in a variety of ways. Some ask patients to write about their trauma first and then talk it through. Others jump right into the talk-it-out stage. Most therapists tape-record exposure therapy sessions so patients can use the tapes in their homework.

When you write or talk about your trauma, your therapist asks you to describe it as if you're actually in the middle of it. For instance, a patient who survived a fire doesn't say, "Then I ran away" — she says, "I'm running now, and I can feel my heart pounding. It's very hot, and I hear fire trucks in the background." Your therapist asks you to describe the sights, sounds, odors, and sensations you recall. Even more importantly, she asks you to zero in on how you felt as the trauma unfolded.

Confronting your horror in this way is scary, but your therapist's job is to make sure you're safe. She keeps an eagle eye on your emotions and makes sure you stay in control as you face this big task together. For instance, she may stop you and ask, "How distressed do you feel right now, on a scale of one to ten?" Or she may remind you to practice stress-relieving skills (see "Step 1: Gaining the Tools You Need to Feel Safe in the Moment," earlier in this chapter).

Here are two major techniques for tackling a trauma; therapists typically base their choice on each patient's needs and resilience:

> ✔ **Systematic desensitization (graduated exposure therapy):** You confront your least-disturbing triggers first and work your way up to your worst memories. For instance, the patient who listed her triggers back in Table 8-1 may start by listening to rap music (a minor trigger) and then — when she can handle that without distress — move on to a more stressful trigger, such as her husband's whiskers. Eventually, she'll be ready to confront the initial traumatic event itself.

✔ **Flooding (prolonged exposure or implosion):** You confront the trauma as a whole, creating as vivid an image of the event as possible. You repeat this process until the powerful emotions linked to the trauma begin to fade. In the process, you gain insight into both your original trauma and the triggers that stem from it.

In some cases, you can confront elements of your trauma directly. For instance, your therapist may ask you to go to a park or restaurant where an attack occurred. If recreating your experience in real life is unsafe or impossible, the therapist asks you to imagine it. Some high-tech therapists are also using computer simulations to create virtual versions of combat or other traumas (see "Virtual reality exposure therapy [VRET]," later in this chapter).

Step 3: Undoing false ideas

Exposure therapy (which I discuss in the preceding section) isn't just about facing your trauma. More importantly, it's about seeing that trauma and its aftermath from a brand-new angle — an approach called *cognitive restructuring.* As you confront your trauma, your therapist can help you spot the false beliefs and thoughts that strengthen the trauma's hold on you and that keep you from breaking free. As you challenge each self-defeating thought, you can replace it with new, positive thoughts and beliefs. The result of this process is a *paradigm shift,* which means that you view aspects of your life through totally new eyes — and as a result, you think and act differently from that point on.

When I talk to groups, I like to explain a paradigm shift like this. I hold up a Federal Express package box, point to the logo that says FedEx, and ask people if they see the white arrow between the *E* and the *x*. Most people squint their eyes as if to say, "How did I never notice that?!" And when I ask them whether they'll notice the arrow every time they see the FedEx logo from that point on, they all nod. Furthermore, they all laugh and say *yes* when I ask them, "If you're stopped in traffic and a FedEx truck stops in front of you, will you point out the arrow to the other people in the car?"

Because the people in the audience see something they didn't see before, they'll never look at the logo in the same way. Similarly — but far more importantly — when you break through the negative thoughts that keep you from seeing your trauma (and yourself) clearly, you'll view your crisis, your reaction to it, your current life, and your own value as a human being in a very different and more positive light.

Here are three examples of how cognitive restructuring works.

REAL-LIFE STORY

Moving ahead by looking back

At age 27, Carol was raped at knifepoint in a large indoor shopping center's parking lot after the stores had closed. She froze at the time, thinking she was going to die, and her screams stuck in her throat.

After the attack, Carol continued work for a few months. She functioned well on the surface, but underneath she was in a daze. After six months, she started having panic attacks. She moved back to live with her parents in another city, started to withdraw from friends, and spent an increasing amount of time in the bedroom she'd grown up in.

Nine months after the attack, the rapist was captured and was then tried and sent to prison. Carol felt some relief, but she was still trapped by her need to avoid a world she now saw as dangerous. Her parents sympathized with her avoidance before her attacker was captured but now urged her go to therapy and try to put the attack behind her.

In therapy sessions, Carol was afraid to talk about the rape in detail. Every time she started, she felt nauseated and lightheaded and said, "I can't do this."

I explained to Carol that at the time of the attack, she froze in order to survive. Because she was still trapped in that frozen state, she hadn't had an opportunity to finish experiencing all the other feelings associated with the attack. Until she returned to that moment in the safe setting of therapy and gradually relived and re-experienced her trauma, she would probably continue to feel like half a person, living in limbo — afraid to look back and afraid to move forward.

After several sessions, when she had a good rapport with me, I gently but firmly encouraged her to describe the trauma in such specific detail that I could see it through her eyes. At the very moment when I *did* see it through her eyes — which gave me the chills — she started to have trouble breathing. In her mind, she was in the past, experiencing a horrific event that she never thought she could survive again.

I continued to have her describe the details, telling her that it was almost a year later and that she was not falling apart or going crazy. Instead, I reminded her, she was finishing feeling all the emotions she didn't have time to feel during and shortly after the trauma because she was just trying to survive and keep from falling apart.

As Carol continued to talk, the tension in her voice began to dissolve and she started to relax. That terrible time she'd spent trapped alone with her rapist had pushed her into a state of frozen terror; now, by reliving the trauma with a supportive and caring person, she could let that terror dissipate and begin to feel and trust again.

Combating concerns about safety (and the underlying need for control)

Before your trauma, you probably felt secure most of the time. You took some precautions — maybe you bought a car with good safety features, installed a deadbolt on your front door, or carried pepper spray with you — but in general, you didn't spend lots of time feeling fearful. What's more, you felt a sense of control over your life. You knew that bad stuff could happen, but you figured that bad stuff was the exception, not the rule.

Danielle's story: Spotless equals safe

Danielle spent hours each day scrubbing every surface of her home, cooking gourmet meals, and manicuring the lawn. By the time her husband, Larry, got home, she'd be exhausted and on the edge of a breakdown. Larry was a mellow guy who didn't mind clutter and thought simple food was fine, but he couldn't get her to relax. He was very supportive, but both of them were tense and upset about the situation.

As Danielle worked through the abuse she suffered at the hands of a violent stepfather, she realized the basis for her actions. Her stepdad used to hit her any time she failed to keep the house spotless, and she now believed she needed to have everything perfect in order to be safe. If anything was out of place, she thought, she could get hurt or even die.

With the help of her therapist, she challenged that idea and replaced it with true and constructive thoughts: "The person who hurt me was impossible to please. I'm safe now because Larry isn't that person. Larry is a good person, and he doesn't expect me to be perfect. I can relax and have fun." As a result, she was able to lighten up and enjoy her life and her relationship with Larry.

After a trauma, those beliefs are turned topsy-turvy. It seems like the universe is out to get you, and you're a helpless pawn in its game. As a result, you may develop negative thoughts like these:

> *I'll never be safe again.*
>
> *The world is frightening and unpredictable.*
>
> *I can't take chances, or bad things will happen.*
>
> *I have to keep everything under control, or else I'll get hurt.*

These thoughts can translate into a fear of taking risks. For instance, you may be afraid to make new friends, change jobs, or even leave the house. They can also lead you to take extreme (and ultimately unsuccessful) measures to regain a sense of control your life. As you identify these thoughts with the help of your therapist and replace them with constructive thoughts, you find that many of your fears fall away and that you can take real steps to take control over your future.

Shedding mistrust and an impenetrable shell

People say that misery loves company, but individuals battling PTSD often lock everyone else out of their lives instead of sharing their pain. This leave-me-alone response can be especially powerful if a trauma involves being hurt by another person (as with a sexual assault) or involves witnessing the death of another person (making the survivor reluctant to get close to another human being and risk being hurt by a similar loss in the future). Often, PTSD packs negative thoughts such as these:

> *I can't trust anyone.*
>
> *Bad things happen to people when I'm around. They're better off without me in their lives.*
>
> *People always let me down.*
>
> *If I get involved with someone, I'll just get hurt.*

These thoughts and similar ones close you off from a world of love and friendship and leave you angry, lonely, and bitter. In addition, they wound other people and often split up once-loving families. As you overcome this type of negative thinking, you'll find a new joy in friendship, family ties, and romantic relationships.

Getting rid of gut-wrenching guilt

Guilt is one of the biggest stumbling blocks on the road to healing because it plants the toxic thought "I don't *deserve* to recover." To give this idea the boot, you and your therapist need to tackle its root causes. Many people with PTSD have to work through five false beliefs that give guilt an iron grip:

- ✔ **"I should've predicted the trauma and avoided it."** If you fall prey to this erroneous thought, called *hindsight bias,* it means you expect the impossible of yourself — because no one can predict the future. Your therapist can help you understand that life is full of risks, and avoiding all of them is impossible.

- ✔ **"I didn't have a good reason for the actions I took before or during the trauma."** This faulty type of thinking, called *justification distortion,* makes you think that perfectly normal actions — such as driving your child to camp or deciding to visit the World Trade Towers as a tourist — were wrong on your part, based on traumatic events that happened afterward. Your therapist can help you understand that it's unfair to judge your actions by their unanticipated outcomes rather than your original intentions.

- ✔ **"It's all my fault."** This form of distorted thinking, called *responsibility distortion,* makes you take total blame for an act in which you played either no role or merely a partial one. Here's an example: You ask your child to climb a ladder to get a ball out of a tree, and the ladder, which turns out to be defective, collapses, causing him serious injury. If you blame yourself for this catastrophe, you're exhibiting responsibility distortion because you're failing to recognize that the ladder manufacturer's error — not your action — is the root cause of the problem. In therapy, you can figure out how to rid yourself of the misplaced guilt you feel as a result of this type of self-destructive thought.

David's story: Mad as hell

David and his friend Nick fought side by side for months in Vietnam. One day, walking through a friendly village, they spotted a little girl waving at them from a hut. Distracted by her smile, David raised a hand to wave in return before he spotted the grenade she'd tossed in his direction. He dived in one direction, and Nick dived in the other. David survived with serious wounds, but Nick died.

Decades later, David refused to talk with his wife about the war. He'd alienated his grown children, and his wife walked on eggshells to keep him from blowing up. When a therapist helped him face that day in Vietnam, David realized that he came away from his terrible experience with several self-destructive thoughts. One was that anybody could be an enemy. Another was "I can never let down my guard." And still another — stemming from the idea that he caused Nick's death by letting the little girl's smile distract him for an instant — was "Even little mistakes are unacceptable."

These ideas made perfect sense in Vietnam, where hair-trigger reactions and constant suspicion saved lives. What's more, the lack of a hero's welcome when he returned to the States — and the red tape of the government, which demanded that every *i* be dotted and every *t* be crossed before David could get any help for his PTSD — strongly reinforced them. But now, he realizes, these ideas are self-destructive. With help from his therapist, he creates new ideas. One is "My family members aren't enemies. Even when they're angry or disagree with me, they love me and want the best for me." Another is "I can relax and nothing bad will happen." And the third is "Most little mistakes are harmless, and some are funny." These new realizations help David to rein in his temper, control his knee-jerk reactions to every little household crisis, and start rebuilding bonds with his family.

✔ **"I did something evil."** This type of misguided thinking is called *wrongdoing distortion,* and it may be the most devastating of all guilt-producing thoughts because it makes you doubt your own goodness as a human being. For instance, if you hurt or killed someone during your trauma, you may feel like a bad person who doesn't deserve to get well. If that's the case, your therapist helps you realize that you're just human — and that no human can always behave perfectly and nobly and heroically at all times or know exactly the right thing to do in any situation. She also helps you see that you probably acted exactly like most people would in your situation.

For instance, if a soldier feels guilt over the emotional rush he felt when he killed an enemy, a therapist may point out, "You were very young and very scared. When people on the other side started firing at you, your body reacted by producing lots of chemicals that triggered your fight-or-flight response, and that's what made you feel such a rush. It didn't happen because you're a bad person. It happened because that's how the human body reacts when it faces and survives a threat. Millions of other soldiers have the same feelings, and they aren't bad people, either."

✔ **"I shouldn't have survived."** Another type of guilt that occurs after a trauma is called *survivor guilt,* a feeling that happens when you feel guilty that you lived through a trauma while another person died. Your therapist can help you get past this misguided guilt in many ways. One is by helping you see that your survival is an achievement, not a reason for shame. Another is by helping you find ways to honor the person who died in the trauma.

Step 4: Putting your new skills into action

The relief you feel when you make a breakthrough in therapy is wonderful, but it's even better when you translate your new skills into real-life successes. As you make progress, you and your therapist talk about ways to put your new awareness into action. For example,

✔ If your trauma involved a car accident and you feel ready to face driving again, your therapist may ask you to get used to sitting in your car, then driving it a few feet, and finally driving it around the block. Eventually, he may give you the homework assignment of driving to the store and back.

✔ If your new skills help you to connect better with family and friends, your therapist may ask you to call a longtime friend and schedule a get-together.

✔ If you're getting anger issues under grips, your therapist may ask you to test your new anger-management skills by handling a longstanding problem with a co-worker in a positive way.

At each session, you and your therapist talk about how well your real-life exercises went and what you need to work on next. Don't be too surprised if you take two steps forward and one step back when you test-drive your new skills in the real world; overcoming bad habits takes patience and practice.

You and your therapist can also talk over ways to tackle any major problems in your life, such as job or housing worries. He can probably show you how the lessons you develop in therapy can help you address these issues in new and more-effective ways.

Variations on a Theme: Offshoots of CBT

You have your own way of doing things, and so does your therapist — and that's why no two CBT sessions are exactly alike. Most therapists who use CBT follow the steps I outline throughout this chapter. Within that framework, however, therapists tailor their approaches to best suit their patients — especially when it comes to the crucial step of confronting your trauma.

Steve's story: Unraveling guilt and accepting human limits

Steve felt crushing guilt when he thought about the accident that occurred when his car swerved out of control and killed a bicyclist on a busy street. His inner thoughts were, "It was wrong for me to drive in a rainstorm. I should've known better and stayed home. I killed another person just because I didn't want to miss work, and I don't deserve to be happy after taking someone else's life."

As Steve and his therapist worked through his trauma, Steve discovered how to challenge these thoughts:

✔ In response to Steve's belief that he should've avoided the accident, the therapist noted that Steve couldn't have known that the accident was going to occur — especially because he'd driven in the rain for years without a problem. Also, Steve couldn't have predicted that his tires were going to slip on a slick spot.

✔ When Steve discussed the guilt he felt for driving in a heavy rain, his therapist pointed out that thousands of people drove to work in the same storm that day — and that the world would come to a standstill if everyone feared driving in the rain.

✔ As for Steve's tendency to blame himself for the accident, the therapist helped Steve realize that thinking that the accident happened solely because of him was unrealistic. The therapist noted that the bicyclist chose to ride in the rain and dressed in dark clothes, making him almost impossible to see until it was too late. Also, a work crew left a slick of oil on the spot where Steve's car skidded. In short, the therapist noted, lots of events came together to cause the accident.

✔ In response to Steve's belief that he committed an evil act when his car killed the bicyclist, his therapist helped him realize that a) he had no intent of causing any harm on the day of the accident; b) he made the best split-second decision he could when he swerved to miss another car; and c) he did everything possible to help at the scene of the accident. All of these, the therapist notes, are the actions of a good person trying to make sense of a bad situation.

By the end of therapy, Steve understood that his accident was just that: a tragic accident that could happen to anyone. Putting his guilt behind him lifted a terrible burden and allowed him to move forward with his life instead of sabotaging his future.

CBT comes in too many different varieties to list, with new methods springing up every year. In this section, I give you a quick sampling of different approaches to give you an idea of how CBT therapists can offer different strokes for different folks.

If your insurance plan is flexible and you live in a big city that's teeming with therapists, you may want to seek an approach that suits your particular needs — especially if you'd like your therapy to address both PTSD and either substance use issues or other psychiatric disorders.

Don't get too hung up on any one flavor of CBT, however. For all their differences, these approaches offer one important message: Facing your problems is the first step in conquering them. And that simple message — rather than the bells and whistles — is what empowers CBT to open the door to healing for so many people.

Tracking motion: Eye movement desensitization and reprocessing therapy

A relative newcomer on the scene, eye movement desensitization and reprocessing (EMDR) therapy combines many steps of traditional cognitive behavioral therapy (CBT — see the earlier sections) with a unique system of eye movements. Like CBT, EMDR asks a patient to confront and work through her original trauma. EMDR therapists also help patients replace self-destructive ideas with beneficial ones. The big difference lies in the eye movements (or other left-right cues) used in EMDR. It's an increasingly popular technique for treating PTSD and one that's supported by many studies. Here's the scoop on what happens in EMDR.

An EMDR therapist starts with the same steps as in CBT. First, you and the therapist zero in on your issues, and you also work on some relaxation and stress-relieving techniques. Next, therapy follows these steps (which may vary depending on your therapist's specific technique):

1. **Your therapist asks you to identify a particular memory associated with your trauma, and she asks you to judge how severely the memory distresses you (usually on a scale of 1 to 10 or 1 to 100).**

2. **The therapist also asks you to identify negative beliefs related to this event.**

   Negative beliefs may include thoughts such as, "I'm weak," or "I can't cope." Typically, you also rate your level of distress as a result of this belief.

3. **The therapist asks you to identify positive beliefs that you'd like to replace the negative beliefs with.**

   For example, you may want to believe, "I'm very strong," or "I'm able to handle stressful experiences." As before, she asks you to rate how strongly you believe these ideas.

4. **Your therapist asks you to identify a "safe place" you can mentally return to at the end of the session.**

   For instance, you may want to visualize a beautiful, deserted beach.

Gaining the strength to face the past *and* the future

In an article in *Behavior Therapy*, Katherine DuHamel and her colleagues describe how CBT helped a 40-year-old cancer patient recover from PTSD following a bone marrow transplant.

Before therapy, the patient reacted with extreme distress to reminders of his cancer treatment. For example, the sound of his microwave oven or the generator at his workplace triggered flashbacks because these noises reminded him of the sounds of the radiation machine used in his treatment. The scent of pine — the same scent as the skin lotion his hospital unit used — affected him so strongly that his family couldn't have a Christmas tree in the house. Even a certain shade of yellow, which reminded him of the color of the antifungal medicine he received during his treatment, triggered strong emotions.

The patient volunteered enthusiastically for CBT, telling his doctors that he feared he was "going crazy." He underwent ten 1-hour sessions of treatment, including both standard CBT techniques and education specific to living with cancer:

✔ In Session 1, the therapist discussed the patient's symptoms with him and explained the steps of his therapy.

✔ In Session 2, the therapist described how a cancer diagnosis and treatment can lead to PTSD symptoms. The therapist also discussed the importance of ongoing cancer monitoring and treatment, explaining that this follow-up care made PTSD triggers unavoidable. The therapist and the patient worked on developing positive coping strategies — for instance, using positive self-statements such as "separate the past and the present." The patient also practiced relaxation techniques (see "Step 1: Gaining the Tools You Need to Feel Safe in the Moment"), using a visualization exercise, self-suggestions, and a relaxation tape.

✔ In Session 3, the patient practiced his relaxation exercises. Then the patient and his therapist created a list of his triggers, organizing them from least to most distressing.

✔ In Sessions 4 through 8, the patient practiced his relaxation techniques and then underwent systematic desensitization (see the section titled "Facing your dragon by your therapist's side"), confronting each of his triggers. These triggers ranged from the mildly distressing sight and smell of vegetable soup (which a relative brought to him in the hospital) to the highly upsetting words *cancer* and *leukemia*. Afterward, he and his therapist talked about ways to help prevent a PTSD relapse.

✔ In the final two sessions, the patient did additional work on confronting his triggers and reviewed his strategies for relaxing and coping when triggers arose. For example, he created a portable "toolbox" containing his relaxation tape, an index card on which he wrote coping statements, and directions for a relaxation exercise.

The man's therapy caused remarkable changes in his life. Afterward, he no longer met criteria for PTSD, he recovered from his depression, and most of his triggers no longer affected him. (Initially, 11 triggers caused him extreme distress. By the end of therapy, 10 of these caused little or no distress, and the 11th caused only moderate upset.) He stopped having flashbacks on the job, avoided a relapse even when he needed re-hospitalization, and told his doctors he felt peaceful, happy, and calm.

5. **You silently remember your trauma while watching the therapist's finger or pen as it moves back and forth from left to right repeatedly (see Figure 8-1).**

   Sometimes a therapist uses right and left finger taps on a patient's knee or musical tones that change from left to right. (**Note:** The tapping used in EMDR is different from the tapping therapies I outline in Chapter 10 because EMDR tapping has nothing to do with the energy points that tapping therapists believe are the key to their therapy.) As you begin this process, your therapist may instruct you to let whatever happens happen and to simply notice the thoughts and feelings that arise.

6. **You repeat this procedure several times.**

   In between, your therapist asks you to discuss feelings that arise or rate your level of distress. Your therapist largely stays in the background and lets you do the talking because EMDR is based on the theory that the eye movements themselves — rather than the therapist's verbal guidance — are the key to helping your traumatic memories become unstuck so you can process them in a healthy way. The session continues until you report that your level of distress is very low and that your belief in the positive idea you identified is very high. At this point, your therapist asks you to visualize your "safe place" and concludes the process.

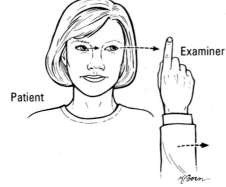

Figure 8-1:
In EMDR, the patient visually tracks the therapist's finger as it moves from side to side.

Examiner

Patient

Interestingly, studies so far can't prove whether the addition of the eye movements makes any difference; some say *yes,* and others say *no.*

REAL-LIFE STORY

The case of the jealous husband

In the *British Journal of Nursing,* psychotherapist David Blore describes a remarkable case that illustrates the power of EMDR — as well as the fact that it's never too late to seek help for PTSD symptoms.

Blore's patient was Maurice, a 75-year-old World War II veteran and a survivor of a Japanese prison camp. An easygoing guy before the war, Maurice came home bitter and angry. Even worse, he became morbidly jealous and was convinced that his wife would cheat on him. He refused to let her have visitors when he was gone or to pay attention to other men — even close relatives.

Maurice's first wife suffered under these rules for decades. He remarried after she died, and his new wife (a woman made of sterner stuff) said, "Get help, or we're getting a divorce." So half a century after his trauma, Maurice sought therapy.

Dr. Blore addressed his patient's problems in three sessions of EMDR. In the first session, the man talked about his fear and anger after his capture and described terrible memories of the guards' making him drag bodies from the water and bury them. Blore notes, "Session 1 was harrowing for Maurice and therapist alike, but a real sense of purpose ensued and the almost immediate relief gained by Maurice after more than 50 years can scarcely be adequately described."

In Session 2, the reasons for Maurice's jealousy came to light. He talked about how the camp guards lined their prisoners up each day and tormented them by saying, "While you are here, your women will be enjoying themselves with other men." Maurice remembered how his jealousy grew over time as the guards' verbal arrows hit their mark. As he relived this memory during EMDR, he realized that he'd been brainwashed and said, "It's so obvious — it's almost as though the war is continuing in my head."

In Session 3, Maurice reported great news: For the first time since the 1930s, he'd entertained a male guest at his home and didn't have a single jealous thought when he saw the man talking with his wife. In this session, he and Dr. Blore handled his remaining issues by exploring his life after the war, his relationship with his wife, and his new perceptions about the effects of his jealousy.

Dr. Blore saw his patient two more times over the next six months. At each, Maurice was relaxed and happy. At Maurice's last visit, Blore says, "He parted by sincerely thanking me for saving his marriage."

Another point of controversy centers on a different question: Is EMDR simply a dressed-up version of CBT? Some researchers say it is. Others say that EMDR differs greatly because instead of requiring intense, prolonged exposure to your trauma — a centerpiece of CBT — EMDR exposes you only briefly during each treatment.

What *is* clear is that EMDR has a good track record — fairly similar to CBT, albeit shorter. A 2006 review of studies comparing the two techniques, published in *Psychological Medicine,* concluded that both treatments were effective and that "the superiority of one treatment over the other could not be demonstrated." So EMDR looks like a good bet — even though researchers don't really know why it works.

Intense but short-lived recollection: The counting method

Patients looking for a rapid CBT intervention that offers some privacy often find the *counting method* (devised by Frank Ochberg) helpful. Here's how you confront your trauma if your therapist uses this method:

1. **Your therapist begins by asking which traumatic memory you want to recall that day.**

2. **The therapist asks you to recall this memory silently while he slowly counts aloud from 1 to 100 (about one second per count).**

   The idea is for you to fill the entire 100 seconds with your memory, letting it peak in intensity and then returning to the present in the last few seconds.

3. **Afterward, you and your therapist discuss what you recalled.**

   For instance, if he noticed you tensing at one point, he may ask, "Do you recall what happened when I was counting in the 50s?" Together, you explore your recalling of the trauma and what you learned by revisiting it.

Counting often works quickly, and Dr. Ochberg reports that about 80 percent of his patients report improvement in symptoms after treatment. The counting technique has three strong advantages:

- ✔ It offers some privacy to a person who may not want to share the full force of a memory out loud.
- ✔ It keeps the person linked to the present through the sound of the therapist's voice.
- ✔ It puts the memory in a box defined by the counting time, making it seem less powerful.

The counting method is somewhat similar to eye movement desensitization and reprocessing (EMDR), which I discuss in the preceding section, because you tackle small bits of your trauma at a time.

Focusing on the present: Rational emotive behavior therapy (REBT)

Is confronting your trauma really a necessary part of triumphing over PTSD? Maybe not, according to rational emotive behavior therapy (REBT).

Instead of focusing largely on your past trauma, REBT looks at your life right *now.* REBT therapists do believe that your past influences your present, but they also believe that you can address your beliefs — no matter when and why they arose — by looking at how they impact your current life and behavior, without taking too deep of a look at the past. As the Albert Ellis Institute (named for the therapy's creator) explains it, "REBT believes that the 'nuttiness' of our past exerts its influence in our current-day thinking patterns and beliefs. Although we cannot change the past, we can change how we let the past influence the way we are today and the way we want to be tomorrow."

REBT therapists focus on what they call the ABCs of your current life problems. The letters stand for

- ✔ **A:** Activating Events
- ✔ **B:** Beliefs
- ✔ **C:** Consequences (emotional and behavioral)

According to REBT, A — in this case, the trauma you experienced — doesn't directly cause C — your PTSD symptoms — unless irrational beliefs (B) enter the mix. So an REBT therapist asks what you think is making you sad or angry or anxious, but she considers that event to be less important than your current beliefs about it. The therapist's goals are to

- ✔ Help you identify false beliefs that are affecting your life in a negative way.
- ✔ Help dispute these beliefs by showing why they're false and how they influence you to take actions that aren't in your best interest.

Here's a brief example of how the dialogue may go in an REBT session:

Diana: I'm just angry all the time.

Therapist: Why are you angry?

Diana: I'm angry at the man who attacked me. And I'm angry that I had a wonderful life, and he ruined it.

Therapist: He ruined everything wonderful in your life? There's nothing wonderful at all left?

Diana: Well, that's not true. My family's really supportive. They're always there for me.

Therapist: You mentioned that you raise horses, and that your horses are very important to you. Did your attacker ruin that part of your life?

Diana: Well, no, of course not. I mean, the attack didn't have anything to do with the horses. So okay, I see where you're going — not everything is ruined. . . .

In general, an REBT therapist focuses on getting you to challenge beliefs that are rigid and inflexible, illogical, inconsistent with reality, and holding you back from accomplishing your goals. For instance, if you say, "I *need* to get back into college right away, or I'm a complete failure," or "I *can't* face driving ever again," an REBT therapist may say something like, "What evidence is there that you'll be a complete failure if you don't go back to school this semester?" or "What would happen if you *did* drive your car again?"

Notice that the therapist isn't zeroing in on past events that contributed to these beliefs (although you and he may talk about them). Instead, he's focusing on what you believe here and now, and he's encouraging you to analyze those beliefs to see whether they're working for or against you.

REBT is a lot like CBT, which also helps a person challenge self-defeating ideas. The advantage of REBT, from some people's point of view, is that it doesn't force you to go through the emotional experience of confronting your trauma. The downside? Researchers aren't sure, but evidence suggests that many people *need* to face down their trauma to get past its effects.

Attacking panic: Multiple channel exposure therapy

Panic disorder (see Chapter 3) and PTSD often go hand-in-hand. One study, for instance, showed that people with panic disorder are more than four times more likely to have a current diagnosis of PTSD than people with no history of panic disorder. Some people with panic disorder are so terrified of experiencing a panic attack when they undergo exposure therapy that they can't face CBT.

These facts led Dr. Sherry Falsetti and her colleagues to develop a special form of CBT that addresses both panic disorder and PTSD symptoms. Falsetti's therapy — called *multiple channel exposure therapy* — starts by educating patients about panic disorder symptoms, teaching them breathing techniques that can stop panic attacks, and having them confront and overcome their panic disorder symptoms through a variety of techniques. For instance, patients may

✔ Breathe through a straw to simulate panicky breathing

✔ Spin in a chair to mimic the dizziness and disorientation caused by a panic attack

✔ Tense their muscles to simulate the stress of a panic attack

When patients figure out how to cope with panic symptoms and no longer dread them, they find exposure to their initial trauma much less scary to face. Early data give the method a thumbs-up: Falsetti evaluated 12 patients using her approach, and found that only about 8 percent still met diagnostic criteria for PTSD after treatment (compared to more than 66 percent in a control group) and that patients undergoing the therapy suffered far fewer panic attacks than the controls.

Confronting your trauma, high-tech: Virtual reality exposure therapy (VRET)

Consider the following scenarios:

A soldier driving down a dangerous road sees the truck ahead of him explode.

A rescue worker runs away from the collapsing World Trade Center towers.

A driver sees another car jump the center divider and head straight for her.

What do all three of these scenarios have in common? For patients undergoing one kind of therapy, they're happening on a computer screen — not in real life. In all three cases, the patients witnessing these events are safe and sound in their therapists' offices. They're participating in a revolutionary new form of exposure therapy that uses virtual reality to recreate traumas.

In virtual reality exposure therapy (VRET), patients sit at a computer or wear a headset that lets them see and hear a computer-generated virtual world resembling the scene of their trauma. The military's test program actually adds some sensory cues that the therapist can trigger at appropriate times, including odors (gunpowder, spices, sweat) and vibrations that simulate being in a tank or Humvee. Some programs also allow the therapist to change the scene — for instance, by triggering gunfire sounds or smoke clouds to match a patient's description of what happened. This form of therapy is a lot like a video game, but this game has a very serious goal: to help participants face and conquer their fears.

VRET follows the same principles of typical CBT, but it adds a layer of realism because patients actually experience elements of the trauma in real life instead of just visualizing these details in their minds. Reliving a trauma in a virtual world can also help patients whose defenses make it hard for them to describe a trauma verbally (for instance, soldiers or police officers, who sometimes find it hard to drop their tough façade and talk openly about their pain). Virtual reality is especially helpful when patients can't physically revisit the location where a trauma occurred because it's too dangerous or far away.

These technologies are so new they're barely out of the box, but two studies indicate that they can be very powerful. Here are some early results:

✔ Six people suffering from PTSD after car accidents completed ten sessions of VRET. Afterward, they experienced marked reductions in intrusive thoughts, avoidance, and numbing.

✔ Nine people who developed PTSD after the World Trade Center collapse underwent 14 sessions of VRET. After therapy, they had a much bigger drop in symptom severity than a control group that didn't receive the treatment.

Undergoing combined treatments if you struggle with substance abuse

If an alcohol problem or drug use complicates your PTSD, treatment can be tricky. Traditionally, therapists ask patients to get clean before they start CBT — but a new trend is to combine treatment for both problems into one package. For example, check out the following techniques:

✔ **Seeking Safety:** This technique uses present-based CBT, which doesn't involve re-experiencing a trauma but instead focuses on a person's current problems, to address both PTSD and alcohol or drug abuse (see the section on REBT for another example of present-based CBT). In some cases, the approach is combined with exposure therapy that does involve re-experiencing the trauma.

The developer of Seeking Safety, Lisa Najavits, says, "Contrary to older views, treating both PTSD and substance abuse at the same time appears to help clients with their substance abuse recovery, rather than derailing them from attaining abstinence." Seeking Safety puts a slightly different spin on CBT because much of its focus is on safety (the reason for its name) — not just safety from substance abuse or PTSD symptoms but also from the dangerous relationships and suicidal or self-harming behaviors that are common in people battling both PTSD and substance abuse. Another feature is its emphasis on positive ideals; each session revolves around an ideal, such as honesty or commitment.

✔ **Concurrent treatment of PTSD and cocaine dependence:** Also called CTPCD, this 16-session approach combines prolonged exposure therapy (see the earlier section titled "Facing your dragon by your therapist's side") with a different type of approach — coping skills training — designed to help people with cocaine problems get a handle on their drug problem. For instance, participants discover how to spot triggers for cocaine craving, identify lifestyle issues that increase the risk of relapse, manage anger control issues, and practice ways to refuse offers of cocaine.

These approaches are still new, but initial results are encouraging. For instance, five men who underwent combined treatment with exposure therapy and Seeking Safety reported drops in drug use, anxiety, trauma symptoms, and hostility, improvements in social and sexual relationships, and a range of other benefits.

Using virtual reality to face the horror of 9/11

A case study reported by Dr. JoAnn Difede and Dr. Hunter Hoffman in *CyberPsychology & Behavior* shows the remarkable power of virtual reality therapy. Difede, an expert on PTSD, and Hoffman, a scientist studying the uses of virtual reality in therapy, treated a 26-year-old executive who was across the street from the north World Trade Center Tower when it collapsed. The woman developed serious PTSD symptoms, including flashbacks of the plane crash, avoidance of any news reports about the attack, and overwhelming feelings of vulnerability. She felt cut off from her loved ones and was often very angry with them. She also developed severe depression.

A few months after the World Trade Center attack, the woman underwent standard CBT. However, she remained flat and emotionless while talking about her traumatic experience (even though she reported significant distress), and she made no progress in therapy.

When the woman tried virtual reality therapy, however, it was a very different story. Wearing a virtual-reality helmet that gave her the sensation of being right in the middle of the attack, she underwent graded exposure to the event. (For example, she first saw planes flying over the building but not striking it. As she progressed, she witnessed the planes crashing with no sound, and then witnessed the crashes with sounds of explosions and screaming.)

The researchers report that the woman responded nearly instantly. She started crying and began to tell the horrifying story of what she'd survived that day. She re-experienced the feeling that she was going to die, remembered the chaos of the crowd around her trying to flee, and recalled needing to leave behind a woman with severed legs who called out to her for help.

Facing her trauma in virtual reality changed the woman's life dramatically. After six sessions, she no longer met criteria for an official diagnosis of either PTSD or depression. Her symptoms of depression dropped by 83 percent, and her PTSD symptoms by 90 percent. Difede and Hoffman say the many different sensory cues provided by virtual reality may explain why some people, like their patient, respond so dramatically to this new technique.

Chapter 9

The Role of Medication in Treating PTSD

*T*hese days we have a pill for just about everything, from balding heads to overactive bladders. Thus, many people are surprised that doctors don't treat PTSD simply by writing a prescription for some new wonder drug. But drugs, although they have their place in treating PTSD, aren't number one on the list of treatment approaches — and often, patients don't need them at all.

Why? One reason is that drugs treat only isolated aspects of PTSD. They can take the edge off certain symptoms, but talk therapy is more effective in banishing PTSD itself. Another reason is that these drugs often come with a steep price tag in the form of side effects.

However, there's a time and place for everything — and that includes PTSD meds, which can sometimes jump-start therapy or even save a life. In this chapter, I look at what these drugs can and can't do, and I give you a quick glimpse at how each one works. In addition, I tell you why your doctor may recommend one or more of them, and I offer a list of questions you need to ask before you say yes or no.

Why Pop a Pill for PTSD?

Patients with PTSD often get better through therapy alone, without ever taking anything stronger than an aspirin. Sometimes, however, PTSD really sinks its claws in, making it hard to handle everyday life and even harder (or sometimes even impossible) to succeed at therapy. The result: slower healing, snowballing job and relational problems, and intense suffering. Worse yet, symptoms can be overwhelming enough to threaten a person's health or life.

If your PTSD causes you serious problems, your doctor may prescribe medications to declaw your most dangerous symptoms and help you handle issues standing in the way of your recovery. Think of these drugs not as a cure-all but as a means to an end — that *end* being successful healing through therapy.

A doctor may recommend medication for you for the following reasons:

✔ You have significant symptoms of depression (see Chapter 3).

✔ You have trouble sleeping nearly every night.

✔ Your anxiety is so strong that you have trouble keeping a job or dealing with therapy.

✔ You're experiencing suicidal thoughts or feelings.

✔ You're dealing with alcohol or substance abuse issues.

Your family doctor may prescribe drugs for one of these reasons, but you typically get a referral to a psychiatrist. That's because psychiatrists, unlike general practitioners, are experts on the best medical treatments for PTSD. In some areas, however, psychologists, nurse practitioners, or psychiatric nurses can prescribe medication for you (see Chapter 6 for more on therapists).

If a professional does recommend a medication, you may be tempted to just say *yes* without giving it too much thought. After all, you have enough on your plate without trying to second-guess your medical team. However, it's a good idea to take a step back and ask yourself, "Is this really the right move for me?" As a psychiatrist, I know plenty of patients who blossomed in therapy after taking the right medication. On the flipside, however, I know many who wound up worse off as the result of a pill. I'm also aware that many doctors prescribe drugs sparingly and wisely, but others pull out the prescription pad a bit too readily.

So before you agree to take a medication, know just what you're saying yes to. The following sections can help you understand how PTSD drugs may help you, how they can harm you, and what information you need to answer the question "To medicate, or not to medicate?"

Accounting for Both Sides of the Scale

Life is full of choices, and often you need to weigh some big pros and cons when you make decisions. For instance, should you buy the pricey car that's fun to drive or the cheaper car that gets better mileage? Vacation in New York City or hit the hiking trails in Yellowstone?

Similarly, deciding whether to include medication in your PTSD treatment plan involves weighing a lot of pros and cons — and the stakes are much higher in this case because your decision can affect your health (and sometimes even your life). In the following sections, I look at the points you need to think over if a doctor recommends a drug for your PTSD or related problems.

The benefits of medications

Medication for PTSD isn't for everyone, but if you're really hurting, it can do a world of good. Here's a quick rundown of the potential benefits:

- **Medication can stop a crisis from escalating.** Sometimes speedy relief is a top priority — especially if your world is spinning out of control. If you're suicidal, unable to work, or in danger of hurting other people, medications may help you regain control.

- **Medication can work fast.** Therapy is a long and sometimes difficult process. If you're not in any shape (physically or mentally) to face that process, temporary treatment with a drug may reduce your anxiety or other symptoms to the point where you can tackle your therapy successfully.

- **Medication can help tide you over if you can't get a therapist right away.** Not everyone lives in L.A. or New York City, where a therapist has set up shop on every block. If you're out in the countryside and help isn't handy, medication may help you stay the course until you can figure out a therapy plan.

- **For some people, medication is highly effective.** Sometimes a drug intervention can turn a person's life around. A trauma survivor who can't sleep, can't focus, can't work, and can't enjoy life occasionally has a remarkable breakthrough as a result of a drug treatment. (The catch is that this improvement is often temporary — something I discuss in the next section.)

- **Medications can treat coexisting disorders.** Sometimes you're dealing with not just one problem but two or more. For instance, you may be battling both PTSD and depression. In that case, you may need medication to get your other issues under control so you can focus on your PTSD symptoms.

- **In some instances, medication works when therapy doesn't.** Studies show that psychological therapies typically work better than medications in treating PTSD — but that doesn't mean they work for everyone. If therapy doesn't do the trick for you, medication could be just the ticket. However, medications work best when paired with therapy — so if a drug helps, go back to therapy and see whether combining the two approaches helps even more.

The cons of meds

TV commercials for drugs that treat psychological problems often make it seem like all you need to do is take a pill, and you'll be running through a field of flowers with a cocker spaniel and an attractive lover, enjoying the heck out of life. Unfortunately, it's not that simple. Drugs can ease symptoms, but they can also cause them — and at their worst, they can cause serious harm. Here's why:

- ✔ **Medications can cause dependence.** Some psychiatric drugs are habit-forming, and one thing you don't need right now is another serious life problem such as drug dependency (especially if you're already striving to overcome alcohol or drug problems). And even if a drug isn't techni-cally addictive, it may cause some severe withdrawal symptoms.

- ✔ **Medications can cause serious side effects.** Many of the drugs used to treat PTSD symptoms are risky. They have the potential to harm your heart, make you suicidal (although this idea is controversial, despite all the news coverage), or even cause diabetes — and that's just for starters. That's why reading up on a drug's possible side effects before you take it is critical.

- ✔ **Drug "honeymoons" often end.** One thing doctors see all the time is the flash-in-the-pan response to a drug. Patients often respond wonderfully to a medication for weeks or even months, only to crash and burn some time later. One reason: Your brain can quickly adapt to a new drug, caus-ing it to lose its effect.

- ✔ **Drugs can lead to denial.** If a drug makes you feel just good enough to get by, it's easy to tell yourself that you don't really need any additional help. But a pill can't substitute for understanding, working through, and overcoming your PTSD — which is why the long-term track record of drug treatments for PTSD isn't all that hot.

- ✔ **Drugs don't always live up to their hype.** For instance, doctors used the drug guanfacine (Tenex) to treat PTSD for years, only to find out recently that the drug isn't any more effective than a placebo.

Knowing How PTSD Drugs Work

You don't need to know how a spark plug works in order to drive your car, and you don't really need to know how PTSD meds work in order to take them. (In fact, even scientists aren't entirely sure what many of these drugs do!) However, it's a good idea to understand the basic mechanisms of these medications if you're thinking about taking one so you know what you can (and can't) expect from them. Later in this chapter, I talk about what specific drugs do — but for now, here's a quick overview.

A tale of two patients

One patient of mine — I'll call him Jack — made slow but steady progress overcoming his PTSD with a combination of two therapy approaches, but his lack of energy continued to frustrate both him and me. At one point, when problems cropped up at work, he started developing sleeping problems and felt even more like he was "swimming through molasses." After six weeks of this, with his job in jeopardy, we both decided that trying an antidepressant may help him.

Two weeks into treatment with the medication, he called me crying. I was worried, but he quickly told me he was crying tears of joy. He told me that he felt "normal" — something that he couldn't ever remember feeling. By *normal*, he meant that things rolled off his back, he walked around with a smile on his face, he felt 20 pounds lighter, and he felt very optimistic about his future — "The way so many other people seemed to be, but that I never dreamed would happen to me." Furthermore, his increased energy gave him the motivation to implement the suggestions we came up with in his therapy for thinking differently about his life and interacting more effectively with other people.

Fortunately, too, unlike many people who turn out to have major depressive disorder and may need to remain on medication indefinitely, he had no problem tapering off his medication six months later and continued his progress without it.

Not everyone, however, reports such success. One of my patients seemed to improve modestly when I put him on antidepressants, but the medications blunted the sharpness he needed to perform in his job. In addition, the withdrawal symptoms he experienced later — feeling tired, not being able to move or think — were worse than the symptoms of PTSD that originally caused him to consult me.

The moral of this tale? Drugs have different effects on different people, and there's no crystal ball your doctor can use to tell whether they'll help you or not. As is the case for much of medicine, doctors can make educated guesses, but they can't make guarantees. So if you take a medication, know its pros and cons upfront — but also watch for side effects and report them to your doctor. Together, you can fine-tune your treatment so it works for you.

Basic brain science: Taking a look at how nerve cells communicate

The drugs that doctors use to treat PTSD come in many different flavors, but all of them affect the nerve cells in your brain, called *neurons*. Your brain has around 100 billion of these busy little cells, and each one has a very big job: to create and send the messages that tell you what your senses detect, what you feel and think, and what you should do. Here's a quick-and-dirty explanation of how they do this (see Figure 9-1 for a picture of this process):

1. **When a neuron gets an exciting message, it wants to share the news with its neighbor; first, it sends a message electrically from one of the branches (*dendrites*) on its receiving end all the way down to its tail (the *axon*) on the sending end.**

2. **The tail then spits out chemicals called *neurotransmitters* (think of them as tiny molecular delivery trucks).**

   These chemicals land in the space — called a *synapse* — that separates the neuron from its neighbor.

3. **The chemicals wander around the synapse, trying to wangle an invite from neuron No. 2.**

   Some of them score — yippee! — and get permission to latch onto a receptor (kind of like a parking place) located on the second neuron's dendrites. When this happens, the neurotransmitter can pass on the exciting news flash from the first neuron, and the process can continue down the line.

4. **A chemical that can't get a parking place at neuron No. 2 keeps wandering around in the synapse, not quite knowing what to do with itself, until the first neuron says, "Oh, forget the whole thing!" and reels it back in.**

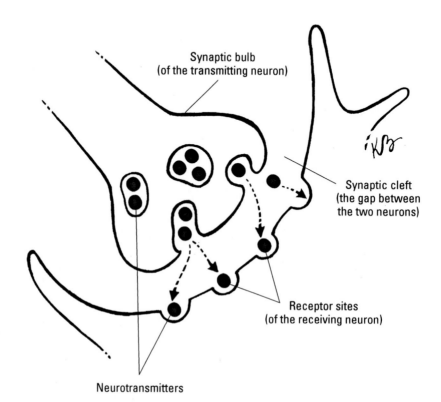

Synaptic bulb
(of the transmitting neuron)

Synaptic cleft
(the gap between
the two neurons)

Receptor sites
(of the receiving neuron)

Neurotransmitters

Figure 9-1:
How
neurons
transmit
messages.

Seeing how meds affect the brain's messages

The drugs that doctors prescribe to treat PTSD symptoms act on different parts of this message-delivery system, and they do it in a variety of ways:

- ✔ **Some drugs act at the receptors of the receiving neurons, either putting out the welcome mat or slamming the door on incoming messages.** They can do this by mimicking the neurotransmitter and triggering the neurotransmitter's usual response from the cell or — conversely — by blocking the door and preventing the neurotransmitter from reaching its target.

- ✔ **Some drugs boost the activity of a neurotransmitter by preventing the sender neuron from retrieving it if it doesn't find a new home right away.** This leaves more of the neurotransmitter floating around in the synapse, where it still has a chance to latch onto a new neuron and send its message.

- ✔ **Some drugs affect several different neurotransmitters at the same time.** For instance, a category of drugs called serotonin and norepinephrine reuptake inhibitors (see the section on SNRIs later in this chapter) increases the effect of both of these neurotransmitters.

The type of drug your doctor may choose depends to a large degree on the specific symptoms you have and which neurotransmitters influence those symptoms. Different neurotransmitters affect different aspects of brain function, including memory, mood, impulse control, motivation, arousal, attention, and wakefulness. Neurotransmitters also affect cells in different ways; for example, some make cells more excitable — that is, more receptive to incoming chemical messages — while others have the opposite effect. And each neurotransmitter has multiple effects; for example, serotonin can affect everything from your emotions and impulse control to your appetite.

Thus, different drugs can have very different effects — and that's true even if they come from the same chemical family. That's why easing your symptoms can take some trial and error (and possibly a combination of medications). That's also why drug treatment can be a lifesaver for one person and ineffective or even dangerous for another — and why you need to carefully weigh the pros and cons of any prescription before you hit the pharmacy (refer to the earlier section, "Accounting for Both Sides of the Scale," for more on that topic).

Surveying Medications Used to Treat PTSD Symptoms

When it comes to picking a medication, your doctor has quite a selection to choose from. Here's a quick look at the primary medications used to treat the symptoms of PTSD.

Antidepressants

As you can tell from the name, *antidepressants* fight depression, but their name is misleading because they can also reduce your anxiety levels and help you get a hair-trigger reaction under control. (In fact, these drugs often work better at reducing anxiety than drugs specifically targeted to combat this symptom.) Antidepressants come in several different types, which work in different ways and have different advantages and drawbacks. Here's the scoop on each one.

Selective Serotonin Reuptake Inhibitors (SSRIs)

SSRIs are currently the medication of choice for PTSD. The initials stand for *selective serotonin reuptake inhibitor,* which is a mouthful but actually not all that complicated (especially if you take a quick peek at Figure 9-1, earlier in this chapter). Here's what the name means:

- ✔ *Selective* means that the drug primarily affects only one messenger chemical.

- ✔ *Serotonin,* one of the neurotransmitters that brain cells use to talk to each other, is the messenger chemical that this type of drug affects. Serotonin is a very important chemical because it can affect mood, anxiety levels, aggression, and impulsiveness — as well as many physical processes including sleep and digestion.

- ✔ *Reuptake* is what happens when a neurotransmitter (serotonin in this case) fails to link up with another neuron and the sending cell then vacuums it back up.

- ✔ *Inhibitor* means that this drug blocks the reuptake process, thereby making the neurotransmitter (again, serotonin in this case) more effective by giving it extra chances to connect with another neuron.

So in short, an SSRI targets serotonin, making it more available to brain cells by preventing the neurons that crank it out from soaking it back up before it can affect another cell.

According to studies, SSRIs often do a very good job of reducing PTSD symptoms. Some patients respond within a week or two to these medications; others may take 12 weeks or longer to feel better. (In part, this depends on the drug; some SSRIs work faster than others.)

On the downside, in rare cases, SSRIs can actually increase depression and cause suicidal thoughts and impulses (especially in children, teens, and young adults), which is why these drugs' labels now caution users about these potential dangers — although the jury is still out on the suicide risks of antidepressants. In addition, SSRIs can cause reduced sex drive and a host of other side effects — and taking them in combination with other drugs that increase serotonin can be very dangerous. That's because too much serotonin can cause a condition called *serotonin syndrome,* in which very serious changes occur in heart function, body temperature, and other physical processes. Although SSRIs aren't addictive, stopping them abruptly can cause serious (but usually temporary) withdrawal effects.

SSRIs include drugs such as paroxetine (Paxil), fluoxetine (Prozac), sertraline (Zoloft), fluvoxamine (Luvox), citalopram (Celexa), and escitalopram (Lexapro).

Serotonin and Norepinephrine Reuptake Inhibitors (SNRIs) and related drugs

In the same way that SSRIs beef up the effects of serotonin in the brain, SNRIs boost the power of two messenger chemicals, serotonin and norepinephrine. Norepinephrine plays an important role in arousal and alertness (for info on serotonin's functions, see the preceding section on SSRIs). Like SSRIs, SNRIs do their job by stopping the cells that send these chemicals out from sucking them back in again. They're considered a second-line treatment for PTSD, in cases in which SSRIs don't do the trick.

SNRIs can be very effective, but they have adverse effects ranging from sexual side effects to insomnia and weight gain. These side effects vary, depending on which medication you take.

SNRIs include venlafaxine (Effexor or Effexor XR) and duloxetine (Cymbalta). Cymbalta has not been shown to be effective in PTSD.

Can SSRIs help your brain heal?

SSRIs can make you feel better, and they may do much more than that: Doctors report some clues that these drugs can help one brain region bounce back after PTSD lays it low.

In Chapter 4, I talk about the hippocampus, a seahorse-shaped brain region that plays a big role in your emotions and memories. Brain scans show that the hippocampus can shrink (atrophy) when it's hammered by too much stress.

In 2003, researchers treated PTSD patients with the SSRI drug paroxetine (Paxil) for one year. The patients underwent brain scans before and after the treatment, and the researchers saw a big difference in the before-and-after shots. Hippocampal volume increased by 5 percent in the treated patients — which doesn't sound like a lot, but it actually is. In addition, the Paxil-treated patients performed much better on tests measuring a type of memory that relies on the hippocampus (*verbal declarative memory*, which you use when you recall information in a paragraph after hearing it).

This intriguing finding jibes with other reports hinting that SSRIs can actually cause new nerve cell growth in the brain. If that's true, then SSRIs like Paxil may actually help fix the hardware of the brain. These studies and others are overturning the long-held notion that adult brains don't grow new neurons — and they're a good example of how we're constantly learning new information about how the brain works and how to treat problems like PTSD.

In addition to SNRIs, a number of other drugs affect the actions of serotonin, norepinephrine, or dopamine (another neuransmitter) in differing ways. These drugs include buproprion (Wellbutrin or Wellbutrin SR), mirtazapine (Remeron), nefazodone (Serzone), and trazodone (Desyrel).

Tricyclics

Tricyclics are the oldest antidepressants still in use, but they're falling out of favor because they have more side effects (such as confusion, headaches, drowsiness, and blurred vision) than newer drugs. Like SNRIs, tricyclics boost levels of serotonin and norepinephrine; they may also increase levels of dopamine. In addition to inhibiting the reuptake of these neurotransmitters and thus increasing their effects, tricyclics block some cell receptors — which is one reason they often cause so many side effects. These drugs sometimes help people who don't respond to other antidepressants.

Tricyclics include amitriptyline (Elavil), nortriptyline (Pamelor), desipramine (Norpramin), and imipramine (Tofranil).

MAO inhibitors (MAOIs)

As you may guess, MAO inhibitors (MAOIs) stop a substance called MAO (monoamine oxidase) from doing its job, which is to break down monoamine neurotransmitters — serotonin, dopamine, norepinephrine, and epinephrine — in the brain. This leads to greater levels of these chemicals.

Traditional MAOIs have many side effects and interact with cheese, a range of other foods, and some alcoholic beverages. (These foods and beverages contain large amounts of an amino acid named tyramine, which is essential for health but can be very dangerous if high levels accumulate in the body. Traditional MAOIs prevent monoamine oxidase from breaking down tyramine.) Because of these problems, doctors don't use traditional MAOIs much to treat PTSD.

However, the FDA recently approved a low-dose patch form of selegiline (Emsam), which is a newer form of MAOI (called a reversible inhibitor of monoamine oxidase A, or RIMA) that doesn't interact with food and has fewer side effects than the oldies in this category. That's because — as the name indicates — it only blocks one type of MAO (the A type) leaving the other type (B) available to break down unwanted chemicals. Also, its effects are reversible so the A form can get back in the game if tyramine levels start to rise.

Anti-anxiety drugs

The anti-anxiety drugs that doctors use most to treat PTSD are benzodiazepines and buspirone (Buspar), which work in different ways. One is quick but potentially dangerous, and the other is slower and safer:

✔ **Benzodiazepines:** These drugs act by enhancing the effects of gamma aminobutyric acid (GABA), which reduces the excitability of nerve cells. Benzodiazepines work fast, and they may begin to ease anxiety and sleep problems within days — but you can rapidly become dependent on them, and quitting can be a bear, which is why SSRIs and other drugs in that family are often prescribed first. Benzodiazepines can also make you sleepy, cause memory problems and aggression, and impair your coordination to the point where it's dangerous to drive. One more warning: Never take them if you have substance abuse problems.

Benzodiazepines include alprazolam (Xanax), lorazepam (Ativan), triazolam (Halcion), clonazepam (Klonopin), oxazepam (Serax), temazepam (Restoril), chlordiazepoxide (Librium), clorazepate (Tranxene), diazepam (Valium), and flurazepam (Dalmane).

✔ **Buspirone (Buspar):** A different type of drug, buspirone, typically takes two to four weeks to work. However, it has fewer side effects, and it can reduce symptoms such as intrusive thoughts and nightmares. Scientists don't know exactly how it works, although it appears to affect the serotonin system.

Beta-blockers

Beta-blockers are one of the most exciting PTSD treatments on the scene right now because at least one type of these drugs may actually address the traumatic memory itself.

Beta-blockers are blood-pressure medications with a long track record and a relatively good safety profile (although people with certain types of heart disease can't take them). They work by blocking beta receptors on certain cells in the heart, brain, and other organs, keeping adrenaline (and a related chemical, noradrenaline) from stimulating these cells. I talk in Chapter 4 about how doctors are testing one particular beta-blocker, propranolol (Inderal), as a means of stopping PTSD before it even starts by keeping memories from "setting." In addition, patients with longstanding PTSD symptoms report that beta-blockers can often calm pounding hearts, rapid breathing, and other physical symptoms of stress (although it's unclear if beta blockers other than propranolol will directly affect PTSD memories).

But the story is much more interesting than that. At the time of this writing, two doctors, Alain Brunet and Roger Pitman, are trying a new treatment approach for patients with long-term PTSD. They ask their patients to describe their trauma as clearly as they can, reliving the scene detail by detail — and then they immediately give these patients propranolol. The goal: to prevent the patients from "re-storing" the memories they just dredged up. This process allows the memory to decay normally instead of staying as fresh as the day it happened.

Remarkably, a single dose of propranolol taken after recalling a trauma can sometimes ward off PTSD symptoms for months, according to early data. It's far too soon to tell whether this treatment is as powerful as early research hints, but if so, it may change the face of PTSD treatment.

Sleeping aids

Benzodiazepines and tricyclic antidepressants (see earlier sections in this chapter) can bring on sleep, but they come with major side effects. If you have sleep problems, your doctor may instead prescribe one of several medications specifically designed to be sleep aids. The latter include the following:

- Zolpidem (Ambien)
- Trazodone (Desyrel)
- Zaleplon (Sonata)
- Eszopiclone (Lunesta)
- Ramelteon (Rozerem)

Ambien, Lunesta, and Sonata all work in pretty much the same way, by targeting the brain's receptors ("parking places") for *GABA,* a brain messenger-chemical that helps to regulate sleep. Rozerem works differently, by stimulating brain receptors for *melatonin* (a hormone that also helps to regulate sleep/wake cycles). These drugs have different lengths of action, different risks when it comes to creating dependency, and differing interactions with other drugs — so if you decide to take one, be sure to read up on its effects.

If you have mild sleep problems, your doctor may suggest that you try an over-the-counter sleep aid instead of a prescription medication. Over-the-counter drugs usually contain antihistamines (for instance, diphenhydramine hydrochloride) which, in addition to easing the symptoms of allergies, can make you very drowsy. Typically, these drugs have less effect than prescription sleep aids, although they can cause some short-term memory loss. They also can interact with other medications, so check with your doctor or pharmacist before taking any of them.

Other meds that often work as part of a combination

Because PTSD has so many different faces, doctors use a wide range of drugs to treat its various symptoms. In addition to the medications I describe in the previous sections, you may get a prescription for one of these drugs:

✔ **Anticonvulsants:** These drugs, usually used to treat seizures, can reduce anxiety in some people with PTSD. Side effects vary depending on the type of medication.

✔ **Lithium:** In low doses, this mood-stabilizing drug can sometimes reduce flashbacks and irritability. Major side effects can include nausea, changes in kidney function, dizziness, loss of appetite, diarrhea, or thyroid changes. Starting with the lowest possible dose can help minimize the risk of these side effects.

✔ **Atypical antipsychotics:** These very potent drugs may reduce paranoia or severe flashbacks in cases where other treatments don't help. However, they have some serious side effects, including weight gain, blood sugar fluctuations, and diabetes. (By the way, they're called *atypical* because they work in a variety of ways that differ from earlier antipsychotic drugs.)

✔ **Drugs to treat alcoholism/substance abuse:** Your medical team may prescribe drugs such as naltrexone (ReVia) or acamprosate (Campral — a drug prescribed after a person stops drinking, in order to prevent relapses) to help you kick the habit. These drugs work in different ways — for example, naltrexone blocks opiate receptors and reduces the high caused by drugs or alcohol; acamprosate helps to reduce the physical and emotional distress caused by stopping alcohol consumption. Because of their different mechanisms and effects, one may be more effective for you than another.

Speak Up! Asking Questions before You Take a Medication

Any medication, even an aspirin, has the potential to change your life for better or for worse. That's especially true for the drugs used to treat PTSD because they're some of the most powerful drugs ever invented. If they do their job right, they can help you tame the PTSD monster. If they don't, you can wind up with more problems on your plate.

If you and your doctor agree that medication is a good choice for you, the next step is to figure out which medication will do you the most good — and, equally important, which is the safest in your case. Because taking a medication is a big life decision, be sure to have the necessary facts in hand before saying yes or no. Here some basic questions to ask your doctor to get a general understanding of the drug:

✔ **What does this drug do?** Make sure the drug your doctor prescribes is likely to treat your most troublesome symptoms, and get a realistic picture of what it can and can't do for you.

✔ **How long does this drug take to work?** Some medications act quickly, and others take weeks or even months to start making you feel better. If you know what to expect, you can tell whether the medication is working right.

✔ **How long will I need to take this drug?** Find out whether this drug is a short-term prescription or something the doctor thinks you should take for months or even years.

The following questions are especially important because they can help you ensure your safety and well-being:

✔ **What side effects does this drug have, and how often do they occur?** Any drug (including the ones you buy off-the-shelf in the grocery store) can cause side effects. The important thing is to know how serious these side effects are and whether they happen a once in a blue moon or fairly frequently.

✔ **Can this drug make me suicidal?** It sounds odd, but medications that prevent depression can sometimes raise your risk of having suicidal thoughts or feelings — especially in the early weeks when you first start taking them. Some antidepressants may be riskier than others in this regard.

✔ **Can this drug cause dependency?** If your doctor says yes to this question, ask how long you can safely take the drug — and ask whether the doctor can provide any safer alternatives.

✔ **Can this drug cause serious withdrawal effects?** If so, find out what these effects are. Even if the withdrawal effects are not serious, find out what effects you can expect to have when you stop the medication. Also ask how long it will take for you to get off the medication when you and your doctor decide to do so.

✔ **Can I safely take this drug with the other medications or supplements I use?** PTSD drugs don't always play well with others, so be sure your doctor knows about any other prescription or over-the-counter drugs you're taking. Trouble can also arise if you combine PTSD medications with nutritional supplements or herbs; for instance, combining SSRIs, MAOIs or Buspar with St. John's wort is risky.

✔ **Does this drug interact with any foods or beverages?** In particular, ask whether your medication can interact with grapefruit juice, which makes many drugs — Valium, for example — far more potent. Also, if your doctor prescribes an MAOI, make sure you fully understand any dietary taboos associated with this type of drug.

✔ **(If you're pregnant) Is this drug safe for my unborn baby?** If taking a drug means you're medicating for two, you need to be even more careful about considering the drug. In this case, you need to check with your entire team of doctors — family doctor, obstetrician, and therapist — before agreeing to take a medication. If at all possible, put off any drug treatment until after your baby arrives — and after you finish breastfeeding if you're planning to nurse.

If your symptoms aren't dangerous and don't seriously interfere with your life and you're not quite keen on taking a medication, ask your doctor whether you can try a non-drug alternative first. Improving your diet, reducing your caffeine and alcohol intake, trying relaxation methods (see Chapter 10), exercising, and reducing life stressors can sometimes solve sleep problems or reduce anxiety levels, reducing or eliminating the need for a medication.

Also, do your own research when a doctor hands you a prescription. The best sources for information include your doctor, a pharmacist, package inserts, reliable Internet sources, and the *Physicians' Desk Reference (PDR)* (published by Thomson). You can find an online version of the PDR's info for consumers at www.pdrhealth.com — just click on the *drug information* tab — or you can find the book itself at nearly any public library.

Taking Meds Wisely

To boost the chances that a medication will chase symptoms away without causing new ones, do your detective work before accepting a prescription (which I cover in the preceding section). Then follow a few sensible rules when you start taking your medication:

✔ **Always take the right dosage at the right time.** Double-check the label to see whether the instructions match what your doctor told you.

If you have trouble remembering to take medications, set a reminder on your computer or use a pill container with dividers for each day.

✔ **When you start your new medication, tune in to your body's response.** Your doctor knows what drugs do to most people, but you're the expert on your own one-of-a-kind body — so you're the best judge of how a drug works for *you*. If you spot any symptoms that you think stem from your medication, call your doctor's office — and call *right away* if your symptoms are serious. Serious symptoms include but aren't limited to

• Significant mental symptoms, such as confusion, agitation, aggressive impulses, suicidal feelings, or extreme restlessness

• Serious physical symptoms, such as fainting, severe nausea or vomiting, rashes, difficulty breathing (which can indicate an allergic reaction), weakness, heart palpitations, or seizures

✔ **If you take medications for other conditions, have all your prescriptions filled at the same pharmacy.** Drugs for PTSD can interact with other meds, and most pharmacies have systems that flag potentially dangerous combos.

✔ **Notify your whole team if you start taking a drug for your PTSD.** That includes your primary care doctor, your therapist, and any specialists treating PTSD-related symptoms.

- ✔ ***Never, ever* stop taking a medication without consulting your doctor.** Quitting your meds abruptly can send your brain and body into a tailspin, so ask your doctor how to wean yourself off the drug slowly and safely. And if your symptoms vanish when you're taking a drug, don't assume that you don't need it anymore — most likely, the drug is what's keeping your symptoms under control.

- ✔ **If you're sick with the flu or food poisoning and can't keep your meds down, talk to your doctor immediately about what to do.** This is important even if you think you'll be over your bug in a day or two.

With luck — and some good teamwork on your part and your doctor's — you can pick just the right medication to clear away stumbling blocks to recovery and help you hit your stride in therapy. When that happens, ask your doctor whether it makes sense to taper off your medications or if continuing to combine therapy and medication is the right one-two punch to knock out your PTSD.

Chapter 10

Additional Paths to Wellness: Drawing on the Power of Mind and Body

*P*eople aren't like gingerbread men, all shaped by the same cookie cutter. Instead, everyone has a history that's his alone, a one-of-a-kind personality, and even a unique biology. Similarly, no one-size-fits-all therapy works for people with PTSD. Cognitive behavioral therapy (CBT — see Chapter 8) and its offshoots have the most scientific support, and many doctors also find medications effective (see Chapter 9), but these approaches don't work wonders for every person with PTSD.

Fortunately, you have a lot of other options of therapies to help you heal after a trauma. As you read through the sections in this chapter, you can see that some of the therapies I describe are used as front-line options, while many work best as *adjuncts* — that is, therapies you do in addition to a primary therapy like CBT.

In this chapter, I talk about the considerations you should keep in mind when deciding whether to try any of these therapies, which fall into two broad categories: psychological approaches that differ from typical CBT, and therapies that tap the power of your body in order to heal your mind.

Seeing Your Trauma through New Eyes: Psychological Approaches

In Chapter 8, I discuss cognitive behavioral therapy (CBT), in which you confront your trauma and discover new ways of thinking about what happened to you. (That chapter also covers several other therapies that employ CBT but are present oriented, meaning that they don't involve confronting your trauma.) CBT is the most popular form of therapy for PTSD, but other psychological therapies — some that are kissing cousins of CBT and others that use very different approaches — may help many people gain control over PTSD. In this section, I look at some of the most popular of these therapies, how they work, and what people know about their benefits or the harm they may do.

 As you read these sections, note that although some of these therapies have documented scientific support, others fall into the buyer-beware category because they're relatively new or untested. However, you don't find a thumbs-up or thumbs-down rating for any of the therapies I outline because I can't promise that any therapy in this chapter will or won't work for a given individual. A therapy that I think is unproven and possibly ineffective may prove to be just the ticket for you.

Note: Several of the therapies I talk about here could just as easily go in Chapter 8. Some of them, however, don't include all the facets of CBT — and others do, but their developers say they're *not* CBT. My suggestion: Don't worry too much about it. Labels aren't as important as results!

Neuro-linguistic programming (NLP)

Back in the 1970s, mathematician Richard Bandler and linguistics professor John Grinder created neuro-linguistic programming (NLP) in an effort to combine what they saw as the best features of many different therapy techniques. NLP is a collection of approaches based on these two principles:

- ✔ **Each person has an internal *map* based on his perception of the world and the language he uses to express this perception.** This map is often distorted or limited, and by changing it, you can alter your thoughts and behavior in positive ways.

- ✔ **By studying successful people, you can model their behaviors and become more successful yourself.** Similarly, by identifying the language and behaviors that make you successful in some areas of your life, you can begin using them in other areas where you currently have problems.

The power of sharing

One question people often ask me is "Why do different therapies work for different people?" The answer, in part, is that the type of therapy is less important than the knowledge that you and your therapist are a team — and that when you enter the therapy room, *you're no longer alone* with your despair.

Years ago, I experienced an incident that opened my eyes to the power of sharing your despair with someone who understands. It started when a colleague called me a few years ago and asked me to see Gina, a lovely woman so tormented by a violent rape that she'd tried to commit suicide several times. In her last attempt, she'd leaped off a third-floor balcony, shattering her pelvis.

For six months, Gina sat across from me in therapy. She rarely spoke and often didn't even answer my questions — but every week, she showed up on time. It was the only clue I had that our sessions helped her.

One day, I was exhausted when Gina arrived. I'd been awake for 36 hours helping emergency room patients who needed psychiatric evaluations, and I could barely keep my eyes open. But my exhaustion couldn't explain what happened next. As Gina talked, I saw all the color disappear from the room around me, replaced by waves of gray. At first, I thought I was having a stroke or a seizure. Gina wasn't looking at me, so I quickly checked my reflexes and vision but detected no problems.

And then I realized the truth: Somehow, I actually *felt* the pain Gina was trying to convey. Before I could stop myself, I said, "I never knew it was so bad. And I can't help you kill yourself, but if you do, I will still think well of you, I'll miss you, and maybe I'll understand why you needed to."

I was horrified when I realized what I'd said. In trying to express my understanding of her bleak world, I'd given her permission to kill herself! But her response startled me. Slowly, she glanced at me — the first solid eye contact she'd made — and then she smiled. When I asked her why, she looked me straight in the eye again, and I could see the "no bull" look of someone who's dropped her defenses.

"If you can really understand why I might need to kill myself," she said, "maybe I won't have to." As soon as the words left her mouth, the colors in the room began to reappear in front of my eyes.

My patient changed, too — in far more dramatic ways. Over time, she completed treatment and went on to get married, raise a family, and get a graduate degree in psychology.

I don't know what happened to me that day; perhaps I was so tired I lost touch with my conscious surroundings and became aware of things I might otherwise not sense. My guess is that my exhaustion, combined with the power of my patient's silent despair, broke through my own defenses.

Whatever it was, it forever changed how I listen to patients. And it helped me to truly grasp the fact that training, intellectual theories, and different therapeutic approaches mean far less than letting a person in despair know one simple fact: You are not alone anymore.

NLP focuses on helping people find more successful ways of thinking, behaving, and communicating. In this term, the *neuro* refers to the neurological processes that underlie behavior, and the *linguistic* refers to both verbal communication and body language.

Very little well-designed research exists on the effectiveness of NLP in treating PTSD. What's more, NLP practitioners have a cornucopia of tools to choose from and the length of therapy varies (although it often lasts only two to four sessions), so comparing one therapist's approach with another's is nearly impossible. However, some bits and pieces of NLP are well-established as effective. For instance, NLP uses two well-studied tools of cognitive behavioral therapy (see Chapter 8): It asks you to experience your trauma again, and it helps you to reframe what happened in a different way.

Common techniques used in NLP

NLP is a toolbox of techniques designed to help you achieve these goals. Several that are relevant to PTSD include the following:

- **Reframing:** In this technique, also used in CBT (see Chapter 8) and many other approaches, you discover how to look at an event in a different way and thus give it a different meaning.

  For example, a person who initially thinks that she failed in a crisis because she couldn't save a friend's life can use reframing to gain the understanding that she tried heroically to save her friend and did the best she could given her lack of medical training. Thus, the message "I failed" becomes the message "I was heroic and did the best job anyone in my shoes could do."

- **Swish:** In this technique, you spot the cues that lead to unwanted behaviors and figure out how to give them the boot by visualizing a desired goal instead. The *swish* involves rapidly pushing the undesired image away from you mentally while pulling the positive visualization toward you.

  For example, if the sight of the bedroom where a robber attacked you brings on panic attacks, you may replace this image instantly with a mental picture of yourself happily redecorating the room with the fancy bedspread and furniture you always wanted.

- **Anchoring:** This method stems from the fact that you associate emotions with certain stimuli. For example, you may associate the smell of candles with happy holidays in your childhood — or with the traumatic memory of a fire.

  Most anchors are unconscious, but in NLP, you discover how to *create* anchors intentionally. For example, by repeatedly recalling a time when you felt strong or happy or calm and associating that memory with an anchor — a ring on your finger or even a touch on a knuckle — you can use this anchor later to trigger the emotion you want to experience.

One key technique of NLP: Separating yourself from a memory

One tool of NLP — visual/kinesthetic dissociation (V/KD) — is particularly important in treating PTSD. This special visualization technique is designed to help the person separate (dissociate) herself from a traumatic memory by viewing it as though she were outside her body. (*Kinesthetic,* by the way, is just a fancy word referring to the sensory input provided by your body — for instance, your perception of gravity or motion.) The idea behind V/KD is that by changing how you view your trauma, you can detach yourself from it and process it from a rational perspective.

Practitioners say that this disassociation is different from *traumatic dissociation* (see Chapter 3), not only because they're spelled differently (although that's true too!), but also because in the therapeutic technique of dissociation, the person remains in control of the process.

A typical V/KD session (patients may undergo a single session or several) involves the following steps, although the steps vary for different therapists:

1. **You first dicsover and use relaxation techniques.**

2. **When you're calm and relaxed, your therapist asks you to picture yourself — as if in a photo — as you were before your trauma.**

3. **Your therapist asks you to visualize your trauma from the viewpoint of an outside observer.**

   Typically, he asks you to imagine that you've stepped out of your body and into the projection booth of a movie theater, where you can watch yourself sitting in a seat below, viewing a movie of your trauma. (This process puts you several steps away from the trauma.)

4. **As you visualize your trauma, the therapist encourages you to alter your movie in different ways.**

   For example, you may view your imaginary film in black-and-white and then in color, run it backward, or make it louder or quieter. You repeat this process until you feel a sense of control over your memory.

5. **The therapist asks you to return to your body, think about the new meaning you gained from the experience, and share your insights and positive emotions with the "younger self" in the photo you initially visualized in Step 2, as if that younger self is in the room with you.**

One variant of V/KD that's also popular is the *rewind technique,* developed by David Muss. In this approach, you first watch your film from the projection-booth point of view and then view it as though you were actually in the film rather than simply observing it. The second time, however, you view the film backwards.

V/KD has little formal research to prove or disprove its usefulness, but it does use several validated techniques, including a version of exposure therapy (more about this in Chapter 8). The few studies published on the technique indicate that it helps some people quite dramatically but provides little or no benefit to others.

One caution if you're considering V/KD: Patients who are vulnerable to dissociation (a type of defense mechanism — see Chapter 3 for a description of this symptom) shouldn't undergo this therapy because the voluntary dissociation technique may trigger involuntary dissociation.

Traumatic incident reduction (TIR)

Traumatic incident reduction (TIR) looks a little bit like cognitive behavioral therapy (CBT) but is really a very different approach. Like CBT, this therapy asks patients to confront their trauma. However, it uses a different method than CBT does and has different goals. (It's also different from visual/kinesthetic dissociation, which I discuss in the preceding section, and other rewind techniques, even though it uses a similar mental-movie technique.)

TIR is a short therapy (usually one session per trauma) in which the therapist acts more as a facilitator and the patient does the majority of the work. Here's how a typical TIR session goes:

1. **The patient (typically referred to as the *viewer*) identifies a trauma he wants to confront.**

   A key principal is that the patient decides what he wants to confront — and how intensely he wants to confront it — in this intervention.

2. **The patient mentally views the trauma as if it's a videotape.**

   First, he "rewinds" it to the beginning. Next, he views the entire trauma from start to finish.

3. **Afterward, the therapist asks what happened, and — with little or no guidance from the therapist — the patient describes what happened and how he felt about it.**

   Typically, the therapist offers no advice and doesn't evaluate or question the patient's insights.

4. **The patient repeats the process of rewinding and watching the mental video of his trauma, talking about the experience after each viewing.**

TIR sessions typically last one to two hours. Overall, therapy can last anywhere from a single session (which is common for PTSD stemming from a single trauma) to a dozen or so (which can occur when a patient has complex PTSD and needs to address multiple traumas). According to TIR practitioners, patients typically experience increasing emotion during the first few viewings, and then this emotion fades until they hit a point where they have no negative reaction to the trauma. The process continues until the patient actually experiences positive emotions (or calmness at a minimum). Therapists who use this approach say that virtually all patients achieve this state at the end of a session.

Although it shares a few features with CBT, TIR involves very little input from the therapist and is a much shorter procedure. It also focuses more intensely on encouraging patients to search for earlier (pre-trauma) similar incidents that may influence their thoughts and behavior. Patients may address these incidents in a somewhat different process called *thematic TIR,* which focuses on a particular symptom. For example, a person with anger issues may choose to use the mental video-tape procedure outlined in Step 2 of the list earlier in this section to work through each remembered incident in which he experienced extreme anger, until he reaches the earliest incident of extreme anger he can remember.

In the absence of any well-designed research on TIR's effectiveness, it's impossible to say whether the approach works for most patients. Its proponents point to case studies indicating that it can achieve quick cures, buts its critics say its techniques — based to a large degree on methods used in Scientology — are unproven.

Psychodynamic therapy

Psychodynamic therapy looks at the unconscious dynamics that play a role in emotions and behavior. In this type of therapy, just as in CBT, a therapist helps you to address the unconscious thoughts and conflicts that arise from a trauma. However, your therapist also explores maladaptive thoughts and behaviors that *don't* necessarily stem from the trauma, and you may spend time exploring pre-trauma events that possibly created a vulnerability to PTSD.

For instance, a psychodynamic therapist may be interested in any feelings of abandonment you feel as a result of your parents divorcing during your childhood, and how these feelings may impact your current PTSD.

Psychodynamic therapy, a great-great-grandchild of Freud's techniques, is a shorter version of psychoanalysis. (If you watched *The Sopranos,* you saw a good representation of long-term psychoanalysis conducted by Tony Soprano's therapist; in fact, the American Psychoanalytic Association gave her an award for her performance!) Unlike long-tern psychoanalysis, which can last a year or more, psychodynamic therapy typically lasts only a few months. This therapy involves lots of talking on your part, as you and your therapist seek to break down the *unconscious psychological defenses* — think of them as barriers to reality — that can get in the way of your healing from PTSD.

One cornerstone of psychodynamic therapy is *transference,* meaning that you may transfer feelings about your trauma or about other people to your therapist. For example, you may become angry at the therapist when you're really angry at a person who hurt or betrayed you during your trauma. Addressing this transference helps you and your therapist to identify the unconscious maladaptive feelings, motivations, and thoughts you have about yourself and other people, so you can bring these out into the open and defuse them.

It's hard to know just how well this approach works in treating PTSD, because psychodynamic therapists use many different approaches. Also, most studies of this technique are single-case studies — not very useful in revealing the big picture. However, the Cochrane Collaboration, a group that reviews medical research to help professionals determine what's effective and what isn't, did include psychodynamic therapy when it reviewed studies on different forms of therapy for PTSD (more on this study in Chapter 8). Their report concluded that psychodynamic therapy isn't as effective as CBT.

That said, a few studies do show that psychodynamic therapy can help some people a great deal, especially when combined with other techniques. One study of traumatized police officers, for instance, showed that those who underwent a treatment called *brief eclectic psychotherapy* (which combines psychodynamic therapy with CBT) showed significant improvement at a three-month follow-up compared to officers on a waiting list for treatment.

One form of psychodynamic therapy that needs to come with a warning label is *repressed memory therapy.* In this technique, a therapist's goal is to guide you to remember memories that you've buried deep down. For instance, a grown woman may suddenly get flashes of memories about her father abusing her. The problem with repressed memory therapy is that the memories it dredges up are often false. (See the nearby sidebar, "False memories and confabulation: Two tricks your mind can play on you.") So if you choose to explore this type of therapy, read up on it and understand the possible risks — both to you and to your family.

Hypnotherapy

Think of hypnosis, and you probably conjure up a picture of someone clucking like a chicken or lying stiff as a board between two chairs. But hypnosis isn't just a magic act. Used therapeutically, it's a means of achieving deep relaxation and opening your mind to things beyond the here-and-now.

Here's what *doesn't* happen under therapeutic hypnosis:

- ✔ You don't lose awareness of who and where you are.
- ✔ You don't fall under the spell of the therapist and do whatever she bids. (No chicken clucking, honest!)

REAL-LIFE STORY

False memories and confabulation: Two tricks your mind can play on you

Record a TV show, and each time you play it back, the plot will be exactly the same. But people's memories don't work like a video recorder, which is why two people can remember the same event very differently. To make matters even more confusing — and dangerous, when it comes to therapy — you can remember things that never happened at all.

Therapists and patients discovered this the hard way in the 1980s and early 1990s, when an intervention called *repressed memory therapy* became popular. Supposedly, the therapy helped patients retrieve memories they'd buried entirely — often memories of horrific abuse by their parents or daycare providers. But as it turned out, therapists often unwittingly planted these memories in their patients' minds. (I'd need a whole book to describe this process, but a quick explanation is that both therapists and patients are suggestible, and if both become convinced that episodes of incest, molestation, or even satanic abuse underlie a symptom, a patient's mind may obligingly create false memories of such an event.) As a result, many patients wound up breaking their ties with loved ones who'd never hurt them, and a number of innocent parents and daycare workers went to jail.

Repressed memory therapy is no longer in vogue, and therapists using other approaches are extremely careful not to use techniques that may accidentally create false memories. But doctors and patients still have to deal with the fact that memory is faulty even under the best of circumstances.

For example, take a look at a phenomenon called confabulation. In its strictest sense, *confabulation* is a symptom seen in many brain-injured patients who fully believe memories of things that never occurred. (For instance, if you ask one of these brain-injured patients why he's wearing a coat in the summer, he may say, "The nurse told me to put it on," fully believing it, even if it's not true.) But new evidence shows that everyone confabulates to some degree, often to justify a decision when someone doesn't really know why he made it.

In one experiment, for instance, researchers laid out four identical pieces of clothing and asked volunteers to pick the best one. In this type of experiment, people nearly always pick the item that's farthest to the right. Four out of five of these volunteers followed suit, but when asked why they chose that particular item, the volunteers made up all sorts of interesting reasons about the fabric, the color, and so on. Not one said "Because it's on the right side," which was the real reason. In reality, they probably didn't know why they picked it, so their minds happily let them off the hook by providing a reason.

Confabulation can occur inside the therapy room as well as outside. To minimize this possibility, a good therapist is careful to let you tell your memories your way, instead of trying to put words in your mouth (or ideas in your mind) — which is especially important if your trauma involved a crime, and you may need to testify clearly and correctly about what happened.

Instead, a hypnotherapist uses soothing imagery or other techniques to relax you, allowing you to view your trauma calmly and possibly to

✔ Remember important parts of your trauma that are currently blocked from your memory. This can help you process and come to terms with these buried memories.

✔ Revisit times when you experienced good events and positive feelings, helping you to put your trauma in context.

✔ Offer positive suggestions such as "You'll feel calmer when you drive." *Note:* A reputable therapist won't do this without your prior permission.

Be wary of any therapist who claims to use hypnosis to unlock "repressed memories." (See the sidebar in this chapter on "False memories and confabulation: Two tricks your mind can play on you," for more on the risks of repressed memory therapy.) A good hypnotherapist offers you the tools to let your own memories surface, but he won't actively plant ideas in your mind (for instance, by suggesting that your insomnia or anxiety is a likely symptom of abuse, and that you're "in denial" if you can't remember it).

Hypnosis has a long history as a treatment for PTSD, and army hospitals used it as a therapy for shell shock in World War II. However, the Cochrane Collaboration (see the section "Psychodynamic therapy" and Chapter 8 for more info) compared hypnosis (as a primary treatment) to cognitive behavioral therapy and found that CBT was far more effective. So the consensus seems to be that if you use hypnosis, use it as part of a well-rounded treatment plan — not as your only option. As such, it's currently most often used to augment other psychological therapies rather than as a primary treatment. Even then, people question its usefulness because some research suggests that CBT alone is as helpful as the combination of CBT and hypnosis.

Art therapy

Art therapy for PTSD hit its peak of popularity in the Vietnam era but isn't used as much today because treatments such as CBT and medications are replacing it. However, some people find art therapy to be very powerful medicine. It's typically offered in addition to other therapies instead of a sole treatment, except when therapists use it as a primary therapy in treating children (see Chapter 15 for more on this).

In art therapy, which can be either an individual or group therapy, the therapist provides you with the materials you need to express yourself artistically, and then helps you to use these materials to work through your trauma. In some cases, she may offer guidance — for example, by asking you to draw a picture of how you perceive your body after your trauma. In other cases, she may ask you to draw or sculpt anything you wish.

In either case, she talks with you about clues that emerge from your artwork. For instance, if you draw a picture of yourself standing far apart from other people on a hillside, you and your therapist may discuss the reasons why the "you" in your drawing is so distant. The amount of direction, guidance, and interpretation offered by an art therapist varies widely from therapist to therapist.

Art therapy has the following advantages:

- ✔ It offers people who can't yet talk about their trauma a safe way to express their pain.

- ✔ Many people find that describing their trauma in the form of imagery helps them to understand and find new meaning in it. Just as some people find healing in talking about their trauma, others find healing in expressing their emotions in paint or clay. Also, defining a traumatic experience within the boundaries of a painting or sculpture can help a person feel a sense of control over it.

- ✔ Art is a powerful stress reliever, and getting lost in the act of painting or sculpting can give a troubled mind a much-needed rest.

- ✔ Art therapy combines the negative emotions of recalling a trauma with the pleasurable process of creation, which may help in processing upsetting memories.

 Because art therapy can arouse powerful memories, it's best to seek out a certified therapist who's trained in both art and psychology (ask whether the therapist has an ATR-BC certification). A therapist with this training can help you work through any painful emotions that arise.

Little formal research on art therapy is available, but small studies on the use of this therapy for veterans indicate that it's frequently helpful. In some cases, it appears to benefit people with severe PTSD symptoms who don't respond well to other treatments.

And remember: You don't need to be a budding Picasso or Michelangelo to benefit from art therapy — nobody grades your work! However, the art at the National Vietnam Veterans Art Museum — www.nvvam.org — includes some remarkable works by veterans with PTSD. You may want to check it out.

"Tapping" therapy

One of the most controversial therapies for PTSD is *tapping*, which comes in several forms. (Two of the most popular are called *Thought Field Therapy* and *Emotional Freedom Techniques*.) Unlike other therapies, tapping derives from the philosophies of Eastern medicine. Roger Callahan, the developer of Thought Field Therapy, says his technique works by "balancing the body's energy system." Gary Craig, the developer of Emotional Freedom Techniques, likens the process to "emotional acupuncture" and claims that you can use his therapy for "anything from the common cold to cancer" — as well as for PTSD.

The premise underlying both of these therapies, as well as other tapping therapies, is that a trauma causes negative emotions that disrupt the body's energy flow. Thus, practitioners say, it's crucial to correct this energy imbalance as you address your negative memories and emotions. The treatment is brief, sometimes lasting only a few minutes.

Tapping therapies involve the following steps:

1. **You think of a disturbing thought or memory.**

2. **You simultaneously tap your fingers on different energy meridian points on your body.**

   Your therapist shows you how and where to tap and may also ask you to do other simple tasks like humming or counting. Another term for these points is acupoints; see *Acupressure & Reflexology For Dummies* (Wiley) by Bobbi Dempsey and Synthia Andrews for more info.

3. **After each round of this procedure, your therapist asks questions about your feelings and whether they're changing.**

   Tapping therapists say that by tapping on the points where energy is either stored in excess or blocked, you assist the energy in flowing freely, thereby allowing the energy to heal your mind, body, and soul. Some tapping techniques specify different sequences of tapping points for different medical problems; others don't.

Unleashing creativity as a source of healing

People with PTSD can express their emotions and make sense of their experiences in many different ways. One, of course, is by talking to a therapist. Another is through art (see section on "Art therapy" in this chapter). But any creative outlet can offer a sense of peace or catharsis. If you live in a large city, you may find therapists who offer these approaches to healing:

✔ Drama therapy

✔ Dance therapy

✔ Poetry therapy

✔ Music therapy

Each of these therapies is much like art therapy in that it allows you to bring your positive creativity to bear on a negative experience and define your trauma in a new way. No hard evidence supports these therapies as effective treatments for PTSD, but some individuals — especially those who find talking about their traumas too painful — find them very helpful.

A few not-very-rigorously designed studies of tapping therapy's effects on simple phobias indicate that some patients improve. However, one study cast strong doubt on why the therapy helps some people. In that test, researchers divided participants into four groups. One group received no treatment; one tapped on the correct meridian points; one tapped on other body areas; and another tapped on a doll. Because all three treatment groups showed similar improvements, the researchers concluded that tapping has nothing to do with unblocking energy and that any benefits may arise from a placebo effect. (A *placebo effect* occurs when a patient improves simply because he expects a treatment to work.)

The bottom line on tapping therapies: No good evidence indicates that they work. But they're relatively quick, so if you decide to try one of these therapies, you aren't out a great deal of time. The biggest risk is that if it doesn't work — or causes only a temporary placebo effect — you may be discouraged from trying other, more-proven therapies.

Another therapy that sometimes uses tapping, but for very different reasons, is Eye Movement Desensitization and Reprocessing (EMDR) Therapy, which I cover in Chapter 8. EMDR shouldn't be confused with the tapping therapies I describe here.

Enlisting Your Body to Help Heal Your Mind

One thing you know for sure if you have PTSD is that your mind affects your body — and vice versa. For instance, a memory of your trauma can make your heart race and your hands sweat. And it works the other way around: A skinned knee, a burn from a stove, or the twinge from a scar can trigger memories of your trauma.

Luckily, you can also put this mind-body connection to work for you. The therapies I describe in the next sections can sometimes help reduce symptoms of PTSD either a little or a lot when you use them to supplement CBT or other effective psychological therapies. *Note:* In most cases, these approaches aren't enough in and of themselves to effectively address moderate or severe PTSD.

Relaxation therapies

One of the first steps in most therapies for PTSD involves developing simple relaxation techniques so you can confront your trauma and still stay in control.

Relaxation techniques can also play a role in preventing PTSD or in minimizing the risk of relapses after therapy. (For examples of some basic techniques, see Chapter 4.)

Relaxation techniques alone can't treat PTSD, but they can ease symptoms and may help you prevent panic attacks. They don't need to be complicated, either; one 1997 study of Vietnam vets found that doing a simple relaxation technique while sitting in a comfy chair worked as well as more-complicated procedures involving breathing exercises or biofeedback.

One great thing about these techniques is that they're virtually risk-free, and some of them — especially yoga and tai chi — can help you keep in shape as well. That's important, because you're less vulnerable to PTSD symptoms when your body is functioning up to par. Here are some popular relaxation therapies:

- ✓ **Yoga and tai chi:** No hard data support the benefits of either of these approaches in relieving PTSD, but studies do show that they can reduce stress and anxiety in general. Exercise that promotes relaxation and calmness can be highly beneficial. One note, however: If you have medical problems, make sure your doctor okays these exercise approaches — especially yoga, which can be surprisingly strenuous.

- ✓ **Massage therapy:** Some people find massage therapy helpful; however, it can sometimes trigger flashbacks or panic attacks in people whose PTSD stems from a physical assault, so go slowly and find an understanding massage therapist who'll back off if problems arise.

- ✓ **Meditation:** Although it doesn't fit neatly into any category, meditation is gaining scientific support. The Veterans Administration hospital in San Diego is currently investigating the effects of *mantram therapy* (which uses the techniques of meditation and involves repeating words or phrases that help you stay centered in the present) and is reporting some encouraging results.

- ✓ **Breathing exercises:** If you suffer from panic attacks, you may benefit from consulting a therapist who specializes in teaching breathing techniques that can stop these attacks in their tracks. (See Chapter 8 for info on a technique that combines breathing therapy for panic attacks with cognitive behavioral therapy for PTSD.)

Neurofeedback therapy

In neurofeedback (also called *neurotherapy* or *EEG biofeedback*), you get a glimpse of what your brain's up to — and you discover some tricks to control it. The therapy is popular for disorders ranging from attention deficit hyperactivity disorder (ADHD) to substance abuse, and many practitioners offer it for people with PTSD as well.

The link between sleep apnea and PTSD

Want more evidence of the link between mind and body? Look no further than that all-important thing you do every few seconds of the day and night: breathing. When you encounter something that reminds you of your trauma, you can fall into breathing patterns that trigger panic attacks (see more on this in Chapter 8). But disordered *nighttime* breathing also appears to play a big role in PTSD symptoms.

For example, one research team identified 23 people who suffered chronic nightmares (including 15 with PTSD) and also had *obstructive sleep apnea* — a common problem in which an obstructed airway causes people to stop breathing for long stretches many times during the night — or related breathing problems. Some of these people followed through on treatments for their breathing disorders, and others dropped out. Those who finished treatment reported an 85 percent improvement in nightmares (compared to a worsening in those who stopped treatment). In the subgroup with PTSD, people who stayed with therapy for their sleep breathing disorders reported a whopping (75 percent) improvement in PTSD symptoms, while those who stopped therapy got worse.

Bottom line: Talk to your doctor if you have symptoms of sleep apnea. These can include loud and prolonged snoring, thrashing during sleep, and fatigue in the day. Sleep apnea is very treatable, and getting treatment if you need it doesn't just reduce your PTSD — it can lower your blood pressure and reduce your risk of heart attack or stroke as well.

In *neurofeedback therapy,* electroencephalogram (EEG) leads attached to your scalp transform your brainwaves into output you can detect with your senses. For instance, a therapist may show you how to use your "brainpower" to move an object in a video game, change the pitch of musical tones, or increase a vibration.

The external changes you cause in neurofeedback are a way of rewarding your brain for creating brainwaves that can make you feel more calm, alert, or happy. So in a sense, neurofeedback is actually a behavioral therapy — but with some added hardware.

Neurofeedback made its initial appearance in the 1970s, and it gained popularity as a PTSD treatment in the 1990s when Eugene Peniston and Paul Kulkosky tested it as an intervention for combat veterans. The two researchers reported that neurofeedback was highly effective for both PTSD and alcoholism (a common problem for people with PTSD). Since then, a number of small studies have also reported positive findings. However, critics say these studies — as well as the initial ones by Peniston and Kulkosky — have significant flaws that make their findings questionable.

Where does that leave us? Case studies clearly show that some people benefit greatly from neurofeedback, but we don't have any solid stats on its overall effectiveness. Two other considerations: It's not an inexpensive therapy, but it's not a particularly risky treatment, either. So you don't have lots of guarantees that it'll help you, but there's little reason to worry that it'll hurt you — other than in the pocketbook.

Transcranial magnetic stimulation

Transcranial magnetic stimulation (TMS) sounds like something out of a science fiction movie, but it's a promising therapy for depression — and early results suggest that it may help people with PTSD as well. (Another term for this approach is *rTMS,* which stands for *repetitive transcranial magnetic stimulation.*) However, TMS is a newcomer on the treatment scene, so therapists can't yet tell if it'll be a useful addition to the toolbox of PTSD treatments.

TMS uses short pulses of magnetic energy, generated by a device placed near a person's head, to stimulate cells in specific regions inside the brain. Picture a shower head held next to your head — only one that delivers magnetic pulses instead of water! See Figure 10-1. As the magnetic pulses pass through the brain, they change the patterns of electrical firing between cells in targeted areas, which in turn can reduce depression and anxiety. Sessions last about 20 to 30 minutes, and patients typically undergo about ten sessions (although this number varies).

TMS is relatively painless, although some people report headaches or mild discomfort due to the heat produced by the device. Patients stay awake and alert during the entire procedure.

A few studies are reporting the effects of TMS on PTSD, and so far the findings are encouraging. For example, one study reported that ten sessions of high-frequency rTMS reduced the core PTSD symptoms of avoidance and intrusive thoughts in patients as well as alleviated anxiety symptoms. And an earlier study found that TMS treatment temporarily lowered avoidance symptoms, anxiety, and physical symptoms associated with PTSD.

TMS can't be used if you have a pacemaker or any other metal implanted in your body or if you have epilepsy (with one exception). Otherwise it appears to be pretty safe, although researchers are still investigating two possible adverse effects:

- ✔ **Seizures:** Seizures occur in rare cases. Fine-tuning the TMS method may reduce this risk. (Interestingly, TMS is also used as a treatment to *reduce* seizures in some people with epilepsy.)
- ✔ **Manic episodes:** In a 2004 study, two patients developed a *manic episode,* in which they experienced excess energy and abnormal thought patterns, after therapy.

Because these side effects are uncommon, most medical practitioners consider TMS to be a fairly safe — but *not* risk-free — procedure.

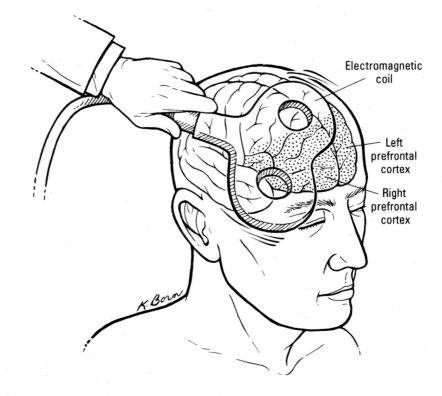

Figure 10-1:
In
transcranial
magnetic
stimulation,
the electro-
magnetic
coil
stimulates
brain cells.

Electromagnetic
coil

Left
prefrontal
cortex

Right
prefrontal
cortex

Considering Supplementary Therapies: What's Best for You?

Experts widely consider CBT to be the first choice for PTSD (see Chapter 8), but you may want to try an add-on therapy if CBT alone isn't handling all your symptoms. If that's the case, I recommend that you carefully consider which therapies you participate in: Do you really need, or want, to do more than one type of therapy? The answer depends on many factors. Here are some of the most important:

✔ **What your current therapist, if you have one, recommends:** Talk to your therapist about how well other therapies mesh with your current one. Many therapists practice more than one therapy, and those who don't can often refer you to other professionals who offer the supplementary therapy you'd like to try.

✔ **How well your primary therapy is working:** If you're getting fantastic results with one therapy, you've no need to gild the lily by trying to add more. One exception is relaxation or exercise therapies, which can nearly always be beneficial as supportive approaches.

✔ **Whether you can afford more than one therapy:** Therapy isn't cheap, even if insurance covers some or most of it. Consider your budget, because adding financial stress to your life may outweigh the benefits of a second therapy added to your primary one.

✔ **How much time you have:** Again, you don't need extra stress — so don't bite off more than you can chew when it comes to therapy. Dedicating yourself to one therapy may do more for you than spreading yourself too thin.

If you're certain you want to try a different type of therapy other than CBT or medication (or in addition to one or both of them), how do you decide which therapy to choose? No two people make that decision exactly the same way, but I recommend considering these points as you read through your options and try to make a choice:

✔ **How much scientific support each approach has:** Initial results are often misleading, so ponder each approach's track record in making your decision. (For info on how to do this, see the sidebar "New Treatments? You be the judge!" in this chapter.)

✔ **The risk/benefit ratio of each approach:** Some approaches (for instance, relaxation therapies) are very low risk, so you're not out much if you try them and they don't help. Others can be expensive or even a little dangerous. Weigh each treatment's benefits and dangers in making your selection. Remember, however, that even a seemingly safe therapy can be harmful if it fails to help and thus discourages you.

✔ **Whether the approach speaks to you:** Everyone has a unique temperament and likes and dislikes — and these traits and preferences play a role in picking the right treatment. As you read through the descriptions of the different therapies, decide which one best fits your personality and beliefs. Researchers look at how much a therapy benefits people *in general,* but factoring your own preferences into the mix is just as important.

If you decide to try more than one therapy simultaneously, be sure to let all your therapists know the different approaches you're using. Better yet, let them communicate with each other so they can plan a coordinated approach that works well for you.

Also, if you're interested in cutting-edge therapies, you can check out clinical trials of new techniques (or, in some cases, combinations of existing techniques). A good place to start is at the Web site of the National Institute of Mental Health, www.nimh.nih.gov. (Just click on the *clinical trials* button at the top of the page.)

New treatments? You be the judge!

Brand-new treatments for PTSD pop up almost as often as flowers in the spring, so knowing what new therapies you'll be able to choose from in upcoming years is impossible. That's why you ought to get the hang of evaluating each new therapy that comes down the pike.

That sounds like a difficult task, but some basic ground rules can help you. The first, of course, is to ask your doctor for his take on any new therapy. Next, do your own homework on the Internet or at the library. Here are some useful things to find out if you're trying to decide whether a new treatment approach is worth your time, hard work, and money:

✔ **How many people the therapy was tested on so far:** The larger the group, the more accurate the findings are likely to be. Case studies involving one or two patients are often very interesting, but they don't mean much in the overall scheme of things. In general, it takes a half-dozen or more studies, involving several hundred patients overall, to get a good idea of a therapy's value.

✔ **How long researchers followed the people treated with the therapy:** Many treatments help for a few weeks, but benefits often fade over time. See whether anyone's done long-term studies to see whether the treatment's effects are lasting.

✔ **Who's promoting the therapy:** If a report saying that a new therapy is amazingly effective comes from a company that makes money from the treatment, be skeptical. If it comes from a less-biased source — say, a university study — then you're on safer ground. Also, be suspicious of too-good-to-be-true claims.

✔ **Downsides that the researchers report:** See whether you can find details on any negative effects of the therapy.

✔ **Use of a control group:** Almost any therapy, effective or not, shows some results simply because patients expect to get better. (That's the placebo effect.) To show how useful a treatment really is, researchers need to compare people getting the therapy to other people who receive either a different treatment or no treatment at all.

✔ **Balanced reports:** If you read glowing reports about a new therapy, search the Internet and see whether you find not-so-glowing reports as well. When you read the opinions of both supporters and critics, you'll be in a much better position to judge the truth.

One good place to get up-to-date info on new therapies is at PubMed (www.ncbi.nlm.nih.gov/entrez/query.fcgi?DB=pubmed), where you can find free abstracts of research papers from thousands of medical journals. Another good resource is the National Center for Post Traumatic Stress Disorder (www.ncptsd.va.gov/ncmain/index.jsp). This center, which operates under the auspices of the Department of Veterans Affairs, offers a wide range of information on the effects of various treatments.

Part III

Choosing the Right Treatment Approach

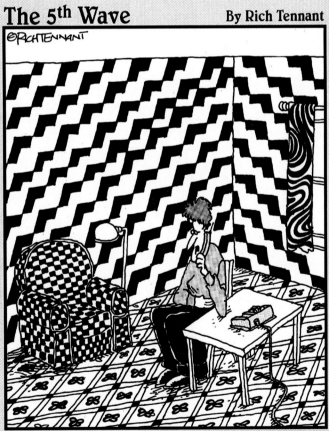

"I've tried Ayurveda, meditation, and aroma therapy but nothing seems to work. I'm still feeling nauseous and disoriented all day."

In this part . . .

Getting treatment is the key that unlocks the door to recovery from PTSD — but it's not as simple as it seems, because different treatments work for different people. In this part, I take a look at the wide variety of treatment options available and offer advice on picking the one that's best for you. I start by looking at the most commonly used approach to treating PTSD, cognitive behavioral therapy (CBT). Next, I describe the medications that sometimes (but not always) play a key role in recovery. Last, I look at a wide range of other PTSD therapies, describing how they work and offering some data on their usefulness.

Chapter 11

The Journey Back: What to Expect

Some life problems are just like a TV-show plot. One minute, you're fine. The next minute, a crisis arises. Then magically, in a few days or weeks (or 30 minutes, if you're in a TV sitcom), your problem gets solved, and all's well again.

PTSD isn't one of those problems. It doesn't come with a tidy script to tell you how long it'll last, when you'll feel better, or how much better you'll feel as you heal. Because no two people with PTSD have the same symptoms or the same life histories, no two people make the same progress or heal on the same schedule.

In this chapter, I look at why recovery is an individual process, explain what the word *recovery* means in PTSD, and offer advice on how to recognize your triumphs and cope with any lingering effects as you heal from your trauma. In addition, I talk about positive ways to handle a therapy setback, an unproductive relationship with a therapist, or the occasional relapses that may occur on your road from victim to survivor to thriver.

Recovery in a Nutshell: What Will and Won't Change

PTSD has no magic cure — no point at which you can declare, "I'll never have a symptom again!" Some people's PTSD symptoms *do* disappear for good, but typically, recovery from PTSD is an ongoing journey toward wellness. In this section, I look at what you can expect on this trek and how you can stay committed by having realistic expectations and keeping your eyes open for the signposts of healing.

Reaching milestones big and small

How do you know that you're getting better? Recovery doesn't happen overnight — but as weeks, months, and years go by, you'll experience large and small victories as your symptoms decrease in intensity, occur less often, and respond more quickly to your stress-management techniques.

As you begin your recovery, be patient and keep an eye out for some or all of these signs:

✔ **You get a better handle on the emotions stemming from your trauma.** You're increasingly able to face your memories head-on, and you experience fewer flashbacks or overwhelming feelings. You may find that you can drive past the scene of your trauma, or see a similar scene on a TV newscast, without spinning out of control.

✔ **You feel a thawing of once-frozen emotions.** You experience more and more moments of feeling more *real* and in touch with your feelings — a sense of true joy when you watch an uplifting movie, for example, or a surge of love when you hug your child.

✔ **You feel a stronger bond with others.** Friendships and romantic ties gradually seem more interesting and enriching and less unpleasant or exhausting. You find social occasions more rewarding, and you become more tolerant of the messy problems that are part and parcel of any relationship.

✔ **You experience new optimism about the future.** You find yourself once again making positive plans and setting goals. You may think about returning to college or applying for a better job, for example. Another sign of healing: You wake up some mornings looking forward to your day instead of feeling like you have a 100-pound rock of dread on your chest.

✔ **You encounter fewer problems at work.** You find your job less stressful and more rewarding as you get better at handling work pressures and relationships with your co-workers.

✔ **You discover that once-overwhelming tasks are easy or even fun.** After months or years of eating fast food or living in a cluttered mess because cooking or cleaning exhausted you, you find yourself picking up a cookbook and flagging an interesting recipe — or putting on some housecleaning music and dusting with gusto.

✔ **You rediscover the joy of truly relaxing.** Instead of being hyperalert 24/7, you begin to experience moments — and sometimes hours or even days — when you're truly calm, both physically and mentally.

REAL-LIFE STORY

Different brains, different healing stories

Why does one person with PTSD heal quickly and completely, whereas another needs more hard work and patience to get well? One study found a clue by peeking inside the brain.

Dr. Ruth Lanius of the London Health Sciences Centre in Ontario, Canada, and her colleagues used a brain imaging technique called functional magnetic resonance imaging (fMRI) to explore why people with PTSD often follow different paths to healing. Their volunteers: a husband and wife who developed PTSD after a multiple-car pileup. The couple spent several minutes trapped in their car during the ordeal and witnessed the death of a child in another car. Eventually, the husband broke the windshield of their own car so they could escape.

After the accident, the husband had flashbacks and nightmares, grew very upset when he thought or talked about the accident, and avoided driving on the highway where it had happened. The wife avoided news about the accident, slept badly, had trouble concentrating, and often became very angry. Her PTSD severely impaired her ability to work, and she sold her business.

A few weeks after the accident and before the couple began therapy, Lanius and her colleagues asked the two to undergo magnetic resonance imaging while they mentally relived their traumatic event. The researchers also measured the couple's heart rates as they recalled the accident.

The husband's heart rate skyrocketed, and stress-related areas of his brain lit up as he recalled breaking the car windshield and freeing himself and his wife. By contrast, his wife's pulse stayed steady and the stress-related regions of her brain showed no increases in signal intensity as she recalled her own experience of feeling numb and frozen during the accident.

The couple underwent therapy, and six months later, the husband was free of PTSD symptoms. The wife still had significant problems, however. Lanius and her colleagues said the couple's different brain and heart-rate patterns and their different rates of healing may support the theory that emotional numbness — a symptom the wife but not the husband experienced in this case — can make the healing process more challenging.

But is that explanation the only one for this couple's different healing pattern? Maybe not. The husband had a happy childhood and supportive parents, whereas the wife experienced the loss of her father early in life and never felt safe with her cold, distant mother. She also had a history of postpartum depression and mild panic disorder. These factors could also make her more vulnerable to developing hard-to-treat PTSD symptoms.

The message: Don't expect to heal from PTSD on exactly the same timetable as someone else, even if you survived the same traumatic event. Your brain, body, and history are different, which means that you'll heal at your own pace.

Viewing recovery as a journey

It's important to anticipate milestones of healing, recognize them when they occur, and have faith that more will come with time, even if they don't happen right away. But it's also important to keep your goals realistic so you don't expect a miracle and feel disappointed if your gains are more modest.

To create realistic expectations, keep these facts in mind:

- ✔ **Healing isn't an all-or-nothing proposition.** You may always have some symptoms of PTSD, especially if you're a combat veteran or if you have complex PTSD stemming from child abuse or other multiple traumatic experiences. Stay positive by celebrating each sign of progress you see instead of focusing solely on the symptoms that stick around.

- ✔ **Healing doesn't mean forgetting.** You'll still remember what happened during your trauma, and those memories may make you feel sad or angry at times. Feelings like those are part of life. Recovery doesn't erase those memories; instead, it helps you deal with them in safe and healthy ways.

- ✔ **Healing sometimes happens in fits and starts.** You may be discouraged when you feel good one day and bad again the next, but these cycles are part of the healing process (for more on this subject, see "The Ups and Downs of Therapy," later in this chapter).

- ✔ **Healing happens faster in some areas than in others.** You may discover that you overcome your flashbacks more quickly than you conquer your relationship problems, or vice versa. That situation is perfectly normal, so be patient if progress is frustratingly slow in some parts of your life; it'll come with time.

- ✔ **Healing skills take time to master.** Remember when you played your first video game? You probably alternated between making great moves and falling flat on your fanny until you got the hang of it and made faster progress. The skills you acquire in therapy take time to gel, too, so you won't always be at the top of your game when you start out. Don't get discouraged; just keep practicing, and your coping and calming techniques will grow more effective with time.

Outlining the Process: Stages of Healing

Recovery from PTSD isn't a straight-as-the-crow-flies journey. It's more like a mountain road on which you wind around, traveling uphill at some points and downhill at others, and you can't always see your destination ahead. At times, you even seem to be moving *away* from your target. But take heart, because the curves and switchbacks are part of your road to recovery. That road takes unexpected twists and turns, but it gradually leads you through three stages of healing.

Progress through these stages can take months, years, or even decades — and not everyone reaches the final stage. But spotting the glimmer of a new stage can give you the hope you need to keep moving on, even when therapy is challenging. In the following sections, I talk about each stage and describe how your progress affects your therapy.

As you read through this section, understand that many factors influence how quickly you heal and how many of your symptoms fade. People with simple PTSD from a single trauma have good odds of recovering fairly quickly and getting most or all of their symptoms under control; however, people with complex PTSD stemming from multiple traumas (for instance, child abuse or combat experiences) need to be more patient and may continue to experience some significant symptoms even after treatment. But no matter what type of PTSD you have, the odds are excellent that therapy will leave you happier, healthier, and more optimistic about the rest of your life.

The first stage: Victim

When your trauma first occurs, it takes over your life. You have difficulty functioning in any area of your life. You're overwhelmed by pain, fear, or anger. At this point, you may have thoughts like these:

> *I'm terrified.*
>
> *My life is destroyed.*
>
> *I'm broken in ways that will never mend.*
>
> *My world will never be the same again.*

When you're in this phase, you need immediate help. In fact, therapists sometimes call this stage the emergency stage. Your therapist will focus right away on supporting you emotionally and handling any immediate health or safety needs. He'll also educate you about the effects of trauma and then help you face your trauma in a way that empowers you to make sense of it. He may also recommend medications to treat your most pressing symptoms; these medications may be either a short-term or a long-term part of your treatment. (See Chapters 8, 9, and 10 for descriptions of the roles that different therapies or medications may play at this stage.)

The beginning is a very intense and emotional time in your therapy. At this point, it's especially crucial to be frank and open with your therapist about the emotions you're feeling. You may experience both big victories and a great deal of tumult at this stage as you stare down your trauma and come to terms with it.

The second stage: Survivor

As you face and overcome your worst fears in therapy, you start to put a terrible event in your past and gain control of your life. Your trauma still defines your life to a large degree, but now you begin to see yourself as being in control of your memories — not as a slave to them. In this stage, you may have feelings like these:

I hate the person who did this to me, but I'm not going to let him ruin my life.

I'm scared, but I'm ready to face driving again.

I'm getting better at dealing with my flashbacks, and I'm not as terrified when they happen.

In addition, you feel new stirrings of interest in your family, friends, and future. You still have bad days, but these days are less likely to make you feel hopeless or helpless.

At this point, you're growing stronger and more confident about your future. Thus, you and your therapist can broaden your work to include long-term goals, such as

✔ Recognizing and defusing toxic emotions (guilt, shame, fear, and so on)

✔ Repairing and strengthening your relationships

✔ Identifying leftover "victim" behaviors and replacing them with healthy beliefs

✔ Developing positive coping strategies for dealing with the lingering effects of your trauma

This phase of your therapy is less intense than the highly emotional work of confronting your trauma, but it's also challenging. At times, you may be tempted to say, "I'm fine now," and quit therapy, but listen to your therapist's advice. People sometimes experience what's called *false recovery*. They stop therapy before they totally process their trauma and master tools for overcoming it — and a too-hasty departure can increase the chance of a relapse.

It's okay at this stage if you decide to take a temporary break from therapy, especially if time commitments or your finances necessitate a pause. But make a definite plan to return within a few weeks or months, and keep an eye out for any symptom recurrences that may mean you need to head back into therapy sooner. Also, look honestly at your motives and make sure you're simply taking a break and not running away.

The third stage: Thriver

You'll never, *ever* forget your traumatic experience. When you make the successful transition from victim to survivor to thriver, however, you no longer live in the shadow of that event. Your trauma still influences you, but it no longer controls you, and you recognize its positive lessons as well as its lasting scars. You may have feelings like these:

It's time to for me to make new friends, have new experiences, and get back in the swing of life.

I want to volunteer as a counselor for other women who are recovering from cancer. I think I can help them because of the lessons I learned myself.

I'm happy with my life and myself.

I'm excited about what may happen tomorrow, or next week, or next year.

At this stage, you no longer need regular therapy sessions, and you'll probably be ready to leave the therapy nest altogether (more on that topic in "Graduation Day: Saying Goodbye When You Achieve Your Therapy Goals," later in this chapter). When you do say goodbye to your therapist, recognize that relapses can happen, and have a plan in hand for coping if they do (see the upcoming section titled "Spotting storm clouds before the lightning strikes"). With that security net in place, you're ready to swing into a sunnier future.

The Therapy Timeframe

Therapy is a major commitment, and it's natural to want to know how long that commitment will last. That question is hard to answer — the general rule about therapy for PTSD is that "it takes as long as it takes" — but here are some general guidelines.

Typically, cognitive behavioral therapy (see Chapter 8) takes 1 to 12 months. Other therapies are shorter. Eye-movement desensitization and reprocessing (EMDR), for example, can take as few as two or three sessions. If your therapy lasts several months, you'll probably start with once-a-week sessions, each lasting about an hour (maybe a little longer), and drop down to one or two sessions per month.

Your therapist can't set the exact number of therapy sessions you'll need to address your PTSD because you're unique, and so are your needs. Here are some of the factors that can affect the length of your therapy:

✔ **Substance abuse issues:** Do you have a problem with alcohol or drugs? (See Chapter 7 for more on this subject.) If so, your therapy will be multi-pronged, possibly involving several therapists and requiring additional sessions to make sure you're well-prepared to handle both your substance abuse problem and your PTSD.

✔ **Difficult life circumstances:** Are you undergoing a life crisis, such as a divorce or illness, that greatly affects your emotional well-being? Or are you living in an unstable or unsafe environment? If so, you and your therapist will have many extra issues to address, which translates into more sessions.

✔ **Complex PTSD:** If you have complex PTSD (see Chapter 2), which typically stems from multiple traumas or abuse as a child, your treatment will be more intense and more long-term.

✔ **Coexisting mental disorders:** Do you have a psychiatric disorder such as depression or an eating disorder in addition to your PTSD? If so, your therapist will probably want to spend extra time with you to make sure you have an opportunity to address all your issues. (See Chapter 7 for more on handling coexisting mental disorders.)

The Ups and Downs of Therapy

On Monday, you feel on top of the world. You handle crises at work with ease, and you feel loving and warm toward your partner. You successfully practice the relaxation techniques your therapist assigned for homework, and you have a nightmare-free sleep.

On Thursday, you're a mess. You have a flashback in the board meeting, disintegrate into a giant hissy fit when your partner pushes your buttons, and spend the night tossing and turning as bad memories take over your dreams. The next day in therapy, you feel angry at your therapist, and your session seems to be going nowhere.

What's going on? You probably feel like you're right back where you started before therapy — or even getting worse. You can easily get scared, angry, or depressed when this situation happens. In reality, however, therapy setbacks are usually temporary and are often stepping stones to big successes.

When these hitches in the getalong happen, reaching the next breakthrough may take extra time and effort. You may be tempted to say, "Forget this!" and give up. But don't! Minor setbacks during therapy are common, and they don't need to stall your progress if you know why they occur and what to do when they happen.

Spotting the causes of setbacks

Therapy is a little like learning to ride a bicycle. At first it's scary, and you wobble a lot (and even have a few tumbles). Then you get your balance, and you grow more confident — until you hit a rock or a puddle. Then you go back to wobbling until you regain control. Eventually, you get your skills down pat, but in the process, you experience a few shakeups.

Here are some of the biggest reasons that setbacks may occur during your therapy:

✔ **An outside event in your life sends you temporarily off track.** A fender-bender or a breakup with a lover, for example, can derail your newfound sense of being in control of your life. In this case, you may lapse into your traumatic patterns of thinking ("Something terrible is always going to happen just when my life starts to go well!"). Thanks to therapy, however, you're gaining the tools you need to regain your confidence. This process may take a few days or even a few weeks, but before long you'll start moving forward again.

✔ **An anniversary triggers symptoms.** You may experience a temporary hit when an anniversary of a traumatic event arrives. If so, you and your therapist can use your reactions to identify and process your feelings. The result: You'll be stronger and better able to cope the next time the anniversary rolls around.

✔ **You're experiencing a normal part of growth.** Sometimes therapists and patients need to create chaos to bring forth order. If you spent the past few sessions probing painful wounds and tackling long-held beliefs, your aroused feelings may take some time to settle into a new and healthy understanding.

✔ **You're letting other things interfere with working hard at your therapy.** Sometimes when life gets stressful or busy, it's easy to let your therapy homework slide or to skip sessions and slow your progress. Ask yourself honestly: Are you fully committing to your healing? Are you following through on your assignments and giving your all in the therapy room? If not, get back in the game. As coaches are fond of saying, "You gotta give some to get some."

✔ **The type of therapy you're undergoing — or your therapist — isn't working out for you.** If a setback lasts for a long time (such as a month or more), perhaps you and your therapist simply aren't meant for each other. In that case, see "Setting a New Course If a Therapist Isn't Working Out," later in this chapter. Changing to a new therapist or a new technique often leads to big breakthroughs.

Although I highly recommend a form of cognitive behavioral therapy called *exposure therapy,* in which you fully relive your trauma in a safe setting (see Chapter 8), some people find this approach too intimidating and leave therapy. If you find that facing your trauma head-on is too much to handle, see Chapters 8 and 10 for information on therapies that don't require this step. Switching to one of these therapies may get you back on track to healing.

Handling your feelings when a setback occurs

Setbacks are a normal part of therapy; the solution is not to dwell on them or magnify them into crises. Instead, think of each setback as a little like a flat tire or radiator problem on a vacation trip. It may slow you down a bit or make you take a detour or two, but it won't stop you from getting where you're going.

Here's what to do if you experience a setback:

1. **Try to identify the source.**

   See the preceding section for some examples.

2. **Don't panic; instead, talk honestly with your therapist about what's happening.**

   If you're following the normal two-steps-forward-and-one-step-back progress that therapy often takes, she can reassure you that you're doing fine. On the other hand, if you're truly stalled, she may want to change tactics and see whether another approach jump-starts your progress.

3. **Renew your commitment.**

   After a setback, take time to think through all the reasons you want to heal from PTSD. Also, review the progress you've made so far. Keeping those motivating thoughts fresh in your mind can prevent you from being stalled if things temporarily go south.

Setting a New Course If a Therapist Isn't Working Out

Successful therapy requires a special chemistry between patient and therapist, and sometimes, that chemistry just doesn't happen. Maybe your therapist's approach is wrong for you, or maybe you're just on different wavelengths. If so, you may want to consider switching to a different therapist.

Before you make that decision, however, answer these questions:

✔ **Did you give the therapist a fair chance?** Unless you're undergoing very short-term therapy, give your therapist at least three or four sessions to get to know you and your issues.

✔ **Are you using your therapist as a scapegoat?** Take an honest look at the situation, and be sure you're not using criticism of your therapist as a way to avoid persisting with the hard work of therapy.

✔ **Is the timing right for a switch?** If you change therapists in midstream, will your insurance cover a sufficient number of sessions for a new therapist to offer real help? A new therapist needs a little time to get in the groove, so switching therapists shortly before your insurance runs out probably isn't a good idea.

If you analyze your answers and decide that switching makes sense, don't feel bad about it. Often, the best and nicest of people just don't click with each other. Your recovery is far more important than the minor discomfort of telling your therapist that things aren't working out.

If you do decide to make a break, call well in advance of your next appointment (at least four or five days) to cancel and let the therapist know that you won't be returning. If the therapist asks to discuss this decision with you, use your judgment. This discussion isn't necessary, but it may be a good idea if you're on the fence.

If you do agree to one more meeting, make a written list of the concerns you have about your current therapy, and go through your list at your meeting. Whether you decide to stay or go, however, be sure that you feel good about your decision, and don't feel pressured by your therapist.

A different situation arises if you feel that your therapist was unprofessional in any way. If so, you may consider filing a complaint. To do so, contact the agency that certifies the professional. (For this reason, I highly recommend selecting a therapist who is certified; see Chapter 6.)

Whatever your reasons for dropping a therapist in midstream, don't let one bad experience turn you off. Instead, plan to get right back into treatment with a new therapist. (After all, you wouldn't quit driving for the rest of your life if your first car turned out to be a lemon, would you?) The faster you get back in the groove, the faster you'll get your healing under way again.

Graduation Day: Saying Goodbye When You Achieve Your Therapy Goals

Adieu. Adios. See ya! You know a lot of ways to say goodbye. But how do you know when the time is right to bid your therapist a fond farewell? In some cases, the answer is simple. A person with mild PTSD, for example, may feel so much better after one or two sessions that he doesn't need any additional therapy. On the other hand, a patient with bigger issues may feel the need for supportive therapy for years after trauma strikes.

How to tell when you're ready to bid adieu

Often, a therapist is the first person to say, "You're ready to tackle life on your own." Good therapists look forward to this day — but not because they want to give you the boot. The goal of therapists is to make themselves expendable, and they're pleased when their work empowers their patients.

Your therapist can tell that it's time to bid you a fond farewell, when she see the following clues:

✔ You're able to look clearly and calmly at your trauma.

✔ You can control your emotions well enough to cope in your daily life.

✔ You're able to use relaxation techniques effectively when issues arise.

✔ You're mastering the ability to reframe your experiences positively so you can handle future problems.

✔ Any problems you have with substance abuse or coexisting mental illnesses are stable and under control.

Typically, both you and your therapist will recognize when you're well enough to say goodbye to the therapy room. Your insurance coverage also plays a big role in how much therapy you receive. Your therapist will factor in your coverage to plan an approach that offers you the biggest benefits in the time you have.

A chance exists, however, that you and your therapist won't say, "All done!" at exactly the same point. If you decide that you're ready to leave therapy even though your therapist isn't bringing the topic up, analyze why you feel that way. Ask yourself the following questions:

✔ **Are you happy that you've achieved your therapy goals?** If so, now may be the time to move on with your life. But listen to your therapist's ideas on this topic, because you don't want to leave unfinished business that can come back to haunt you. If your therapist thinks you have more on your plate that needs addressing, the two of you may agree to lighten your therapy schedule — say, from once a week to twice a month.

✔ **Are you dissatisfied with your progress in therapy?** If you feel that you're getting nowhere, or you and your therapist are incompatible, you may be ready to look for a new therapist. (See "Setting a New Course If a Therapist Isn't Working Out," earlier in this chapter.)

What to expect when the day arrives

When you're ready to leave therapy, you don't need to feel like a boat set adrift. Your therapist or another professional will always be available if you have a relapse or if you just want to return for a few sessions to handle an issue or two. Also, the more you practice your new, positive thoughts and behaviors, the better you get at them, so you'll gain more confidence as each day goes by.

Realize, however, that unlike a sprained ankle or a bout of pneumonia, PTSD doesn't just go away. Therapy ends not when you're magically cured but when you master the skills you need to stay in control of symptoms when they arise. Healing is a lifelong process when you have PTSD, and you take most of that journey after you wave goodbye to your therapist.

Expect to experience both happy and sad feelings as you leave therapy. On one hand, finishing therapy is a powerful affirmation that you're in control of your PTSD symptoms and your life. On the other hand, you may develop a strong friendship with your therapist and feel sad about losing a relationship that means a great deal to you. These conflicting emotions are perfectly normal — and your therapist will experience them, too.

If you have a wonderful relationship with your therapist, it's nice to let her know how much you appreciate her. Be aware, however, that she can't let your relationship turn into an ongoing personal friendship outside the therapy room, because that behavior would be unprofessional (especially if you may return for more sessions someday). So if you say, "Let's do lunch someday," and she says, "I'm so sorry; I can't," don't take it personally. She's doing the right thing.

Also, talk with your therapist about whether attending a support group after you leave therapy is a good way to maintain your gains. (See Chapter 4 for more on this option.) If so, he can help you find a group that's right for your needs.

Bracing Yourself for Relapses While Peacefully Moving Along

When you leave therapy, you close a chapter in your life with PTSD, but you don't necessarily finish the book. A big key to dealing successfully with PTSD is realizing that after you think you've healed, PTSD can pop up again, either in bits and pieces or in a full-blown relapse.

The term *relapse* means that your symptoms are returning in full force or that you feel like you're losing control over them. If you're ready for that possibility and prepared to tackle a relapse with confidence instead of fear, you can ride out a rough patch successfully and get your life back on track in the shortest possible time.

Of course, you may never feel a twinge of trouble after therapy. But it's equally possible that at some point in the future, you'll spot symptoms creeping back into your life (or in some cases, kicking down the door). In the following sections, I look at factors that can put you at risk for a relapse, how to spot the red flags that warn you of a relapse, and how to cope if symptoms pop up again.

Judging your risk for a relapse

Life is unpredictable, and so is your risk of experiencing a relapse of PTSD symptoms after you give them the boot. But here are some guidelines. You may be more likely to experience a relapse if you have one or more of these risk factors:

✔ You're recovering from both PTSD and substance abuse. In this case, you may find yourself sliding back into one or both of these problems.

✔ You suffered from complex PTSD. People with this form of PTSD, which stems from repeated traumas (especially early in life), often encounter some extra potholes on the road to recovery.

✔ You have a coexisting mental illness.

✔ You're living in an unsafe or unsupportive environment.

✔ You suffer additional traumatic experiences following your therapy.

Conversely, you're at *lower* risk for a relapse if you have these protective factors:

✔ You ended your initial therapy only when both you and your therapist felt confident that you were stable and had a full toolbox of coping skills.

✔ Your initial therapy included some intensive work on relapse prevention skills (which is usually part of the therapy package).

✔ You have strong support from a partner or other family members. Support groups (such as Alcoholics Anonymous, if you're battling a problem with alcohol) can also lower your risk.

✔ You actively work on improving your physical health. (See Chapter 12 for tips on healthy life habits.)

✔ You continue to practice the relaxation techniques and positive-thinking strategies you acquired in therapy.

Whether you're at high or low risk for a relapse, being prepared for the possibility of relapse is smart. Think of this preparation as taking an umbrella along on a mildly overcast day; you may not need it, but you'll appreciate it if the raindrops start to fall.

Preparing yourself . . . just in case

Upsetting life changes are a major risk factor for relapses. Unfortunately, you can't go through life sidestepping all the banana peels on the sidewalk. In the real world, stuff happens: divorces, accidents, job losses, and all the rest. You can decrease your vulnerability to a relapse, however, by increasing your confidence in your ability to handle the problems that life sends your way. When you do, you're less likely to react catastrophically when a crisis occurs.

In this section, I give you some tools that can help prevent a relapse by helping you set your expectations in the right place from the start and by making you feel more confident and in control when something doesn't go according to plan.

Avoiding the expectation trap

Why do little kids' birthday parties often descend into chaos and tears? Partly, the reason is the excitement (and all that sugar!). But even more often, the birthday boy is completely convinced that everything has to go perfectly on his big day. When his ice cream cone falls on the floor or the clown shows up late, he can't handle this hitch in his plans — and the tears and tantrums start.

You may think this behavior is childish, but the truth is that adults do it, too. How often do you think, "This *has* to happen (or not happen) for me to be happy or successful"? With PTSD, this mindset is self-defeating because it can prevent you from facing and overcoming a relapse.

To stay in the right frame of mind during healing, you need to be willing to manage your expectations. Keep these principles in mind:

✔ When you *count on* something and it doesn't happen, you're devastated.

✔ When you *expect* something and it doesn't happen, you still feel a sense of failure or loss but are less distressed.

✔ When you *hope* for something while realizing that it may not occur, you can handle your disappointment with relative ease if life doesn't follow your blueprint exactly.

So what do expectations have to do with PTSD?

If you *expect* to stay relapse free (or, worse, tell yourself that you *must not* experience a relapse), you set yourself up for despair or a sense of failure if a relapse occurs. That expectation in turn can create even bigger problems.

Conversely, if you hope for the best (a hitch-free recovery) but plan for the worst (a possible relapse), you'll be ready for either scenario. As a result, you can overcome your setback in a shorter time with less emotional fallout.

Acknowledging mistakes and making plans for a brighter future

Everyone occasionally commits acts that are foolish, cruel, hugely embarrassing, or all three combined. These acts can make you cringe even years later when you think about them. If you're struggling with PTSD, however, the emotions they stir up can be powerful enough to revive old, self-destructive thoughts that can start a spiral down into PTSD-think.

You can't go through life without committing a big mistake now and then. What you *can* do, however, is react in a healthy way instead of wallowing in distress. As I tell my patients, "You can react to failure by blaming others, making excuses, feeling sorry for yourself, or crawling into a hole and avoiding the world. Or you can use your pain to say to yourself, 'I won't let this happen again,' and then create a plan to make good on this pledge."

To follow the latter (and smarter) strategy, first acknowledge that you messed up. Then use what I call the Never Again Tool, which I detail in the following list, to plan how you'll avoid making the same mistake in the future. When you do, you can quash the negative thoughts that can pull you back into PTSD and replace them with positive plans, steering you toward a happier future.

Ask yourself the following questions to analyze the lessons you learned from your mistake and to make positive plans for the future:

- If I had to handle this situation again, what would I do differently?
- *Why* would I do things differently?
- How high is my level of commitment to following my new action the next time? (1 = I won't do it; 5 = I might do it; 10 = I will do it)
- Who can I ask to hold me accountable to following through on my new action? (This person should be someone you respect and trust, because telling him about your plan can give you powerful motivation to follow through.)

Practicing responses to your biggest worries-come-true

If you ever acted in a play, you probably remember the craziness of rehearsals. At first, everyone missed his or her cues, and the rehearsal was utter chaos.

After a few run-throughs, however, everything fell into place, and on opening day, you brought down the house.

Rehearsing for life problems can serve the same purpose. When you actively practice the steps you can take to handle a crisis, you gain confidence in your ability to cope with anything. As a result, you can spend less time stressing out over what the fates have in store for you.

The Dress Rehearsal Tool I offer in this section can help you in this process. To use it, think of four or five problems that you worry about the most — such as losing your job, getting sick, or breaking up with your partner. Then ask yourself these questions to figure out what you can do to take charge and stay in control if any of these problems occur:

✔ What problem am I most worried about?

✔ How am I likely to feel if this problem occurs?

✔ What coping skills do I have to handle these feelings?

✔ What active steps can I take to deal with this problem if it occurs?

✔ Have other people I know handled a similar problem successfully? If so, what can I learn from their example?

✔ Have I survived a similar problem in the past? If so, what positive steps did I take to get through the problem?

✔ Which of my friends or relatives can support me if this problem occurs?

✔ If this problem occurs, how is it likely to change my life one year or five years down the road? How can I react positively to those changes?

✔ Can I take any steps now to reduce the chance that this problem will occur or to lower my stress about the possibility that it will occur?

As you answer these questions for each potential problem that worries you, you'll probably feel your tension drop dramatically. Why? Because you're most fearful when you passively dread the future and least fearful when you walk confidently into it. (That's why the people who make monster movies never let you see the monster right away. The images you conjure up in your mind are almost always scarier than the reality!)

Lowering your anxiety when stress is high

Similar to the Dress Rehearsal Tool (see the preceding section) is the Six-Step Pause Tool. You can use this tool anytime you're upset or under stress. Following these steps can stop you from shooting from the hip when you're under stress (and usually shooting yourself in the foot). These steps help you pause until you're calmer and can think logically, shoot from your head, and make the best choices. The result: wiser decisions, less chance that a new upset or trauma will occur, and lower risk of a relapse.

Here are six steps to follow when a life problem crops up:

1. **Practice *physical awareness.***

   Where do you feel the tension? Pinpoint it (a knot in your stomach, tight shoulders, and so on) and give the sensation a name.

2. **Practice *emotional awareness.***

   Attach an emotion to the physical sensation (for example, "I'm very angry" or, "I feel afraid").

3. **Practice *impulse awareness.***

   Complete this sentence: "This feeling makes me want to . . ." Fill in the blank with your immediate emotional reaction (for example, ". . . tell my boss that he's a jerk and that I quit").

4. **Practice *consequence awareness.***

   Answer this question: "If I respond this way, what's likely to happen?" Think through all the possible consequences.

5. **Practice *solution awareness.***

   Complete this sentence: "A better thing to do would be . . ."

6. **Practice *benefit awareness.***

   Finish this sentence: "If I try that strategy, the benefits will be . . ." List as many benefits as possible.

This tool is a highly effective way to talk yourself out of acting impulsively and doing something you'll regret.

As a bonus, you can teach this technique to your children to help them gain better control of their emotions and impulses. Fewer upsets on the kid front translate into fewer upsets in your own life — another way to avoid a relapse.

Spotting storm clouds before the lightning strikes

Even if you do everything possible to keep your recovery on track, a relapse can occur. If so, you can get the upper hand by spotting the signs of trouble and taking quick action. Here's how to spot the warning signs of a relapse:

✔ Your symptoms start to occur more often.

✔ The intensity of your symptoms increases.

✔ The techniques you've used successfully to control your symptoms aren't working anymore.

✔ If you have substance abuse problems, you begin to lose control of your drug or alcohol use.

✔ You experience a return of depressive or suicidal thoughts.

✔ You begin engaging in self-destructive behaviors, such as excessive gambling or unsafe sex.

If you spot a relapse red flag, make your move quickly! Here's how to nip a relapse in the bud:

✔ **Pick up the phone.** Call your doctor or therapist for an immediate appointment — time is of the essence. Getting back into treatment quickly is the best way to stop a relapse in its tracks.

✔ **Consider medication.** Talk to your doctor about trying a drug treatment (see Chapter 9 for more on this subject) if therapy alone doesn't get a relapse under control.

✔ **Redouble your self-help efforts.** Eat well, exercise, practice your relaxation techniques, and take steps to foster healthy sleep. (For help with all these steps, see Chapter 12.)

✔ **Call in your backup team.** Tell trusted friends and relatives that you're experiencing a relapse and let them lend you moral support and a helping hand.

✔ **Avoid catastrophic thinking.** Relapses happen, and they're not the end of the world. Don't think of a relapse as a brick wall that stops you cold; instead, think of it as a patch of rugged terrain you need to cross to get back on your road to healing.

Chapter 12

Helping Yourself Heal Your Body, Mind, and Soul

*F*or a long time, you've probably felt like a tree in a terrible thunderstorm: battered on every side, bowed low by strong gales, and attacked by forces that threatened to bring you down. Now, just like that same tree when the storm ends and the skies clear, you're once again beginning to grow, blossom, and open yourself up to the joys of the world around you.

As therapy empowers you to put the past behind you and look to a better future, you're getting stronger each day — and as you gain more and more control over your life, you can take a bigger role in healing your body, mind, and spirit. That role becomes even more important as you reach the end of your therapy and start the next stage of your journey into wellness.

In this chapter, I talk about the many steps you can take to enhance your healing both during and after therapy. Among the topics I explore are improving your physical health, rediscovering intimacy and sexuality, and regaining your appreciation for the simple joys of daily life.

Regaining Your Physical Health and Strength

PTSD takes your body on a rough ride. One reason is that PTSD directly affects many systems, from your heart to your immune system (see Chapter 3 for more on this). Another reason is that when you're wracked by anxiety and can't picture a happy future, putting good nutrition, exercise, and other health-enhancing practices on the back burner is easy. Drugs or alcohol can take their toll on your physical well-being as well, and nightmares and insomnia can steal the shut-eye you need to stay healthy.

As you begin taking more control of your life, you can start to undo the damage PTSD did to your body — and getting back in shape can, in turn, make it far easier for you to keep the PTSD blues at bay. In fact, each step you take to improve your physical health can make your mind and spirit stronger as well. In the following sections, I look at how you can take charge of three of the most vital areas of your health: diet, exercise, and sleep.

Eating healthy to keep your brain and body happy

PTSD can throw a wrench into your dietary habits for several reasons. Here are some of the biggest ones:

- ✔ When you feel awful, finding the energy or enthusiasm to cook for yourself is hard. As a result, you're likely to turn to nutrient-poor fast food or TV dinners.

- ✔ Food is a powerful comforter. You may find yourself putting on weight because you're turning to ice cream, mashed potatoes, and chips as a way of numbing your emotions.

- ✔ Your body may crave carbs when you're in the grip of PTSD because high-carb foods can raise levels of the brain chemical serotonin — and higher serotonin levels can make you feel happier and less stressed. In short, you may unconsciously use high-carb foods to self-medicate your painful emotions.

- ✔ Drugs and alcohol can complicate the picture, creating nutritional deficiencies that can severely affect your thinking.

In the following sections, I explain why establishing healthier diet habits can aid in healing your brain and body — and why it's not as hard as it sounds.

Making the food-mind connection

The expression *food for thought* takes on new meaning when you think about the connection between food and your brain. Here are some examples of the food-mind connection:

- ✔ Your body needs high-quality raw materials from food to build the chemicals that transmit messages via your brain cells and to keep the cells themselves healthy. A chronic shortage of these dietary building blocks can put a serious whammy on brain chemistry and function. The result: fatigue, depression, or even aggressive feelings. Shortages of any vitamin, mineral, or other nutrient can affect your thoughts and actions dramatically.

- ✔ In the form of glucose, food provides the energy your brain cells need to work. Too low on this fuel? If so, you may feel tired, depressed, hostile, or spacey.

Getting your diet in shape

The first step to take when you decide to address dietary glitches is a simple but powerful one: Offload any guilt you feel about your eating habits. If you gained weight during your low times or ate in ways that harmed your health, blame PTSD — not yourself.

The next step is to realize that you don't need to overhaul your diet drastically (although you can if you want to). With nutrition, even small positive steps can give you a big boost as you begin your recovery from PTSD. Here are some simple ways you can improve your eating habits to get your body and mind into shape:

- ✔ **Set the table.** If possible, set regular mealtimes and stick closely to them. If you've been eating over the kitchen sink or at the fridge, try setting the table (and maybe even lighting a candle). Eating regular meals — and taking the time to savor them — can reduce your stress and set the stage for better eating habits. Regular eating habits also help you sleep better.

- ✔ **Put the basics in place.** Is your current diet light years from perfect? If so, try making one positive change at a time. Adding an extra fruit or veggie each day, or switching from white to whole-grain bread at breakfast, can supply crucial nutrients. You don't need to become Captain Health overnight; just keep moving in the right direction, and each week, try to eat a little healthier than you did the week before.

✔ **Get the facts about your personal nutrition needs.** Talk to your doctor, dietitian, or other healthcare expert about tailoring your diet to address specific problems that may be linked to your PTSD. If you're overcoming a long-term problem with alcohol, for example, you may have deficiencies of B vitamins and other nutrients, and you may need extra supplements. If you're taking an antidepressant that's causing you to put on pounds, talk to your doctor about this common side effect and see whether you can switch to a different medication.

✔ **Take a good multivitamin-multimineral supplement, and add some fatty acids.** If you chow down on doughnuts for breakfast and takeout food for dinner, taking a basic supplement is good insurance (and not a bad idea even if you eat well). Many doctors recommend supplementing your diet with fish oil, which provides essential omega-3 fatty acids that tend to be scarce in today's diet. Omega-3 fatty acids appear to play a powerful role in brain health and can help your heart as well.

One thing I *don't* really recommend, especially when you're in the middle of therapy, is starting a fad diet. Typically, fad diets cause you to lose a lot of weight in the first few weeks but quickly prove unworkable, and you usually gain back more weight than you lost. Going off the diet (as just about everyone does) can steer you right back into the "I'm a failure"/"I'm weak" frame of mind that's a big trap for people with PTSD.

Instead, if you have a weight problem, simply make gradual changes toward a healthier diet and increase your exercise (see the next section). Slow-and-steady weight loss is a far healthier approach than crash dieting, and it's a low-stress approach that won't trigger the negative thoughts you're trying to chase out of your life.

Exercising to soothe your nerves and relieve tension

Just as PTSD can freeze your emotions, it can freeze you physically. You may find yourself tensing up for no apparent reason or clenching your jaw or grinding your teeth — and you may not even realize what you're doing until you're in serious pain at the end of the day. Backaches, headaches, and other problems related to muscle tension can also make you miserable.

Melting away the tension in your body can ease these problems and make you feel better physically. Thanks to the powerful mind-body connection, relaxing your body clears your mind and reins in negative emotions, too. In this section, I look at the best tools for accomplishing this mission.

Reaping the benefits of moving your body

A good workout relaxes tense muscles and generates feel-good chemicals called *endorphins,* which calm and soothe you. But these are just two of the benefits for someone who's healing from PTSD.

In your case, exercise also offers these bonuses:

- ✔ When you're stressed and that extra adrenaline is flooding your system, exercise is an outstanding way to turn that fight-or-flight response to your advantage by burning off your chemical overload in a health-enhancing workout.

- ✔ Exercise can be a wonderful distracter. When your mind is working overtime to turn molehills into mountains, a 20-minute workout can sweep exaggerated worries away and help you put your life back in perspective.

- ✔ Exercise helps you feel in control of your life and your body — a big plus when you're recovering from the feelings of helplessness that PTSD can generate.

Equally important, exercise offers you these big health benefits:

- ✔ It helps counter the elevated risk of heart disease and high blood pressure that's associated with PTSD.

- ✔ It aids you in getting a handle on a weight problem if your PTSD contributed to a problem with overeating.

- ✔ It's good for your brain function and memory.

- ✔ It promotes sound sleep.

- ✔ It can significantly reduce symptoms of depression and anxiety.

Selecting the right activities for you

You're much more likely to stick with an exercise program if it's fun, so pick an activity you enjoy. Don't think that exercise needs to be strenuous; a daily walk or bike ride can ease your stress just as effectively as an hour of lifting weights.

Exercise is one of the world's best do-it-yourself approaches for chasing away the blues and worries, and it works for any lifestyle. Don't feel like seeing other people? Then pop a disc into the DVD player and exercise by yourself. (You can even find free discs or tapes at your library.) Trying to reach out to new friends? Joining a gym offers a low-stress way to meet new people. Have health problems that rule out vigorous exercise? Your doctor may approve a walking program or steer you to a chair exercise program that can improve your flexibility, strength, and overall fitness. (Chair exercise is a type of work-out that allows you to exercise all your muscle groups while sitting down.)

Try aiming for 20 to 30 minutes of exercise at least three times a week, and schedule a regular routine so you're more likely to stick with this healthy habit. (See "Following Through on Your Wellness Plans," later in this chapter, for more tips on sticking with an exercise plan.)

A few cautions before you start an exercise program:

- ✔ If exercise could trigger hyperventilation and panic attacks, talk to your therapist about breathing exercises and other techniques for preventing or managing these attacks.

- ✔ Get your doctor's okay before undertaking any strenuous exercise program, especially if you have significant health problems.

- ✔ Avoid the urge to bite off more than you can chew. If you're a health nut, go ahead and train for a marathon. But if you're in average or iffy shape, setting unrealistic goals can lead to frustration and trigger negative feelings of failure. Pick an activity that relaxes and de-stresses you, not one that's overly challenging.

Exercise: Strong medicine for clinical depression

Doctors always knew exercise was good for you, but now they know that its benefits go far beyond six-pack abs and a strong heart. Recent studies show that in terms of mental health, spin cycling or kickboxing may even beat out drug therapies.

In one study at Duke University, researchers divided patients with major depression (a problem that often tags along with PTSD) into two groups. They treated one group with exercise and the other with Zoloft (sertraline), an antidepressant drug. Both groups did equally well, but the people in the exercise group had better luck keeping their symptoms from returning after their initial depression lifted.

Recently, a different group of researchers at Wake Forest University Baptist Medical Center in North Carolina did a similar study with depressed

seniors. Again, they found that both exercise and Zoloft treated depression effectively. What's more, the seniors who exercised showed gains in physical functioning, so they got an added boost that the drug group didn't enjoy.

Exercise doesn't always affect depression, and some people experience bigger benefits than others. If you're depressed, the gains you experience with exercise may depend on how longstanding your depression is and on whether it's mild, moderate, or severe. (Short-term mild or moderate depression may respond better than long-term or severe depression.) But just about everyone enjoys physical benefits from exercise, so adopting some form of exercise routine has almost no downside.

Freeing your mind

In Chapter 4, I offer a few of the most basic techniques for relaxing. If you're in therapy, you've probably mastered additional relaxation techniques. Make these strategies part of your life outside the therapy room, too — whether you're stuck in traffic, upset by an argument with a friend, or just feeling overwhelmed by the pressures of life.

Giving painful thoughts the boot

If flashbacks and intrusive thoughts continue to intrude in your life, try these imagery techniques:

- ✔ **Toss out the trash.** Picture your unpleasant thoughts, images, and emotions as untidy junk piling up in your house. Now clearly picture yourself picking up each unwanted piece of trash — a frightening flashback, a negative emotion, and so on — and tossing it into a big trash bag. When you're done, look around the house. Is all the trash gone? If so, visualize yourself sealing the trash bag, putting it in the trash can, and taking the trash can to the curb. Picture the trash truck coming and carting off all that trash. Watch the truck as it disappears from your life.

  Alternatively, visualize putting your negative thoughts and feelings in a box marked "To handle at therapy" and setting the box out in the garage.

- ✔ **Mop up the memory.** Picture your intrusive thought, image, or emotion as a spill on your kitchen countertop. Now visualize yourself getting a paper towel and mopping up the spot. Picture the spill getting smaller and smaller until it disappears; then imagine throwing the towel away.

- ✔ **Shred a sad picture.** Write a description or draw a picture of your flashback. Then run the paper through a shredder (or toss it in the fireplace).

- ✔ **Watch your thought fly away.** Imagine your troubling thought sitting next to you; then imagine it sprouting wings and taking flight. Picture the thought moving farther and farther away, getting smaller and smaller, until it's just a speck — and then it vanishes. (Or picture it shooting into the sky like a rocket, getting smaller and smaller, until it reaches the sun and goes "poof.")

These imagery techniques are very potent because they help you remember that you're in control of your bad memories. One caution, however: Some people, particularly those prone to very vivid flashbacks, can find relaxation techniques that use imagery counterproductive. If imagery techniques trigger flashbacks or emotions instead of calming you, switch to techniques that don't use imagery.

Meditating to keep yourself centered and grounded

When you have PTSD and get stressed out, your first urge may be to shoot from the hip, venting your anger on anyone in your path — an act that creates *more* stress, not less. Suppressing your feelings, on the other hand, leads to burnout, depleted energy, and health problems. (They aren't called *tension headaches* for nothing.)

Instead, try this approach: meditate. Meditation is one of the most powerful ways to trigger what physician Herbert Benson, a famous pioneer in the field of mind/body medicine, identified as the *relaxation response* — a response that's opposite to the fight-or-flight response that can send your anxiety skyrocketing. In the relaxation response, your heart rate, metabolism, rate of breathing, and brain waves all slow down. These changes translate into dramatic reductions in stress and anxiety, and increased power to handle life problems calmly and efficiently.

Here's one meditation technique that can help you achieve the relaxation response; it's a tool called *mindfulness meditation,* which many people with PTSD find extremely useful (for more on this technique, see the sidebar on "Turning off the alarm with mindfulness meditation or 'talk therapy'"). When your world starts to spin out of control and you sense your fear or anxiety or anger coming to a boil, stop what you're doing and sit down, and follow these steps:

1. **Close your eyes and breathe in and out slowly through your nose.**

   Many people find repetitive activities such as humming or saying a particular word to be helpful as well.

2. **Quietly take note of the world around you (perhaps note the sound of the wind outside or the feeling of your body as it relaxes).**

3. **Let your thoughts and emotions arise naturally without judging them in any way.**

4. **Identify and acknowledge your thoughts or feelings as they arise, and then gently let the thoughts go, bringing your attention back to your breathing.**

   For example, if you're frightened, simply identify and acknowledge the feeling — "I'm afraid" — and then, just as gently, let the thought go. Relax and be in the moment, peacefully and nonjudgmentally. As you achieve this state, you eventually experience something remarkable: the quiet. (As I tell my patients, it's located between the noise in your head and the noise in your life, and right now it's screaming out to be heard.)

A bigwig breathes a sigh of relief

I once asked a high-powered CEO who was overwhelmed by the pressures in his life to do the simple quieting exercise I discuss in the section "Meditating to keep yourself centered and grounded." He stopped his rant about job pressures and relationship problems; he simply sat with his eyes closed, breathing slowly. After a few minutes, I saw tears in his eyes. He cried for five minutes and then slowly opened his eyes with a smile on his face.

"What was that about?" I asked. He replied that the sense of peace he'd felt was what he'd been seeking his whole life — something he'd felt slipping further and further away as he frantically pursued the brass rings of fortune and success.

When he simply exhaled, lowered his defenses, and opened his mind to the quiet — and to just letting his emotions be present without entertaining them with an internal debate — he found that elusive peace for the first time.

Just like this CEO, everyone needs to step out of the rat race when the pressure gets too great — even if it's just for a ten-minute break. Exhaling is an excellent way to cast off your stress and find the inner peace that's so hard to capture when life is filled with stress. Think of your exhaling strategy as the little valve on the pressure cooker of your life with PTSD: It allows dangerous steam to escape in a safe way so you won't blow sky-high.

Another good relaxation technique that doesn't use imagery is *grounding,* which places you in the here and now. Here's how to do it:

1. **Sit on the sofa or in a comfortable chair.**

2. **Place your hands on the arms of the chair or on your clothing.**

   Feel the fabric, noticing its texture and color.

3. **Notice the position of your body.**

   Rub your neck, stretch your fingers, stomp your feet, and tense and relax your muscles.

4. **Notice the sights, sounds, and aromas around you.**

5. **Slowly name 20 things you can see from where you are.**

   You may see a window, a door, a cat, and your shoelace, for example.

6. **As you continue looking around, tell yourself, "The flashback/emotion I felt is a part of the past; this is now, and I'm safe."**

Turning off the alarm with mindfulness meditation or "talk therapy"

New data from a 2007 study by two research groups helps explain why two different types of interventions for PTSD — practicing a form of meditation called *mindfulness meditation* and talking about your trauma-related emotions with a therapist — can make you feel much better.

Matthew Lieberman and his colleagues at UCLA conducted the first part of the study, which investigated the effects of verbally identifying emotions. In this part of the study, they asked 30 people to undergo brain imaging while viewing images of people showing different facial expressions. Below each picture were two words, and the researchers asked the volunteers to pick the word that best described the expression in the picture. In some cases, the words described emotions such as "angry" and "fearful." In other cases, the words were male or female names; for instance, the words under one woman's picture said "Sally" and "Harry."

Looking at angry or fearful faces activated the amygdala, a brain region that sends an alarm when a person perceives a threat. This response stayed strong when the task involved picking the correct male or female name for a photo, but it dropped significantly when people labeled the photo with an emotion. That task caused a different part of the brain — the right ventrolateral prefrontal cortex — to spring into action. This part of the brain may inhibit emotional responses, allowing a person to think calmly about a situation.

Lieberman says that when you put feelings into words — as you do in a therapy session —

"you're activating this prefrontal region and seeing a reduced response in the amygdala. In the same way you hit the brake when you're driving when you see a yellow light, when you put feelings into words, you seem to be hitting the brakes on your emotional responses."

In part two of the study, David Creswell and his colleagues (several of them also involved in the first study) asked the same volunteers to fill out questionnaires measuring their mindfulness — the ability to identify and pay attention to thoughts, emotions, and body sensations without judging or reacting to them. (This ability is a key aspect of mindfulness meditation.) Creswell and his colleagues compared the data on their questionnaires to the brain-imaging data that Lieberman collected in part one of the study.

The researchers found that the more mindful participants were, the more activation they showed in the right ventrolateral prefrontal cortex and the less activation they showed in the amygdala. Creswell says, "This suggests people who are more mindful bring all sorts of prefrontal resources to turn down the amygdala. These findings may help explain the beneficial health effects of mindfulness meditation, and suggest, for the first time, an underlying reason why mindfulness meditation programs improve mood and health."

If you're overcoming PTSD, these findings are important because they indicate that combining treatments like cognitive behavioral therapy (see Chapter 8) and mindfulness meditation can add extra horsepower to your healing efforts.

Fostering sleep to refresh your mind

If you've lived with PTSD a long time, you've likely suffered more than your share of wide-awake nights or sleep-destroying nightmares. Now that you're getting your life back on track, get back into the groove of restful sleep.

Therapy for PTSD often leads to better slumber, and you can increase your odds of getting a good night's sleep by trying the suggestions in Chapter 4. If you still have problems, talk to your doctor or therapist. Your doctor may recommend prescription sleep aids (see Chapter 9 for info on the advantages and disadvantages), and your therapist may have some specific sleep-enhancing tricks up her sleeve.

Many patients report good results with two nightmare-reducing techniques:

- ✔ **Image rehearsal therapy:** In this therapy, you write down your nightmares, change their endings, and rehearse these new endings before bedtime. (For details, see Chapter 4.)

- ✔ **Lucid dreaming treatment (LDT):** This technique teaches you to gain a degree of control over your dreams while they're happening. The treatment involves a range of techniques (for instance, dream recall, dream rehearsal, self-suggestion, and changes in sleeping schedules) that help you achieve *lucidity* — that is, the knowledge that you're dreaming — so that nightmares have less power over you.

You can practice steps on your own to take control of your dreams. Here are some ways to defang nightmares:

- ✔ **Tell someone else about them.** For some reason, sharing your dreams with a trusted person in the daytime takes much of the sting out of them.

- ✔ **Walk through your dream mentally in the daytime, and as you reach a scary or upsetting part, put your hands out in a *stop* position and say, "This is just a dream."** Doing this each night before bedtime may empower you to take the same action when you're asleep and thus stop a bad dream in its tracks.

- ✔ **Write about your nightmare as though it's a fiction story you're creating — and then change how the story turns out.** Try three or four different plot twists, all with positive endings. This is much the same as what a therapist asks a patient to do in image rehearsal therapy (which I discuss in the preceding bulleted list), and you may find that you don't need your therapist's guidance to have success with this method.

✔ **Sit down in a calm moment and ponder your dream.** How would you change the events of the dream if you could? What message would you give yourself if you could be another character in the dream? By analyzing the dream rationally and calmly, you can often rewrite its contents in the future.

Also, remember the body-mind connection and prepare your body during the day for the sleep it needs at night:

✔ Eat regular meals; a predictable meal routine helps establish a predictable sleep pattern.

✔ Exercise early in the evening at least three hours before you go to bed so you can burn off stress but still have enough time to wind down.

✔ Take a soothing bath or shower before going to bed.

In addition, have your doctor rule out any physical causes for your sleep problems, such as sleep apnea. (See Chapter 10 for more on the link between this medical problem and PTSD.) Also talk to your doctor if pain from an injury stemming from your trauma interferes with peaceful sleep.

Simplifying and Organizing Your Life

Do you ever get the urge to yell "Stop!" as your chores and obligations pile up? The all-too-common scenario always seems to happen at the worst times (or all the time). Your boss asks, "Can you work overtime?" Your kids say, "We're late for soccer!" Your church wants your help with a fundraiser. The dentist's staff calls to say you're overdue for a cleaning. The dog wants a walk. The bills are overdue. The lawn needs mowing. The floor needs mopping. And somebody *really* needs to get to the grocery store before that last roll of toilet paper runs out.

When you're healing, avoid big stressors that can make you feel out of control and trigger anxiety or flashbacks. But in the real world, avoiding stress is often nearly impossible — and even harder if PTSD-linked memory problems make it hard for you to stay on top of all your responsibilities.

Here's encouraging news: If you can't get rid of stress, you can at least tame it. Start by taking these simple but powerful steps:

✔ **Figure out how to say no.** Decide what tasks are necessary and which aren't and stop agreeing to every request. Getting a sick child to a doctor's appointment is necessary, for example, but baking cookies for the same child's school fundraiser isn't. The world keeps revolving if you occasionally say, "I'm so sorry. Can I help another time?"

✔ **Call for backup.** Take a look at your list of obligations and see whether you can call for reinforcements to help you with them. Is one of your kids old enough to take over some of the yard work? Can a co-worker take over some of your overtime work? (See Chapter 13 for advice on asking for and accepting help when you're healing from PTSD.)

✔ **Relax your standards.** Do you think more highly of a friend just because she waxes her garage floor or trims her lawn with manicure scissors? Neither do I. Often, people get stressed out because they hold themselves to impossibly high standards for tasks that aren't really all that important. If you feel rushed and overwhelmed, ask yourself whether you can cut corners on yard work, housework, or routine tasks at the office without creating any problems.

✔ **Think about your long-term goals.** As you decide which responsibilities to keep on your list and which to throw overboard, ask yourself where you want to be in one year, five years, or ten years. Then ask yourself whether a specific responsibility (such as agreeing to work overtime at a job you dislike) will further those goals. Free yourself from dead-end obligations and focus on the ones that will stand you in good stead over the long run.

In addition to simplifying your life, implement some strategies to get organized. If you're running in all directions, trying to remember dozens of tasks and coping with PTSD-related memory lapses, you can easily forget important chores — which in turn can cause the stress monster to rear its ugly head. ("Oh, my gosh — I forgot to pay the credit card bill!") To keep an ever-growing pile of chores under control without losing your cool, try these tricks:

✔ **Go high-tech.** Use your computer or cellphone to set up reminders for daily, weekly, monthly, and yearly chores.

✔ **Go low-tech.** Do you have scribbled notes taped all over the house? Hang up a bulletin board, chalkboard, or whiteboard in a handy central location (the kitchen is good) and post all your reminders there. If everything's in a central location, important appointments and chores are less likely to slip through the cracks. Day planners and organizational tools can help as well — and if you're still stressed because things fall between the cracks, check out *Organizing For Dummies* (Wiley) by Eileen Roth and Elizabeth Miles.

If your PTSD-related memory problems make it just about impossible for you to stay organized and on top of your responsibilities, talk to your doctor. Certain medications, such as the antidepressant Paxil (paroxetine), appear to reduce memory impairment in many people with PTSD.

Rediscovering Physical Intimacy and Sexuality

Intimacy and sexuality are among the deepest forms of sharing people can experience, and physical closeness with a trusted partner is a source of great pleasure and emotional bonding. But achieving physical and emotional intimacy can be a struggle if you're healing from PTSD, especially if your previous relationships didn't survive the strain of your trauma and its aftermath. Sexuality can be an even bigger problem if your trauma involved rape or sexual abuse, leaving you frightened or disgusted by the idea of physical intimacy.

If you're in either of these situations, the road to sexual healing may be long — but with time and patience, you can enjoy the closeness and joy of a physical relationship with someone you love.

Identifying your fears about intimacy

The first step in the recovery process is talking openly with your therapist about your issues with intimacy and sexuality. He can help you understand that these problems are common in PTSD, as well as help you (and your partner, if you're currently in a relationship) reestablish positive, healthy feelings about your sexuality. Among the fears your therapist can help you address are

- ✔ **Fear of losing control:** If your trauma occurred at the hands of another person, it caused you to feel powerless. As a result, accepting the loss of control that's a natural part of a sexual relationship is very hard for you.

- ✔ **Fear of betrayal:** Being sexually assaulted by a date or abused by a parent can leave you feeling that no sexual partner can be trusted.

- ✔ **Fear of flashbacks:** The intense emotions awakened by intimacy and sexuality can trigger strong emotions or even flashbacks, and you may avoid physical contact to protect yourself against this possibility.

- ✔ **Fear of being touched:** If your trauma involved rape or sexual abuse, the touch of another person can physically repulse you.

- ✔ **Fear of being unguarded:** You may keep your guard up because you fear that letting it down may open the floodgates of pain — both from your trauma and from a lifetime of holding in your feelings. (This may explain why people often start to cry when someone is suddenly kind to them for no reason. It catches them off guard — or rather, without their guard up — and the relief they experience often feels painful.) But in reality, this pain is a good kind that comes from healing, not the pain that comes from being hurt.

Realizing how a therapist may help

Your therapist can help you understand that your fears aren't weird or crazy. Instead, they're your mind's perfectly normal protective response to the trauma you experienced. Now that the trauma is over, these feelings no longer serve a purpose — and with time and patience, you can put them in the past.

Your therapist can help you address feelings of shame or disgust about your sexual identity by

- **Helping you replace negative thoughts about sex with positive affirmations:** For instance, your therapist may help you spot the distorted thought "sex is painful and disgusting" that results from a sexual assault so you can replace it with accurate thoughts such as "The person who attacked me caused me pain and did things that disgusted me. That was a physical attack, not a loving sexual experience. That incident is in the past now. My current partner is very kind and gentle and can help me experience sex in a way that won't be painful. I know that I found sex enjoyable before I was attacked, and with time, I'll be able to enjoy it again."

- **Helping you visualize your body as being worthy of respect:** People who experience rape or childhood sexual abuse may view their bodies as dirty or disgusting or develop a condition called *body dysmorphic disorder,* in which they see themselves as physically unattractive or grotesque. If you have issues like these, your therapist can help you see that these beliefs stem from the trauma you experienced and don't reflect reality. With this guidance, you can view your body as strong, attractive, healthy, and worthy of your respect and the respect of others.

- **Aiding you in developing relaxing and calming tools that can help prevent flashbacks during intimacy:** Techniques involving slow breathing, imagery, and massage can be especially helpful.

- **Empowering you to say either yes or no to a decision about having a sexual relationship — and to be in control of either decision:** This control is especially important if you suffered childhood sexual abuse — a trauma that can create distorted ideas about who controls your body. Childhood abuse may also cause you to use sex as a weapon or a means of manipulation, habits that lead to serious relational problems. Your therapist can help you to identify the roots of these behaviors and to create healthy boundaries that allow you to have safe and satisfying sexual relationships.

In addition, if you're a man, your doctor or therapist can help you address fears of leaving your partner unsatisfied. If you have these fears, you're not alone; erectile dysfunction and premature ejaculation are relatively common in men with PTSD. PTSD itself appears to cause sexual problems for many men, and antidepressant use and alcohol abuse are also major contributors. Fortunately, your doctor can offer medications that may correct problems with sexual performance, and a therapist can help you work on the mental blocks that can lead to physical problems in bed.

Becoming comfortable with your sexuality

One key to preparing for intimacy is making peace with your body. Make a point of engaging in activities that can help you get in touch with your sexuality and reduce feelings of numbness or disgust.

Some excellent healing activities include the following:

- **Massages:** Start slowly, and tell your massage therapist ahead of time to stop if you encounter any issues. Gradually increase the amount of massage you're able to handle.

- **Physical activities that make you feel physical pleasure:** In addition to exercise (which I discuss earlier in this chapter), pleasurable activities may include ballet and other forms of dance, swimming, or spa days.

- **Self-affirmations:** Picture a person you love deeply — a partner, a friend, or a parent. Now picture yourself walking up to that person and saying something like this: "Wow, you have big hips. It's just disgusting to look at you. And your legs are too short. Ick! How can you even go out of the house looking like that?" Wouldn't you feel terrible if you said hurtful things like these? Yet you may give yourself hurtful messages about your body all the time.

  Now's the time to spot those messages ("I'm fat as a pig," "I'm ugly and scrawny") and replace them with healing and self-affirming messages ("I love having my grandmother's hair color," "My body is beautiful," or "This scar is a sign that I'm brave and I came through my ordeal").

Above all, be patient as you discover how to reexperience the joys of intimacy and sexuality. Because we're all very hung up on our bodies and sexuality, healing in this area of life often takes longer than healing in other areas. It's important to go with the flow instead of stressing out and trying to take steps before you're ready. In this race, the tortoise almost always wins out over the hare — no matter what you've heard about rabbits and sex!

Working with your partner to expand your boundaries

Your mind and your body may not reach the point of readiness for intimacy at the same time. As a therapist who treats individuals who suffered molestation or rape, I'm convinced that the body has a memory that's separate from the mind's. Your skin remembers both good touch and bad touch, and these memories can be strong even after your mind comes to terms with a trauma. Thus, your mind and heart may say yes when your body continues to say no — and your body may trap you into thinking that the desperate loneliness of no touch is better than the horror of bad touch. Getting past this point is important. Otherwise, you may spend your life missing out on the good touch that's so crucial to your healing.

To help your body rediscover the joy of good touch, try some simple but powerful healing approaches:

- ✔ If you're not ready to touch yet, consider this boundaries exercise: Stand facing your partner and walk toward her. Keep walking, one step at a time, until you begin to feel uncomfortable. Stop at that point and note how you feel. Is your pulse faster? Do you feel a little queasy? Each day, try this exercise again to see whether you can get a little closer without feeling scared or trapped. Before the exercise, be sure your partner knows the importance of remaining still and not moving toward you.

- ✔ If you have a loving and caring partner, practice simple, nonsexual touching. (Think of it as foreplay without the afterplay.) To do this, find a quiet, peaceful time and simply touch or massage each other gently on a spot that's not strongly linked to your sexuality. Do *not* progress to sexual intercourse. Instead, merely enjoy the pleasure of simple touching and the joy of being in each other's company.

- ✔ Close your eyes and have your partner lead you around your house. By putting yourself in your partner's hands in a nonthreatening and non-sexual situation, you can learn to let go of your fears of intimacy.

When you reach a point where you're ready for sexual intercourse with a trusted partner, talk openly with your partner about the flashbacks you may experience and how to deal with them. It's important for both of you to realize that overcoming the aftereffects of your trauma may take time and that you may experience feelings of disgust that have nothing to do with your partner's attractiveness. Both of you should be prepared for the possibility — indeed, the probability — that your first few times together may be less than stellar successes. With luck, sensitivity, and a dash of humor, you can overcome your fears and negative emotions — but be prepared for this process to take months or even years.

If you don't currently have a partner and your issues with sexuality are holding you back from seeking a committed relationship, work with your therapist to address these issues.

Enjoying Life's Pleasures

When you have PTSD, you can easily view the world as a menacing place full of constant threats, broken promises, and frightening shadows. As you recover, it's crucial to reopen your eyes to the joys and wonders of the world instead of focusing solely on its terrors. Here are some important and possibly life-changing healing steps to put on your to-do list.

Stop and smell the roses

The famous philosopher Søren Kierkegaard said, "Most men pursue pleasure with such breathless haste that they hurry past it." That's even truer in the modern era, when people spend so much time rushing from Point A to Point B that they rarely have a chance to enjoy where they are right now. All that hurtling around can hurt you if it keeps you focused solely on your stressors — work deadlines, undone laundry, lawns to mow — and turns your eyes away from the life-affirming pleasures that surround you (including the smell of those roses).

If you're chronically stuck in overdrive, make a resolution to shift gears. Take full advantage of the healing power of the world around you and work actively at slowing down in a speed-of-light world.

Here are some good, unhurried activities to try:

- **Take a walk every day.** Instead of dashing around the block, take the time to look around. Spot the big wonders — the trees changing color, the snow on the mountains — and the little wonders, such as a spider web or a flock of birds. To help yourself appreciate your surroundings, try picking out five beautiful (or funny, or unusual) things on each walk.

- **Bury your nose in a book.** Read a novel you've always wanted to read. Don't read it in haste, snatching a few seconds in the bathroom or at bedtime to read a page or two. Instead, make a cup of tea, settle into a big chair, and just read for an hour or two. (Do you have trouble concentrating on a book because of your anxiety? Then try this trick: Set a timer next to your reading chair and tell yourself, "I can get back to those anxieties in 30 minutes — but right now, I'm reading." Often, this trick can give you temporary control over your stress.)

✔ **Put your chef's hat on.** If you're the family cook, join the "slow food" craze. Once a week, forgo rushed meals and spend an hour or two preparing something new and fun. Even if the meal's just for you, enjoy treating yourself to a nice meal and all the preparation that goes into it. If you have leftovers, bring them to work the next day, wrap them for another single friend, or just save them for a few days' lunches.

✔ **Make yourself slow down.** Set aside a few hours each week for mandatory relaxation — time when you don't *allow* yourself to work. These enforced mini-vacations can discharge your stress and recharge your batteries so you can head back into the fray stronger and more confident. If possible, find a calming spot — a lake, a park, or a bubble bath with soothing music — where you can tune out the world.

✔ **Do something creative.** People think of painting, gardening, or restoring old cars as fun, but these activities are also healing — and they require a focus that can take your mind off the daily grind.

Spread some sunshine

Something I suggest to most of my anxious, depressed PTSD patients is to smile and say hello to three strangers each day — grocery checkers, bank tellers, post-office clerks, waiters, and parking valets, for example. You'll often bring a smile to these people's lips as you lighten their load of stress (especially if you follow on the heels of a rude or angry customer). In addition, you can help yourself by cracking the shell of self-involvement that PTSD can build around you. Putting a smile on a stranger's face can make you realize that you care about the people around you, and it makes you feel better about yourself as well.

Of course, every once in a while you'll run into someone who greets your smile with a sullen look or ignores you altogether. If so, don't take it person-ally. That person may be dealing with her own life issues. Instead, give a spare smile to the next stranger you meet.

Try something brand new

PTSD tends to make you *reactive* — always on guard, ready to defend yourself against a new threat. When you're in that frame of mind, you find it easy to retreat from new experiences and relationships that challenge the status quo. Now's the time to reverse that trend, because new people, places, and events are part of your prescription for putting your trauma behind you and discov-ering a brighter future.

To find new and positive directions in your life, try these exercises:

- ✔ **List five new skills you want to master.** They can be big skills such as playing the violin or little skills like playing poker.

- ✔ **List five places you want to go.** Pick places that are realistic given your current budget. It doesn't matter whether they're exotic and far away or just a few miles from your house.

- ✔ **List five experiences you want to have.** Your list can include things such as scuba diving, going to a concert, climbing a mountain, owning a cat, or taking a gourmet cooking class.

Pick any one item in any of these lists and put plans in motion to achieve it. As you expand your horizons, continue to add items to your wish list of new adventures and accomplishments. Each new experience you enjoy can become a healthy memory that helps push the bad ones into the background.

Join in

When people are troubled, they turn inward. They develop tunnel vision and zero in on their own crises and problems and let the rest of the world fend for itself. Turning inward is a necessary part of protecting yourself immediately after a trauma occurs, but it's unhealthy long term because you're healthiest when you're a loving, caring member of your community.

When you're well on the way to healing, you're ready to rejoin that community, and one of the best ways is by helping others. Reaching out to people in need benefits you as well, in the following ways:

- ✔ **It puts your own problems in perspective.** As the old saying goes, "I felt sad because I had no shoes, until I met a man who had no feet." No matter what your troubles are, you're likely to find that other people have woes that are equally bad or even worse — and that knowledge can help you value the good things in your life.

- ✔ **It helps you transform a negative event into a positive force.** Many people find healing by helping other people who are undergoing the same trauma they experienced or by working to prevent others from suffering that trauma. For instance, Mothers Against Drunk Driving (MADD) was founded by Candy Lightner, who lost her own child to a drunk driver.

Many people choose to volunteer for organizations that have some connection to the type of trauma they experienced (something you should consider only if you're sure that it won't trigger out-of-control memories or emotions). Others pick very different outlets. No matter what form your outreach takes, giving of yourself can help you discover new meaning and purpose in life.

For ideas on ways to volunteer in your community, check out these sites; all three let you enter your zip code to find activities near your home.

✔ **Network for Good:** www.networkforgood.org

✔ **VolunteerMatch:** www.volunteermatch.org

✔ **Do Something:** www.dosomething.org

Harness the power of play

The next time you're at the park, watch the kids playing ball, the teenagers rollerblading, the 80-year-olds pondering their next moves in chess, and even the dogs playing Frisbee. They're all intensely *alive* — because nothing is more mentally, physically, and spiritually awakening than the simple act of play. Whether you're a kid or a grownup, play has the power to clear out the cobwebs, get your creative juices flowing, and give stress the boot. It's also a great way to reach out to other people and bring new friends (and possibly new loves) into your life. The simple act of play can even improve your memory, ease depression, and — no kidding — make you live longer. You're never too young for play, and you're never too old for it, either.

One family's road from grieving to helping

Charlotte and Robert Hullinger's happy lives fell apart in 1978, when their daughter Lisa's ex-boyfriend stalked and killed the 19-year-old woman. Rocked by their loss, the Hullingers turned to the only people who understood their pain: other parents of murdered children.

In 1978, the Hullingers and two other couples held their first meeting. Talking and crying together in the Hullingers' living room, the grieving parents immediately felt a powerful bond. That simple beginning led the Hullingers to create a national group, Parents of Murdered Children (www.pomc.org), which now offers support and advocacy for thousands of families trying to come to terms with this terrible trauma.

No family should ever need to endure the pain that the Hullingers experienced, but the harsh reality is that many families will suffer the same unspeakable tragedy. Those who contact Parents of Murdered Children can find loving, caring people to help them through their loss — the powerful legacy of a couple who turned their own pain into a mission to help others. As Charlotte Hullinger says, "If life experiences are not used, they are wasted."

PTSD can be a grim business, so when you begin healing, you may have to make a conscious effort to stretch out those rusty "fun" muscles and get used to kicking up your heels again. To get your groove back, think back to the time before your trauma and remember the playful activities you enjoyed. If you loved a pickup basketball game at the gym or a game of bridge with the neighbors, see whether you can take up these activities again, or look for new outlets. If you have kids or grandkids, get into the habit of tossing a football with them or set up a backyard badminton net.

Other avenues for locating playful outlets as well as new friends include the following:

- ✔ Your town's parks and recreation department
- ✔ Local gyms, which often offer a wide range of activities
- ✔ Groups offering activities for singles, mothers of preschoolers, and so on
- ✔ Your local senior citizens' center if you meet the age requirements (many centers offer activities for people as young as 55)
- ✔ Local colleges and universities (many schools offer just-for-fun activities, especially in their adult education catalogs)

Remember, too, that you can play on your own. Put on some salsa music and do a crazy dance in your own living room — or head outside and play a rousing game of fetch with your dog. Fly a kite, buy yourself a pair of rollerblades or a new video game, or build a sand castle at the beach. What form of play you choose doesn't matter; if it makes you feel like a kid again, it can restore your mind and spirit.

Following Through on Your Wellness Plans

Throughout this chapter, I offer many ways to promote healing. But as a fellow human being, I know that it's easier to say, "I'm going to change!" than to follow through when daily crises distract and frustrate you.

Stay on course with these strategies:

- ✔ **Be realistic.** Set goals you can meet so you don't add to your PTSD stresses. Don't confuse reasonable expectations with realistic expectations. *Reasonable* means "makes sense." *Realistic* means "likely to happen." It may be reasonable to stop smoking, start a new diet, and begin exercising, for example, but making all three changes at the same time may not be realistic. Instead, pick one goal (starting with the easiest one may be best) and focus your energy on it.

✔ **Set specific goals.** Often, picturing how you want to feel — less stressed, more healthy, more calm — is easier than figuring out the steps you need to follow to achieve that feeling. To keep yourself on target toward your wellness goals, create a step-by-step plan to achieve those goals. If you want to incorporate exercise into your healing plans, figure out what equipment you need, which gym you want to join, or what times of day you can fit exercise into your schedule.

✔ **Write down your goals.** You write reminders to buy coffee or give the dog a bath, so write down your wellness goals, too. Outline exactly what you need to *stop* doing and what you need to *start* doing to reach your goals. Writing down your goals increases your commitment to do them.

✔ **Tell your friends about your plan.** Sticking to a commitment is easier when you tell people whom you like and respect — and whose respect you value in return — that you're making a positive change.

✔ **Use the buddy system.** Scheduling a weekly visit to the gym with a friend who's trying to improve his own health or joining Habitat for Humanity (www.habitat.org) with a buddy who's also seeking a soul-renewing outlet can help both of you stick to your new goals. Joining a support group can also be a big help in keeping you on track; see Chapter 4 for info on how to locate groups in your area.

✔ **Don't let negative people knock you off course.** See Chapter 7 for info on how to keep the emotional vampires in your life from discouraging you when you set out to improve your health and well-being.

✔ **Give it time!** You need somewhere between 21 and 30 days for a new behavior to become a habit, which means you've mentally internalized it (which is probably why Alcoholics Anonymous gives out 30-day chips for maintaining sobriety); it takes about 6 months for that habit to become second nature, which means it's engrained in your personality. So stick with your new healing behaviors, and give them time to become part of the fabric of your life.

Chapter 13

Caring for Your Loved Ones While They Care for You

****

In This Chapter

▶ Seeing how PTSD affects your loved ones

▶ Understanding the role of secondhand stress

▶ Figuring out how to help your family help you

▶ Reaping the benefits of therapy for family members

****

*I*f you're coping with PTSD, you're fully aware of your hurt and just want to feel better. You can't handle the screaming kids, your partner's complaints about the bills, your parents' nagging, or the pressures at work. The nightmares keep you awake. The flashbacks leave you drenched in sweat. Maybe you're struggling every day with a drug or alcohol problem. You're scared, you're angry, and you don't know how much more you can take. In short, your life's not a day at the beach.

But here's another fact: Life's no picnic for your loved ones right now, either. As you probably already know, keeping your family together when you have PTSD isn't easy. To have a fighting chance, you have to start by facing facts — and the fact is, your PTSD is hurting everyone you know. It's not your fault that PTSD makes your life so hard, but it *is* your responsibility to deal with your symptoms, especially when they affect your family.

In this chapter, I look at how your PTSD can affect your loved ones (with extra attention to wee ones due to their special needs), why therapy can help all of you get on the same team, and how you can help your family understand and help you.

Stepping Outside Your World: Common Feelings Your Loved Ones Face

Just for a minute, think about what life's like for the people you love. In some ways, your PTSD is as hard on them as it is on you; for example, your partner may be overwhelmed by your emotional meltdowns, your parents may feel deep heartache when they witness your suffering, and your children may feel tremendous insecurity about their own futures as well as yours. What's more, your parents or partner may have taken on the primary job of offering moral, financial, and practical support, which can be a whole lot to handle.

The good news is that together, you and your loved ones can take many practical steps to keep your relationship on track. In this chapter, I show you what you can do to foster a healthy healing environment for yourself and your family. I also devote a whole chapter (Chapter 16) to guiding your loved ones and helping them support you through this tough time.

Before you start thinking about a solution to heal your loved ones' hurt, though, you need to know just what PTSD is doing to their lives — because that insight, although painful, can give you empathy for what they're going through. It can also motivate you to ease their burden, which in turn can give them added strength to support you. The end result: Everyone wins.

Here's how relatives or close friends of people with PTSD often feel:

- ✔ **Helpless, which may lead to feelings of frustration, depression, or guilt:** Your loved ones care deeply about you, and if they're knowledgeable about the reality of PTSD, they sympathize with the pain you feel. Watching you suffer is hard, especially if they can't make the problem go away.

- ✔ **Overwhelmed and confused by the emotional rollercoaster ride:** As you cycle through the heights and depths of PTSD, you take your family members along for the wild ride. For instance, one day you give your partner a big hug and say, "You're beautiful" — and the next day, you say you're thinking about a divorce. Or you reach out to your parents for help, only to pull away and say, "Leave me alone — I can handle this myself." Or you scream at your brother about some trivial matter, apologize two minutes later, and then turn your back on him when he tries to hug you.

These emotional twists and turns leave your loved ones feeling like a tightrope walker crossing a pit of alligators. As a result, they may be tense, unsure of themselves, and often angry. They may feel — with good cause — that they're sacrificing their own emotional needs just to keep you on an even keel. (If they are, that effort can eventually spell bad news for both of you; see the next section to find out why.)

✔ **Scared about the future:** PTSD hits families in the pocketbook, so your partner may lie awake nights worrying about how he'll pay the bills, or your parents may wonder how long they can chip in on your bills without jeopardizing their retirement. If you have a drug or alcohol problem, your loved ones may also worry about the risk you'll get into trouble with the law.

To complicate matters even more, you likely have trouble planning for the future — a common problem for PTSD sufferers. (I talk more about this problem, called *foreshortening,* in Chapter 3.) Big problems arise if you're thinking, "I doubt I'll even be alive in ten years," and your partner's struggling with thoughts about how you'll pay the mortgage, put money in the IRA, or put your kids through law school.

✔ **Insecure about your love:** PTSD can put the chill on your warm-and-fuzzy feelings for a partner, and she's likely to respond to this frigid blast by thinking you don't love her anymore. You reinforce this fear every time you turn away from a hug, avoid a kiss, or say, "Not tonight, okay?" PTSD can also cause your sex drive to plummet and lead your partner to think, "I'm not attractive anymore."

Worse, if you're like many people with PTSD, you *do* have one foot out the door. You're afraid to commit and too numb to respond to your partner's romantic feelings. You love her, but you can't show it — and right now, you can't handle the emotional needs of another person. At the same time, you expect her to love you, care for you, and be available sexually when you *are* in the mood. Unless her hometown is Stepford, handling this kind of one-sided relationship is tough for a partner.

✔ **Scared about your safety or their own:** A far worse situation arises if you have an out-of-control temper and abuse the people close to you either physically or emotionally. In this case, loved ones live with the constant fear of your violence and chronic worries about your future and their own. That's especially true for a partner, who may not be sure which is scarier: a future without you or a future as a punching bag. If your PTSD leads to depression, or worse yet, to suicidal thoughts, your loved ones may also be terrified that you'll hurt yourself.

✔ **Overburdened, which may lead to resentment:** If you have PTSD, life is a hard slog, and even little crises can seem overwhelming. You can all too easily avoid handling problems or making decisions by making statements like these:

  • "I don't *know* how I'll pay my credit card bill, okay? Just leave me alone."

  • "I can't talk about Jason's bad grades right now. You handle it."

  • "You know I can't deal with my sister when she's upset. *You* talk to her."

If you're married, your PTSD can make your partner feel like your parent, because she's the one who needs to make all the big decisions. (One wife said, "It's like raising a teenager. He wants me to do everything, and then he complains about being bossed around and second-guesses my decisions.") If you're living with your folks, over time, their compassion and caring can turn to frustration and even resentment if they wind up saddled with your responsibilities.

✔ **Guilty for adding more stress to your life:** Are you still in denial about your PTSD? If so, you probably blame other people for your problems when PTSD is the real culprit. Like a crime-scene detective following the wrong set of footprints, you may do things like these:

- Accuse your partner of being too clingy when you're actually too numbed by PTSD to show him the affection he needs

- Criticize your kids for being too noisy or messy, when your hyper-vigilance makes you supersensitive

- Complain that your parents are nags, when they have legitimate concerns about how you're acting

This blame game works for you in the short run because it lets you avoid facing your problems head-on. (As they say, "Denial ain't just a river in Egypt.") At the same time, blaming saps your loved ones' confidence and makes them feel tremendous guilt when they're actually innocent bystanders at an emotional train wreck caused by PTSD.

✔ **Deeply conflicted:** This is a variation of guilt that your partner may feel. If you have PTSD, you can't run away from it — you're stuck with it like Velcro reinforced with superglue, and it follows you around wherever you go. But your partner or family members aren't necessarily stuck with it. In fact, if they were to leave you, they'd leave your PTSD behind as well. That conflict — feeling loyal to you one moment but at their wits' end and on some level, wanting to escape the next — can make many loved ones feel wracked with guilt and frustration.

Seeing How Secondhand Stress Plays Out in Adults

PTSD can have a host of negative effects on your loved ones — and on their relationship with you. Here are two of the most common ways in which your PTSD can affect a loved one's physical and mental health (and can affect *your* healing as well).

How stress over your PTSD can affect a loved one's health

The problems I discuss in the preceding section all too often lead the loved ones of people with PTSD to take it on the chin health-wise for two primary reasons:

✔ They don't have time to take care of themselves because they're shouldering more than their share of the family's responsibilities. This can be especially true for elderly parents trying to juggle your life problems and their own or for a partner trying to raise children while coping with your symptoms.

✔ They're trying to cope with unmanageable stress on too many fronts, from unpaid bills to emotional upheavals.

Here are some of the most common health-wreckers I see in people coping with a loved one's PTSD:

✔ Excessive drinking or use of prescription, nonprescription, or street drugs to relieve anxiety

✔ Overeating or eating disorders

✔ Neglecting health problems such as diabetes or heart disease

✔ Giving up exercise because "there's just no time"

✔ Seriously lacking sleep (for example, if you wake up screaming from a terrible nightmare, that shot of adrenaline goes right to the heart of everyone else in your house as well)

Codependency: How others' responses can affect your healing

One word families often hear in therapy is *codependency,* which means that a person reacts to problems in a relationship in a way that enables another person to keep behaving in unfair or self-destructive ways. Anyone can develop codependent behaviors, but people coping with a loved one's PTSD are at higher-than-normal risk (especially if substance abuse enters the picture). Here are some signs of codependency in a partner, parent, or other loved one:

✔ **She lets you escape responsibility on a regular basis, even if she knows you're capable of handling it.** Deneesha asks Jamal to mow the lawn because company's coming over. He blows his top and says, "Can't you see I have enough on my mind right now? I'll get to it! Quit whining all the time!" First, Deneesha has a long cry in the bathroom. Then she mows the lawn. The next time the lawn needs mowing, she does it without even asking Jamal.

✔ **He covers up for you if you do self-destructive things.** Bob comes home to find his daughter Sarah passed out on the couch and an empty Scotch bottle on the floor. The paper she desperately needs to finish for her graduate class is on the computer screen, barely started. Bob's angry, but he thinks, "At least she's majoring in the same field as her old man — I know this topic, so maybe I can bail her out." He tosses out the Scotch bottle, sits down at the keyboard, and starts typing.

✔ **She makes decisions for you.** Li comes home from a therapy session to find his wife Keiko painting the living room green. "I know how hard it is for you to make decisions right now," she says, "so I picked the color myself."

✔ **He accepts out-of-whack dynamics in your relationship.** For example, a codependent partner may fall into the role of Mom or Dad — "Do you *really* think you should have another beer, Jack?" — instead of expecting you to take responsibility for your own behavior. Similarly, a parent may let you slip back into patterns of selfish, irresponsible, or childish behavior.

Codependency seems like kindness, but it actually barricades the road to recovery. A codependent partner, parent, or friend keeps you from facing reality and acting like an adult, instead letting you slide ever deeper into helplessness. In effect, a codependent person sends you the message that you're not capable, which is why getting out of this rut is so important for your own healing as well as for your loved one's emotional health.

If codependency is the pattern in your relationship, a therapist can help you turn things around. But change is going to be painful for both you and Captain Codependent. Your loved one's used to feeling like a martyr; you're used to handing your responsibilities over to her; and changing that setup will rattle both your cages. But the reward is big: You'll both come out of the process stronger, happier, and less burdened by anger and resentment.

Helping Your Loved Ones Help You

No matter how hard PTSD is battering you, sometimes you need to take time out to care for your loved ones. As much as you need them right now, they're still human, and they need love and reassurance, too — especially when they're supporting you and aren't tending to their own needs as much as they should. You can take plenty of simple steps to ease your loved ones' path and, indirectly, foster your own healing.

As you read through the following sections, you may notice that most of these steps involve one thing: loving communication. Sure, talking is easy; a 2-year-old can do it! But *talking* and *communicating* are often very different things — something you've probably learned the hard way since PTSD took hold of your life. The negative thoughts and emotions that PTSD causes may lead you to utter hurtful or destructive words that fray friendships and strain loving bonds to the breaking point. As you heal from PTSD, you can begin mending your relationships (or keep them healthy and strong if they aren't broken).

To establish effective habits of communication, you need to break old patterns of defensiveness and anger and create new patterns in their place. These positive patterns can allow you to get your own needs met effectively without trampling on your loved ones' emotions. In the following sections, I offer positive communication strategies to keep or help make your relationships strong and mutually supportive.

Bringing your PTSD out into the open

One of the most important things you can do for your loved ones is simply talk to them. Don't try to hide your PTSD symptoms; instead, get them out in the open where you can face them together. If these loved ones include a partner, open communication about your sexual relationship, your kids, and your family finances is especially important.

As you talk about your PTSD, here are some healing things you can say:

✔ Tell your loved one, often, that you appreciate his sympathy and concern.

✔ Let your loved one know that she's not to blame for your problems.

✔ Help the person "exhale" by communicating to him that you understand what he's going through. Here's how:

- During a calm time, say, "You sometimes feel really burdened by me, don't you?" Pause and let him respond, even if he just asks, "Huh?" Then say, "Sometimes, you wish you could run away, or that I'd go away and never come back. Isn't that true?" (Don't say this accusingly. Instead, make it clear that you understand.) Pause and give the person time to reply.

- At this point, the person may start to cry as he feels you understanding him rather than judging him the way he judges himself. If so, you can ask, "How bad does it get for you, having to deal with me?" This question may really cause the tears to pour, after which you can say, "I'm so sorry that you have to deal with my problems, and I appreciate your hanging in there with me."

• If you've touched a nerve, the person is likely to cry for a while. Then he may lighten up and even give you the first real smile you've seen in a while. He may say something like, "It's okay. It's not your fault. If it happened to me, you'd hang in there, too. That's what love's all about."

Making efforts to show love and responsibility

Actions truly *can* speak louder than words, so don't just offer lip service to your loved ones; put some body language behind it. If you realize that they're carrying too heavy a burden, take steps to ease their load. When you do this, you accomplish three goals: you make their lives a little easier, you encourage them to offer you support in return, and you get a step closer to taking charge of your own life again. Here are ways to show your loved ones that you care:

✔ **Do your best to shoulder your household responsibilities.** Even if PTSD makes it impossible for you to handle some parts of your life, pitch in wherever you can. If your partner takes over the job of earning a living, for example, reciprocate by doing more of the yard work or laundry. (And if some jobs are beyond you, explain this clearly and lovingly instead of just neglecting these chores or becoming defensive when your loved one mentions them. See the upcoming section titled "Keeping anger in check and defensiveness at bay" for info on defusing arguments.)

✔ **Show your commitment to seeking help and healing.** Ignoring PTSD doesn't make it go away; instead, you can make it even worse. So do everyone a favor and get in the healing game. If you need therapy, get therapy. If you have a problem with alcohol or drugs, face up to it and take steps to deal with it. These steps can reassure your loved ones that you're actively working to get your life — and by extension, theirs — back on course.

✔ **If your loved ones don't know much (or anything) about PTSD, supply some information and give them time to learn the ropes.** Nobody becomes an expert on this disorder overnight, so forgive them if they have some misunderstandings. For instance, if your girlfriend doesn't understand why you have trouble being intimate right now, show her the section in Chapter 3 about how PTSD can cause this problem. With time, most friends and family members go from being clueless about PTSD to being knowledgeable and supportive.

✔ **Once a day (at least on your good days), focus on your loved ones and do something nice for them.** You don't have to do something big — just something that lets them know they count. For example, bring home your kids' favorite flavor of ice cream, take your friends out to lunch, give Mom a bouquet of flowers, or surprise your partner by doing one of her chores.

> ✔ **If you're in therapy, ask your therapist for specific ways to improve your relationship with your loved ones.** A therapist can offer ideas tailored to your own family dynamics and relationship issues.

Offering your undivided attention when it counts

Everyone in your life competes for time, but nobody should need to compete for importance. Nothing makes an important person in your life feel more *un*important than hearing something like this: "Yeah, that's interesting, dear. Just a sec — I need to get this call. . . . Okay, hold that thought while I take this laundry upstairs. And could you call Bobby for dinner? . . . Now, what were you saying?"

Making time for the important people in your life isn't always easy, especially when the minutes are ticking by and your to-do list is long. Making time is even harder when you have PTSD and extra worries and stresses are pulling you in different directions. But remember: The *amount* of time you offer a person is less important than the *quality* of that time. Remember, too, that if you make an active effort to tune in to your family's and friends' needs — something that doesn't always come naturally when you have PTSD — you improve the chances that they'll return the favor by tuning in to *your* needs.

To show another person that he's important, let go of other thoughts and concerns when he's talking and focus your attention totally on him — even if just for a few minutes. I like to use the model of the guy at the beach in Venice, California, who juggles chainsaws. He knows how to focus on one saw while the others are flying, which is why he still has all his fingers! Keep the same focus when you're talking to someone you care about, and you'll strengthen bonds with your family and friends.

Letting loved ones express themselves

Right now, your loved ones have a lot of intense thoughts and feelings about what PTSD is doing to both your life and theirs. Letting them share these pent-up feelings can clear the air like a summer shower, and it can defuse the tension that can get in the way of your healing. Here are some good communication strategies to help you accomplish this goal.

Really listen

Does this situation sound familiar? A loved one says, "We need to talk," and you instantly throw up your defensive shields. Right off the bat, you start thinking of a killer retort or plan an escape route so you can avoid the conversation altogether.

Instead, try this revolutionary approach: Simply listen.

Wilfred Bion, one of the greatest psychoanalysts of the past century, said, "The purest form of listening is to listen without memory or desire." Simply put, that means to clear your mind, open your heart, and hear what another person is saying — without thinking, "Jeez, here she goes again," "I don't want to hear this," or anything else. Just . . . listen.

True, you may not like what you hear. But when you break down your defenses and hear the words coming straight from another person's heart, you often discover two remarkable things:

- ✔ The other person's anger or frustration often drops instantly, simply because you're *hearing* him for the first time.

- ✔ Addressing the other person's concerns is easier when you're not all tied up in knots trying to deny or deflect them.

Talk with your loved one — not over, at, or to her!

Often, people forget that communication is a dialogue, not a monologue. Here's an example: Bob's wife says, "I know Uncle Charlie drives you crazy, but I'd really like to invite him over to . . ." Bob can respond in many ways:

- ✔ **By talking *over* her.** Before she gets the rest of the sentence out, he says, "Forget it. The guy's a jackass. No way am I going to his house ever again, and I don't want him here, either. By the way, have you seen my tennis racket? I'm going to the gym."

- ✔ **By talking *at* her.** He lets her finish her sentence but then goes right into high-school debate-class mode and outlines the ten reasons going to see Uncle Charlie is a bad idea. Then he heads out for his tennis game.

- ✔ **By talking *to* her.** This time, he says, "I know you like Uncle Charlie, but I don't. So let's just skip it. Thanks," and grabs his tennis racket.

- ✔ **By talking *with* her.** In this case, Bob says, "Let's sit down and talk about it. I really don't like how Uncle Charlie makes me feel. He always brings up how my business went under, and that bothers me. But help me understand why you'd really like to see him, and let's see if we can work out a solution that works for both of us."

Clearly, the last strategy is the best. Communication is a two-way street, not a one-way avenue. Say your piece, but leave the door open for discussion. Cutting off another person's communication is a hard habit to break, especially if the other person typically lets you get away with it because of your PTSD. Realize that your loved one has an equal stake in the outcome of your communication, and that she may have info that changes your outlook.

Give your loved one permission to say the unspoken

PTSD can leave your loved ones with a toxic legacy of unvoiced hurts, invisible scars, and hidden anger. Sunlight is the best disinfectant for these hidden wounds — but be prepared, because it can sting.

If you're feeling strong and you're in a good place in your healing, here are some questions to ask to start a cleansing conversation that can wash away many of the secret aches in a loved one's heart:

- ✔ "Have I ever made you feel that you weren't worth listening to?"
- ✔ "Have I ever made you feel that I don't admire and respect you?"
- ✔ "What was the hardest part about living with me when I was at my worst?"

When your loved one answers these questions, do your best to listen without becoming angry or defensive. By simple hearing her out, you can defuse her negative emotions and allow positive ones to take root in their place.

These questions are hard to ask, and the answers aren't easy to hear. But the conversations you start with these simple words have astonishing healing power, both for you and for the loved one who's stood by you through the worst of the storm. In fact, they may be the most powerful relationship-saving questions of all time, whether you have PTSD or not.

Accentuating the positive

Therapists who work with severely troubled kids have a saying: "Find a good behavior — *any* good behavior — and reward it." This rule is great in any relationship. People tend to take positive behavior for granted and to notice only the bad stuff, and when you ignore good behavior, you get less of it.

You'll strengthen your relationships with other people — especially kids — if you keep your eyes open for good deeds and acknowledge them in words. If you and your teenager spend most of your time arguing about her nose rings or creepy boyfriends, for example, catch her off guard by saying things like, "I like the way you treat your little sister. Not everyone would have that much patience" or, "Thanks for taking Grandpa his groceries. I know you're busy, and it was a big deal for you to volunteer."

Also, if you do need to criticize someone, see whether you can start with a positive remark. If your son's garage band is too much for your PTSD-frayed nerves, don't say, "Knock off the noise *now!*" Instead, try saying, "You know, you guys are really pretty good. I like those bass licks you're experimenting with. But tell you what — the noise is pretty rough on my nerves, and I think we need to cut down on your practice hours a little." You'll still hear some whining, but it'll be mixed with pleasure at your praise.

Keeping anger in check and defensiveness at bay

Even the happiest, most stable relationships have their bad moments. Right now, there's a good chance that your relationships aren't all peaches and cream, so there's also a good chance that hot words will start to fly on a regular basis.

Losing your temper occasionally isn't necessarily a bad thing, because a little honest anger can clear the air. But if you're recovering from PTSD, you need to control your anger for two very good reasons:

- ✔ Your loved ones are your strongest allies in your recovery, and they can't help you if you alienate them.
- ✔ PTSD can cause your anger to spiral out of control, harming both you and the ones you love. (For more on this topic, see Chapter 14.)

For both of these reasons, you should learn strategies for putting the kibosh on your angry outbursts and defusing rather than escalating the arguments that pop up in any relationship. The next section offers some of the best strategies for accomplishing those goals.

If you recognize that you have trouble keeping your temper under control and you're still in therapy, ask your therapist to work with you on this problem. This topic is also a good one to bring up if you participate in a support group for PTSD or substance abuse issues.

If your anger makes you physically violent or verbally aggressive to the point that you regularly frighten people, recognize this behavior as an emergency and seek professional help.

Here are additional ways to keep your temper under control:

General anger-management techniques

If your anger isn't dangerous but is upsetting the people you love and straining the bonds of your friendships, the communication skills I describe throughout this chapter can help you simmer down when things heat up.

- ✔ **Pause before you act.** The Six-Step Pause, which I describe in Chapter 11, is both a tool for preventing relapses and a highly effective anger-control technique.
- ✔ **Leave the scene.** Time-out isn't just a good strategy for kids; it's also helpful for an adult who needs a little cooling-down time. Simply say, "I need to take a walk, and then we'll talk about this." Or excuse yourself and go to the bathroom so you can get a handle on your temper.

✔ **Practice your reactions.** If you can predict an event that's likely to make you angry — such as your teenager's staying out too late and then giving you lip — walk through this event mentally, and figure out

- How you'd respond if you were to let your anger take control of you

- How you'd respond if you were to react firmly but calmly

By trying out each scenario, you can prepare yourself to make the right choice if the situation actually arises.

✔ **Get plenty of exercise.** Opt for the kind that wears you out and works off the excess adrenaline that PTSD can create. (See Chapter 12 for more on the benefits of exercise when you're recovering from PTSD.)

Count to three — seriously

I know: "Count to three" sounds like something your kindergarten teacher used to say. But guess what — she was right!

When you feel like you're under attack, your first urge is to fire back instantly, particularly if you have PTSD, because this disorder keeps your anger level set on max. But here's a better idea:

1. **Think of the first thing you want to say, and** *don't say it.*

2. **Think of the second thing you want to say, and** *don't say that,* **either.**

3. **Think of the third thing you want to say, and this time,** *say it.*

Why go with the third comment that crosses your mind? The first thing you want to say is about defending yourself. The second thing is about retaliating. But the third thing is about finding a solution. Start with #3 first, and you'll often put the brakes on an argument that otherwise could turn vicious.

Imagine how the other person feels

You're across the room from each other, arms gesturing, fur flying, tempers flaring. You're both saying hurtful things, and you're both spiraling out of control. How can you stop this train from barreling down the tracks to disaster? The answer is surprisingly simple. Try this three-step strategy:

1. **Stop talking.**

2. **Admit that you and your partner (or parent, or friend) have a problem.**

3. **Ask yourself, "What's it like for the other person right now?"**

When you make this switch in perspective, you discover that it defuses your own anger. What's more, you can defuse the other person's anger as well simply by following through with a comment like this: "I realized that I don't like what we're saying to each other, and I realized that you don't like what's happening, either. Why don't we start over again and figure out a way we can work together to solve this issue?"

Nine times out of ten, you can turn a nasty argument into a positive conversation when you try this approach. If the other person doesn't respond positively and continues to ramp up the argument, try the next approach.

Look at yourself through the other person's eyes

Here's a powerful exercise that can help you prevent an angry outburst. The exercise is based on the fact that *you can't feel anger and empathy at the same time*. Here's why:

- Anger is a motor response (from you to the world) in which you lash out at someone who hurts or disappoints you.
- Empathy is a sensory function (from the world to you) in which you emotionally understand and experience another person's feelings.

Like matter and antimatter, anger and empathy can't exist in the same place simultaneously. As a result, if you open the window to empathy, anger flies out. Here's how to do this exercise:

1. **Think of someone close to you.**

   For purposes of this exercise, call him Bob.

2. **Visualize something Bob does that frustrates, angers, hurts, or disappoints you.**

3. **Score your anger about this behavior on a scale of 1 to 10, where 1 is "not at all" and 10 is "I want to punch him right in the nose."**

4. **Now imagine what Bob would say if someone were to ask him what frustrates, angers, hurts, or frustrates him most about you.**

   This step is uncomfortable because you need to be honest about the negative things you do. You might picture Bob saying, "He doesn't listen," or, "He doesn't do what he says he's going to do."

5. **Imagine what incident Bob would bring up if someone were to ask him to describe something hurtful that you did to him.**

   Unless you're a saint, some uncomfortable memories are likely to come to mind.

6. **Pause and feel the emotions that Bob probably experienced as a result of your hurtful actions.**

7. **On a scale of 1 to 10, rate how frustrated, angry, or hurt you are *now* about Bob's behavior in Step 2.**

After you trade places with Bob and look at your relationship through his eyes, your upset should go down in intensity. As a result, you're far more likely to forgive him the next time he hurts or frustrates you — and far less likely to head straight into a temper tantrum.

Repeat the message you're hearing

Often, a person who's upset is angry because he thinks you're not really hearing what he's saying. He may be right if you're too busy parrying his arguments or venting your own anger to really pay attention to him.

The next time this situation arises, take a deep breath and resist the urge to fight back. Instead, listen to what the other person is saying. Then rephrase it and say it back to him — not in a snide or sarcastic way but gently and caringly.

Suppose, for example, that your father says, "Sometimes I think you're a selfish jerk, and you don't give a @#$% about me or your mother!" Your urge may be to say something like, "Why should I? You don't give a @#$% about me, either." And you're off to the races.

Instead, try saying something like this: "It's important for me to know why you're feeling so bad. You're saying that you think I've been behaving selfishly and that I act like I don't care about you or Mom." If he agrees, you can say something like, "Do you *really* believe that I don't care about you?" or, "Can you tell me what I did that made you feel that way?"

Saying these things calmly is tough, especially if you're still in PTSD mode and your emotions are on a hair trigger. But if you can short-circuit your attack reflex, you can stop a spat in its tracks. The big payoff: You'll prevent a big fight that could send you spiraling back down into PTSD mode, and you'll strengthen your relationship with someone you need to have on your side.

Use "I" messages

"I" messages focus on how you feel, not on another person's faults. Often, a simple change in perspective can mean the difference between a nasty argument and a thoughtful discussion. For example, compare these two statements:

> **Version 1:** "You stomp around here, screaming and yelling like some kind of lunatic, and you expect the kids and me to respect you?"

> **Version 2:** "When you lose your temper, the children and I feel like it's not safe for us to be here. We want to support you, but your anger is frightening for all of us."

Notice the difference? Version 1 is just about guaranteed to generate a hostile reply. Version 2, however, allows you to express your feelings without putting the blame on the other person. It also gives him deeper insight into your feelings, increasing the odds that he'll listen to what you're saying.

Find common ground

No matter how unfair another person's anger seems, you'll probably spot a grain of truth in her complaints if you're willing to listen. If you find even a single point of agreement and can start from there, you can often nip a potentially stressful confrontation in the bud. Consider these two scenarios:

Scenario 1:

Your partner: "We never talk anymore. I might as well be invisible. It's like you and the TV live in this house, and I'm not even here. I think I made a big mistake when I moved in with you."

You: "If you think I'm such a jerk, why don't you move out?"

Scenario 2:

Your partner: "We never talk anymore. I might as well be invisible. It's like you and the TV live in this house, and I'm not even here. I think I made a big mistake when I moved in with you."

You: "I can see why you're unhappy with me. I've been pretty much glued to the TV during the playoffs, haven't I? That wasn't fair to you, and I'll try to do better. But are you really sorry you moved in with me? I know I'm not perfect, but I'm really happy you're here, and I thought you were happy, too."

Scenario 2 is clearly smarter because by agreeing on a single key point, you pave the way for discussing other issues in a sane and constructive way. Often, you'll also stop the other person from blowing a minor problem out of proportion — something that can easily happen if a loved one who's stressed out from dealing with your PTSD symptoms doesn't get some acknowledgment of her issues.

Communicating your needs and accepting help when you need it

One thing that quickly goes out the window when PTSD flies in is honest, heart-to-heart conversation. As a result, many important things — both good and bad — go unsaid, especially when you're in the depths of your suffering. Now's the time to reopen the lines of communication and to start sharing your thoughts and feelings with your loved ones.

That's especially true when it comes to getting your own needs met. You may hesitate to talk openly and honestly about these needs for several reasons. Here are some of these reasons and why they're misguided:

✔ **You equate asking for help with weakness.** Often, people with PTSD — especially if they're veterans, police officers, firefighters, or rescue workers — feel uncomfortable admitting that they need help. That's because they're used to giving help rather than receiving it, and the role reversal is hard to accept.

If you feel that way, here's an illustration to help you put things in perspective: Picture a rescue worker rushing up to help two people trapped under a burning car. The first person says, "Thank you!" and cooperates fully, allowing herself to be rescued quickly and safely — situation handled. But the second person forces the rescue worker into a long, dangerous argument by saying, "No thanks, I'm just hunky-dory — leave me here, and I'll be fine. Really!" Clearly, this person is way off-base, and he's complicating everyone's life — just as you are, if you refuse to let your loved ones help you overcome PTSD. Like the rescue worker in my story, your friends and family know full well there's a problem, and they want to help — so let them!

✔ **You don't want to be a burden.** You may think that by keeping your suffering to yourself, you're protecting your loved ones and shielding them from your misery. If so, you're wrong. That's because your loved ones feel your pain even if you try to hide it — and in addition, they feel terrible frustration because they want to help and you won't let them.

✔ **You're hamstrung by guilt.** The toxic effects of post-traumatic guilt can make you feel like you don't deserve to call on family or friends to help you when you're hurting, because somehow you "deserve" the pain you're experiencing.

If that's the case, read Chapter 8 for info on getting rid of guilt — and if you're in therapy, discuss this issue with your therapist. Misguided guilt can poison your family's life as well as your own, so don't let it stand in the way of seeking and accepting help

✔ **You can't stand the idea of losing your independence.** If this is your hang-up, you think that asking for help reduces your control over your life. In reality, however, getting help in battling PTSD will speed your healing — and the faster you heal, the faster you can handle all aspects of your life on your own again. In other words, asking for help makes you *more* independent in the long run.

✔ **You're angry about needing help.** Many things you used to do easily are now hard or impossible, and you're furious about that — and rightfully so. However, this anger creates a double burden for your loved ones. One woman, for example, talked in an Internet group about her husband's anger when she took over driving their son to ball games — even though he couldn't face being in the car after his accident. Putting your loved ones in this kind of losing situation makes much less sense than facing reality, acknowledging that right now you can't do everything on your own, and graciously accepting a hand.

One good way to enlist your loved ones in your healing is to make a written list of the things you need help with. For example, you may need financial help, moral support, transportation to therapy sessions, or simply a quiet place to relax or do your therapy homework. After you identify your needs, approach your most supportive friends and family members and ask for their assistance.

When you ask your loved ones for help, be open and honest about your symptoms and how they affect your life. If your loved ones aren't knowledge-able about PTSD, be sure to offer them some basic info so they can better understand what you're going through and how they can help.

Seeking Outside Help through Family Therapy

Not all families need professional therapy when they're dealing with PTSD. If you're in therapy yourself and your symptoms are under control to the point that your family life is usually calm and happy, don't fix it if it ain't broke. If the cracks in your family are starting to look like earthquake fault lines, however, you need to call for outside help.

In the following sections, I focus largely on the most common scenario: family therapy involving a partner and possibly children. But family therapy can involve anyone who's close to you — not just a partner or child but also a parent, brother or sister, or grandparent — so feel free to be flexible in defining "family." In the next sections, I offer some clues about when to seek therapy for the whole gang (or at least some of it) and what therapy options you have.

Deciding whether your family would benefit

In just about any family — not just one that's coping with PTSD — spouses sometimes get annoyed, children argue and whine, and teenagers seethe and act weird. Those occurrences are everyday events, and you can't always tell when emotions cross the line from normal to problematic. So how do you decide whether your flock can benefit from professional help? Here are clues that everyone (not just you) may need therapy:

- Major blowups occur in your household on a regular basis — once a week or even more often.

- Your family members sneak around like quiet little church mice, afraid to ask you about anything.

✔ Your partner is talking about leaving you, even if he's just making vague threats.

✔ Your partner (or a parent, if you're living with Mom or Dad) is exhausted and says she can't handle your problems anymore.

✔ Your child is exhibiting dangerous behavior, such as driving under the influence, hanging around with a bad crowd, taking drugs, or failing in school.

✔ You think your partner or your child is developing an eating disorder.

✔ Anyone in the family is suffering from depression or may be suicidal.

✔ Anyone in the family has alcohol or drug problems.

✔ You're going through a rough patch in therapy, and you want your family to understand why you're not as supportive as usual.

If nothing in this list applies to you but you still have a gut feeling that therapy can help your family, go for it if your tribe is willing. If they're reluctant, see whether you can get them to commit to a single session. A good therapist may be able to use that session to help them see why continuing with family therapy is a good idea.

Understanding what family therapy is all about

Family therapy is a specific type of therapy in which a therapist helps your family members, both separately and as a group, understand your PTSD and the different roles they can play in helping you overcome it. The therapist also tells you how you can help your family.

Some people fear that if family members talk to the same therapist, the tales they tell in confidence will become front-page news for the entire family. But that's not how family therapy works. Instead, therapists typically see each family member individually and then ask each person if it's okay to talk about certain topics as a group. If everyone agrees, the whole family can put those issues on the table for joint discussion. If not, secrets stay secret.

So don't worry that your daughter will find out what you *really* think of her purple hair and her boyfriend's tattoo. On a more serious note, don't worry that your husband will find out that you're unsure of your feelings for him or that your son will discover that you're disappointed in his lifestyle. Confidentiality is the lodestone of therapy, and telling tales without permission is strictly forbidden.

Helping everyone benefit from therapy

Family therapy is a great option for teens and older preteens, but younger children may benefit more from other approaches, such as art or play therapy. These approaches allow a sensitive therapist to find out what's troubling a young child and to work out solutions.

The label *family therapist* is used somewhat loosely. See Chapter 6 for tips on finding a therapist who's truly qualified to help a family dealing with PTSD.

Combining family therapy and CBT

Family therapy is excellent, but it may not be the right choice as your primary therapy. Cognitive behavioral therapy (CBT), which I discuss in depth in Chapter 8, is considered to be the gold standard for treating the person who has PTSD, whereas family therapy has a less-stellar track record as a front-line treatment (see Chapter 6). Thus, it may make sense for *you* to have a CBT therapist and for *your family as a whole* — including you — to see a family therapist separately.

You may find it helpful to complete trauma-based CBT therapy (see Chapter 8) before the rest of your family enters therapy. CBT can reduce your symptoms to the point where you can focus more on your family's needs and less on your own problems.

Knowing your options

A professional therapist may suit your family to a tee. But if professional therapy is too expensive, not covered by your insurance, or not available in your area, here are some other options. (For more ideas, see Chapter 6.)

- ✔ Families who are religious often find pastoral counseling (provided by a minister or other religiously oriented counselor) to be useful. A benefit of pastoral counseling is that it's often free or inexpensive.

- ✔ If you're a military veteran, your family may be able to receive counseling at one of the many Vet Centers across the country. In this case, professional therapy is available free of charge. For info on what's available in your area, go to www.va.gov.

- ✔ If neither of the preceding two options works out for you, consider steering your family to online support groups where they can vent their frustrations, talk with other families battling PTSD, and even have some stress-relieving laughs. These groups can be appropriate for older teens as well as for partners. Chapter 16 lists several of these discussion forums.

Be extremely careful if your child participates in one of these groups. Preteens shouldn't be involved in unsupervised chats at all, and adolescents need to know the dangers of online wolves posing as friendly, sympathetic sheep.

Little People, Big Hurt: How PTSD Affects Your Children

If you have kids, right now they're both the lights of your life and arrows through your heart. You love them more than life itself — but most likely, you spend too much time yelling at them, and they spend too much time yelling at you (or hiding from you).

No matter how mature they are, kids can't fully grasp how PTSD changes your life. As a result, there's a limit to how much you can expect them to understand about your troubles. But here's the good news: If you try hard to understand what *they're* going through, they're likely to cut you some slack in return. So just for a minute, put yourself in their shoes.

Understanding what your children may be feeling

Your kids care about your pain (even if they don't always show it), but they also may be feeling plenty of their own. Here are some of the emotions kids can feel when they live with a parent with PTSD:

- ✔ "I'm sad. I want my house to be happy like my friends' homes, but everyone here is angry or upset all the time."

- ✔ "I'm scared. What if Mom leaves us? What if we can't pay the bills? What if things get really out of control?"

- ✔ "It's my fault. I made too much noise, and it set Dad off. Now Mom is crying, and I'm to blame."

- ✔ "I'm angry. Being a kid is supposed to be fun. Instead, I have to be the parent while the person who's supposed to take care of me acts like a baby. It's not fair."

- ✔ "I'm trapped. There's nowhere I can go till I'm older, so I have to live in this mess."

- ✔ "I'm jealous. My friend's dad coaches his baseball team and takes him fishing. My dad just sits in his chair and drinks."

✔ "I'm embarrassed. My mom does weird things when my friends come over, and I think they're laughing behind my back. Last week one of my friends turned on the news, and my mom started crying. I wanted to crawl in a big hole and die."

Identifying unhealthy behavior

The feelings PTSD stirs up can make you act in some strange ways. The same is true for your kids, who have their own boatload of big emotions as a result of living with your PTSD. No two kids are alike, but children often fall into one of three unhealthy patterns when a parent has PTSD:

✔ **The perfectionist:** This kid simply seems too good to be true. He excels at school, never raises his voice around the house, and spends his time trying to keep everyone else happy. What's wrong with this picture? This kid really *is* too good to be true. Underneath, he's scared that if he makes a single wrong move, his family will fall apart. He's afraid to feel, afraid to question, and too scared to ask for help. Worse, he thinks it's his job to "rescue" you — an impossible task for a child.

✔ **The scapegoat:** Everybody in the family blames this child for their problems to deflect attention away from the real problem. ("Of course your dad is angry! He wouldn't yell if Cheryl didn't set him off. Did you see the note from her teacher?") This child acts out because the pressures in her house make her angry and upset — and then she gets blamed for *causing* those pressures.

Hand-me-down PTSD

Can your PTSD rub off on your children? Studies of Holocaust survivors suggest that their children may be more vulnerable to developing PTSD. Other studies hint that this may also be true for children of traumatized combat veterans.

Scientists are investigating the idea that PTSD can affect multiple generations. Here's what they suspect happens:

✔ If a parent's trauma is a huge problem but the family treats it like the proverbial elephant in the room ("Don't ever mention that again, Bobby. We don't talk about it"), a child may become terribly anxious about this taboo incident and about keeping it hidden. This anxiety may make him vulnerable to PTSD.

✔ Conversely, a child exposed to all the gory details of a trauma may take in more than she can handle and be traumatized herself.

Either theory worries parents because they're afraid of either saying too little or saying too much. The best approach is to give your child basic info about your PTSD and its causes but not keep rubbing it in his face. Also, skip the most frightening details.

Another excellent way to prevent intergenerational PTSD is to make sure your trauma isn't the sole focus of your family's life. Invest time and effort in creating fun family activities and traditions to offset family problems.

✔ **The copycat:** This type of child is so affected by a parent's PTSD symptoms that he begins exhibiting similar symptoms himself. (Doctors call this behavior *overidentifying.*) Some children even develop full-blown PTSD; see the nearby sidebar "Hand-me-down PTSD" for more info.

If your child falls into any of these patterns — too good, too bad, or too much like you when it comes to PTSD symptoms — recognize that she needs help. Here again, a therapist can provide your child a safe place where she can express her fears and anger and learn to deal with them in a positive way.

Reaching out to help your children

Knowing that your children have negative feelings about your PTSD and its effects on your family can upset you, especially when you know that many of your symptoms are out of your control and that you're doing your best.

The good news is that you can soothe some of your children's concerns and heal the rifts between you. Here's how:

✔ Find a therapist who knows how to help kids who are dealing with a parent's PTSD. As you interview potential therapists, ask them about their specific experience in treating children coping with this issue. Also, check with your family pediatrician to see whether she can offer good leads.

✔ Talk about what's going on with you in simple terms that a child can understand. Say something like this: "Remember how you fell off your bike and didn't want to get on it for a week? Something really bad happened to me a long time ago, but it didn't involve a bike. Instead, it involved a bad man who hurt me. He's in jail now, so he can't hurt us — but I still get scared when I drive by the place where he used to work. My therapist is helping me learn to get over being afraid, just like you got over being afraid to ride your bike." It's especially important to explain symptoms that can terrify a child, such as a parent's nightmares or violent startle responses.

✔ If you have specific triggers that your child should know about, give him this info, which may help him understand why a siren or a TV newscast sets you off and what to do if this happens. For example, you may say, "I know you were worried when I started shaking when I saw you watching the car race on TV. When I see cars going fast, it reminds me of my accident and makes me feel all shaky. You don't need to feel bad about watching that show, because my symptoms aren't your fault — it's part of my PTSD, and I'm working on getting it under control. If you see me getting upset by something on TV in the future, here's a good idea: You can help me by reminding me to practice the relaxation techniques my therapist taught me."

✔ Tell your child that it's okay to express her feelings — both positive and negative. Then do your best to avoid getting defensive if she takes this advice, because she probably will. If she says, "You're never there for me," don't respond, "Hey, I'm busy, and I can't handle everything." Instead, say, "I'm really sorry that I didn't make it to your soccer game. I was feeling really overwhelmed and couldn't go, and I know that it really hurt you when I didn't see you make that goal." (See "Bringing your PTSD out into the open," earlier in this chapter, for the exhale approach, which can work wonders with kids as well as adults.)

✔ Let your child know that your PTSD isn't his fault. Tell him, "Sometimes I get mad if you drop something. The chemicals in my body make me over-react to loud noises. It's not your fault, and I'm very sorry it happens."

✔ Make sure your child knows that solving your problems is your job — not hers. But let her find age-appropriate ways to help if she can. For example, maybe she can help feed the pets on nights when you're worn down by your struggles with PTSD.

✔ Tell your child often that you love him. Your love may seem obvious to you, but it's probably not obvious to your child.

✔ Create a soothing environment. If you can, give your child her own room and fix it up with a good study area so she has a haven where she can hide out when things are tense. Also, make sure she has recreational outlets, such as a new pair of rollerblades or a good supply of books. (A teen may appreciate exercise tapes, which can keep her in shape and help burn off stress at the same time.) If you sense tension rising, try putting on some soothing or perky music.

✔ Another gift you can give your child is simply to let him escape once in a while. If he likes summer camps, see whether you can afford to send him to one — or if he loves his Grandma, see if he can sleep over at her house once a month. Getting away can help a child decompress and gain a little perspective on the situation.

If you have the opposite problem — that is, if your child doesn't see enough of you because of a divorce or separation from your partner — make a point of getting together with her regularly. Even if you're in a bad spot and you feel like you're just going through the motions, your child needs to know that you're there and that you care.

Chapter 14

Getting Your Life Back on Track

*W*hile you're living in the shadows of PTSD, you often have trouble coping minute-by-minute. But as you step into a better future, you can start thinking ahead — to next week, next month, or even next year and beyond.

In this chapter, I help you answer the $64,000 question: "Where do I go from here?" To start, I offer tips on analyzing your current life situation and charting a course for the future. I also share ideas on asking forgiveness from the people PTSD made you hurt, strengthening your ties with the loved ones who stood by you, and handling anger issues that can damage relationships. In addition, I look at whether it's time for you to go back to work (and what financial options you have if you can't). Last but not least, I talk about adding joy and meaning to your life by recognizing what you've gained in your struggle to overcome PTSD.

Taking Stock of Your Life As You Enter the Future

For a long time, you went in any direction that PTSD pushed you, and as a result, you probably took some wrong turns. As you heal, PTSD has less power to steer your life in bad directions, and you have more power to steer it in good ones. But life doesn't come with a built-in GPS unit. So how do you know which way to head?

That question is tough to answer, especially if PTSD caused you to put your future on hold for a long time. To help you get back on track, here are two handy self-help tools. The first helps you evaluate your goals in life, and the second helps you reflect on the past to identify the people and situations you want to play more — or less — of a role in your future.

Lookin' on down the road

Before PTSD struck, you had hopes, dreams, and goals. At this point, you may feel adrift because you've focused so intently on healing from the past that you put your plans for the future on the back burner. Now that you're ready to head into that future, the following activity can aid you in

- Identifying your most important life goals
- Identifying specific goals that PTSD thwarted and getting them back on track
- Recognizing the steps you need to take to accomplish those goals
- Overcoming any negative PTSD-think that could hold you back from achieving your goals

Set aside some quiet time for this exercise because these questions aren't the kind you can answer on the fly. Also, don't worry if you're not sure exactly what direction you want your life to follow. PTSD knocked you off track, and getting your bearings again can take time. Think of this exercise not as a cast-in-stone life plan but as a free-form tool to get you thinking about your future direction. The exercise has no right or wrong answers — it's just food for thought. Answer the following questions:

- What do I feel is my purpose in life?
- What am I passionate about doing?
- What are my strengths, gifts, and talents?
- What limitations do I realistically need to factor into my life plans?
- Are my life goals different now from what they were before I developed PTSD? If so, am I happy with this change, or did I get sidetracked from goals I still want to pursue?
- Do I feel fulfilled doing what I'm doing now, or am I ready for a change?
- Do I have specific goals for the next year? For the next five years? For the next ten years?
- What steps can I take to accomplish these goals?

✔ What fears may hold me back from reaching these goals?

✔ What coping skills can I use to keep these fears from interfering with my progress toward my goals?

✔ What obstacles stand in the way of my achieving these goals, and what specific steps can I take to overcome those obstacles?

These answers can help set your feet on the right path to achieve your goals and dreams. If your answers suggest that you can benefit from additional guidance, here are some good books that can help:

✔ *Life Coaching For Dummies* (Wiley) by Jeni Mumford

✔ *Zen and the Art of Making a Living: A Practical Guide to Creative Career Design,* by Laurence G. Boldt (Penguin)

✔ And — if you don't mind my blowing my own horn! — *Get Out of Your Own Way: Overcoming Self-Defeating Behavior* by Mark Goulston and Philip Goldberg and *Get Out of Your Own Way at Work . . . And Help Others Do the Same* by Mark Goulston (both books published by Perigee).

Revisiting the path you've traveled

PTSD makes you view the past as an enemy to overcome, but instead, you can see it as a friend and a guide to the future. The following exercise helps you use your past experiences to recognize which aspects of life you want to embrace as you move forward and which ones you want to leave behind.

Here are the steps:

1. **Look at your calendar or schedule for the past six months.**

   If you don't have one, ask someone in your family to help you recall various events you experienced during that time, as well as people who influenced your life during that time.

2. **Mark the positives.**

   Without thinking deeply about your responses, put a blue plus sign (+) next to the people, events, and meetings in the past six months that you enjoyed and that left you feeling energized and wanting more afterward.

3. **Mark the negatives.**

   Now put a red minus sign (–) next to the people, events, and meetings that you didn't like or enjoy — the ones that knocked the energy out of you and maybe even put you out of commission for the rest of the day.

Make a distinction between reactions influenced by your PTSD and reactions not related to PTSD so that you don't rule out a potentially positive person or event just because your symptoms got in the way of your enjoyment.

As you look at your plus and minus marks, you become more aware of which people and situations you like and which ones you dislike. This awareness can help you keep positive activities and people in your life — and give negative ones a nudge out the door.

Healing Relationships That PTSD Frayed

As an old Portuguese proverb says, "Friends are the flowers in the garden of life." But when PTSD has you in its grip, you can all too easily crush those flowers into the dirt by seeming aloof, uncaring, angry, or self-destructive.

While you're healing is a perfect time to repair broken ties with any people you wounded emotionally during your struggles with PTSD. In addition, it's a good moment to strengthen your bonds with the people who stood by you through thick and thin, even when PTSD prevented you from giving your fair share in a relationship. In this section, I offer advice on how to accomplish both of these goals.

Repairing damaged friendships

Did you ever disappoint, injure, or even betray someone because of your PTSD? If so, you may fear that you've burned your bridges. However, with some hard work and luck, you can repair broken bonds and possibly even make your relationships stronger than they were before PTSD struck.

To repair a damaged relationship, you need to address the four *h*'s you may have triggered in the other person:

- **Hurt:** Hurt can result from any thoughtless or cruel acts you committed when PTSD had you in its grip.

- **Hate:** This emotion is powerful but also normal when you violate a person's trust or sense of safety.

- **Hesitation to trust:** The person fears that you'll cause him more pain if he lets you back into his life.

- **Holding onto a grudge:** Resentment is another defensive wall a person uses to avoid lowering her guard and being wounded again.

That list is pretty daunting. But here's the happy news: You can overcome all these obstacles if the person you're asking to forgive you is willing to open the door even a tiny crack. To set things right, you need to practice what I call the four *r*'s:

- ✔ **Remorse:** You need to show your friend or loved one that you know you damaged your relationship and that you're truly sorry.

    Here's how Margery approached her former best friend: "Peggy, your friendship is so important to me, but I acted like you didn't matter at all. When I didn't even come to your mother's funeral, I know I hurt you badly. I'm so sorry. Now that I'm getting my PTSD under control, I can be a much better friend to you."

- ✔ **Restitution:** Payback time is here because you need to make amends for the damage that your PTSD caused you to do. If you hurt your mom by missing the past five family get-togethers because social pressures triggered your PTSD symptoms, make amends now by asking whether you can treat her to a spa day or even a mini-vacation with you.

- ✔ **Rehabilitation:** Actions really *do* speak louder than words, so let your friend or loved one see that you're working hard to change your behavior. If you hurt someone as a result of an alcohol problem stemming from your PTSD, join Alcoholics Anonymous or a similar group — and don't miss meetings.

- ✔ **Requesting forgiveness:** Don't expect your friend or loved one to forgive you immediately. Instead, practice the first three *r*'s for a minimum of six months. Then go to the person and ask, "Are you able to forgive me for hurting you?" With luck, your good track record will prove to him that you're worthy of a second chance.

Not every person you've hurt will forgive you. The people who hang onto their grudges may say some cold or hurtful things, and you need to be prepared for this reaction. But even if you get the cold shoulder, you'll find that making the effort to repair your relationship causes you to feel far better about yourself. (Also, unforgiving people aren't the best of friends when you're mending from PTSD and are still vulnerable to self-doubt or self-blame. You're probably better off without them in the long run — even if your parting reopens some wounds.)

You can't always restart a relationship on the same footing, of course. People change, and that goes for your loved ones as well as you. But even if your ex-spouse remarried and you can't get together again, or if differing interests are taking you and a once-close friend on different paths, you can defuse toxic anger and replace it with warmth and respect. When people are willing to hear your message and say, "I forgive you," you empower them to go from being angry to trusting, liking, or even loving you again, and that's a wonderful feeling.

Say, "I forgive you" — to yourself!

When you make a list of everyone you'd like to forgive you, put one name at the top of the list: your own.

Consider the results of a 2007 study by Dr. Mark Leary and his colleagues at Duke and Wake Forest universities. The researchers reported in the *Journal of Personality and Social Psychology* that self-compassion — that is, the ability to be kind to yourself, which can include forgiving yourself for perceived mistakes — plays a central role in healing after a negative experience.

Leary and his colleagues reported that

✔ People with high levels of self-compassion reacted less negatively to real, remembered, or imagined bad events.

✔ Self-compassion enabled people to take responsibility for any part they played in a negative event while controlling their bad feelings about it.

✔ Self-compassion helped neutralize the effects of poor self-esteem. In this study, people with low self-esteem who were able to treat themselves kindly fared as well as people with high self-esteem after an unpleasant life event occurred.

✔ Self-compassionate people are less at the mercy of negative life events than self-scolders are because they respond kindly to themselves whether their lives go well or hit a rough spot.

The moral: Instead of kicking yourself when you're down, treat yourself with the same kindness that you try to show others. You'll be rewarded by reduced risk of a PTSD relapse — as well as by the happier face you see in the mirror.

Creating healthy relationship dynamics

PTSD can run roughshod over your relationships with the most important people in your life: a partner, parents, children, other relatives, and friends. While you're healing, you can work on making your relationships strong and mutually beneficial once again. One good way is by brushing up on your positive communication skills. You can find some specific advice in Chapter 13 on strengthening ties and communication with a life partner or child. And here's an additional way to get your relationships back on track as you heal: Make sure that they're in balance.

Understanding how PTSD tips the scales

The term *quid pro quo* is Latin for *something for something*, which is what a good relationship should be: a pact in which you give of yourself and gain something valuable in return from the other person (love, loyalty, support, caring, and so on). That balance of give-and-take often gets out of whack when you have PTSD — and here's why:

✔ PTSD can cause you to withdraw and feel out of touch with others, so you can't give them the emotional support they need.

✔ PTSD can cause physical aches and pains, depression, and fatigue, all of which can cut down on the practical help you're able to offer your loved ones.

✔ PTSD can make you a ticking time bomb, meaning that loved ones can't count on you for emotional support.

✔ PTSD often takes a bite out of your budget, especially if you can't work, so loved ones can't count on you for financial help.

✔ PTSD can make it hard to care about yourself or your future, or to go to the effort of asking people to respect your needs. As a result, other people — even those who love you — may fall into the pattern of neglecting your needs.

✔ PTSD can anger the people who love you, making them withdraw the emotional support that's crucial for your healing.

Assessing the dynamics of your relationships

Spotting the ways in which PTSD threw your relationships out of whack can help you restore the balance. The simple tool in this section, called the Self-Other Inventory, can help you take a critical look at what you're giving and getting in each important relationship in your life — in particular, with your partner, mother, father, child(ren), sibling(s), and friend(s). This tool helps you be more precise about what you expect from others and about what you need to be willing to give in return. Here's how it works.

As you think about each person you're close to, consider whether you mutually share each type of support that follows:

✔ **Practical assistance:** Making a genuine effort to help

✔ **Emotional support:** Listening with empathy

✔ **Psychological support:** Taking other people's needs and desires seriously

✔ **Financial support:** Being willing to help in a real time of need

✔ **Prompt help:** Keeping promises and meeting important deadlines

Here are some of the not-so-healthy relationship patterns this list can help you identify:

✔ **The others-can't-count-on-me pattern:** Do you see an area in which your loved one can't depend on you for help or support? If so, your PTSD may have created behavior patterns that prevent you from pulling your weight in a relationship.

If you spot this problem, take active steps to remedy it. For instance, if your answers indicate that your partner can't count on you for practical assistance or prompt help, offer to take over two or three of his chores — and make sure you do these jobs on time, without any reminders.

✔ **The I-can't-count-on-others pattern:** Do your answers indicate that you can't turn to the people you love and say, "I need help?" If so, PTSD probably deflated your self-esteem and led you to think that you're not worthy of asking other people for assistance. In the long run, this pattern can leave you feeling used and can deprive you of the support you need to keep your healing on course.

Change this pattern by being open about your own needs and by asking your friends and family members for help when you need it. If your partner tends to ignore you when you talk about your problems, don't just sigh inwardly and walk away. Instead, say, "Can we sit down and really talk for a few minutes? I'm very worried about this problem, and I'm really hoping you can help me find a way to solve it." Also, if a loved one routinely takes advantage of you, see Chapter 13.

Relationships don't always balance out neatly like two sides of an equation, of course. Any relationship has an ebb and flow. Sometimes — if you're caring for young children or aging parents, for example — you need to give more than you get in return. But in general, you should give as much as you get from a relationship. Don't expect to achieve this balance overnight if PTSD threw your friendships or family ties out of kilter. But do keep working to make your relationships fair, satisfying, and emotionally healthy for everyone involved.

Thinking about Work and Finances

Some people manage to keep their careers under control even when their PTSD is in full swing. Many others, however, need to reduce their workload or leave their jobs. If you're in that big second group, you may be wondering, "When — if ever — can I go back to work?"

In this section, I offer advice about deciding whether you're ready to return to work. I also talk about some alternatives to the 9-to-5 routine if your PTSD symptoms make that leap too challenging. In addition, I discuss your options if work isn't in the cards for you.

Preparing for a successful return to work

If you're getting the itch to get your career back on track, that itch is a healthy sign. Congratulations! But you don't want to head back into the workplace jungle too quickly and risk a setback. Here are tips on timing your return to work correctly:

✔ **Talk with your therapist.** She has a good feel for your progress and can offer an educated opinion about whether you're completely ready to head back to the office. If you've completed therapy, you may want to schedule a refresher session so you can brush up on your relaxation and coping skills before you head back to the rat race.

✔ **Talk with your doctor.** Your physician can tell you whether you're physically up to the challenge of going back to work. Also, if you're taking medication for your PTSD, you can take this opportunity to talk with him about any side effects that may interfere with work. If you'll be asking for special accommodations at work, you may also need your doctor (or your therapist) to document the reasons for these accommodations. (See the legal protection sidebar in Chapter 5.)

✔ **Talk with your supervisor.** If you're returning to the job you had before PTSD struck, get back in touch with your boss. If you think you'll need special accommodations to do your job — such as an office where you won't be exposed to loud or sudden noises that could trigger panic attacks — you need to explain why. You may qualify for these accommodations under the Americans with Disabilities Act (ADA). If you don't want special accommodations, it's completely up to you whether to discuss your PTSD with your supervisor.

✔ **Talk with your staff if you're the supervisor or boss.** If you're a manager or the boss of your company and your PTSD symptoms are likely to be evident at times, give your employees the info they'll need to put these symptoms in context. You don't need to say, "I have PTSD" (although that's often the simplest way to handle the situation). Instead, you can say something like, "As a result of my accident, I tend to jump out of my skin if I hear a loud noise. I may also get more upset than I should if I'm startled. So don't take it personally if you drop a plate and I bite your head off — it's just taking me a little while to get over that reaction. I appreciate your understanding — you're a great bunch."

Smoothing your way with a powerful thank-you

Here's a helpful hint: If your supervisor does welcome you back and goes out of her way to make your return smooth, acknowledge her efforts with what I call the Power Thank-You. This tool helps you solidify her support in the event that your remaining PTSD symptoms cause problems down the road. Here are the two steps of a Power Thank-You:

1. **When you say thanks, acknowledge the extra effort she made to help you.**

You may say, "I know you went to a lot of extra trouble to find me a quieter location in the office, and I really appreciate it."

2. **Tell her what a difference her actions made to you.**

You may say, "It was so helpful of you to talk with my coworkers about understanding my flashbacks. I feel much less worried about the reception they'll give me."

Handling the demands of the job

If you plan to return to the job you had before your PTSD struck, you have the advantage of knowing the routine already. Because you know what to expect, you can think about potential stressors and plan ways to defuse them. Here are a couple of examples:

- ✔ If certain machinery sounds trigger unpleasant memories of your trauma, try listening to music or nature tapes through headphones while you work; use a white noise machine to distract yourself from the noises; or record the sounds at work and then play them back at home so you can desensitize yourself to them.

- ✔ If certain sights at work upset you, you may want to ask ahead of time whether you can move your desk to a different area.

In the following sections, you can take a look at some other techniques.

Packing a stress-management toolbox

You can prepare for your return by creating a toolbox of coping and relaxation aids that you can take to work with you. This toolbox can be a small carton or envelope that you can tuck away in your purse, desk, or wallet. Items to put in your toolbox can include

- ✔ **Affirmations:** Write out several positive statements, such as these:

  - *I'm very talented, and I have the tools I need to do my job well.*

  - *I have the confidence to remain calm during any tense situation.*

  - *I have the power to respond to criticism in a positive way.*

- ✔ **Relaxation exercises:** Make a list of relaxation techniques you can use quietly at your desk. (Even if you know the techniques by heart, keeping a written list at hand can remind you to put them into action.) You can find some good examples in Chapter 12.

- ✔ **Anchors:** Include one or two objects that remind you of your strengths or favorite aspects of your life — for example, a medal from a contest you won or a photo of your kids or Fido.

- ✔ **Jokes:** Humor is one of the best ways to defuse stress and short-circuit a blowup. Clip out a funny cartoon or write down a couple of jokes that always make you giggle.

Getting help from co-workers

If one of your co-workers is a trustworthy friend, ask him to give you a heads-up if he sees you getting tense or reacting to a situation in a PTSD-think way. One way to do this discreetly is to come up with a code word or phrase she can drop innocently into a conversation. (One person used the phrase "Is it warm in here?" to remind a colleague to chill out when things got tense.)

If your symptoms are still significant, you probably need to clue in your boss and co-workers about your PTSD. Otherwise, you may prefer to keep this part of your life private.

Dealing with discrimination

When you return to work, you may encounter what you feel to be unfair discrimination on the job because of your PTSD symptoms. In such a case, you can turn to several sources of help or information:

- A union representative (if you belong to a union)
- Your company's human resources department
- The U.S. Equal Employment Opportunity Commission's disability discrimination information Web site at `eeoc.gov/types/ada.html`, where you can find information on the ADA

Explaining your PTSD to a new employer

That first day on a new job is stressful, and you're even more likely to have butterflies if you're overcoming PTSD and you're worried about how your condition will affect your career. Of course, if you're asking a company to make specific accommodations for your PTSD, your employer needs to be aware of your symptoms early on (for info on how to handle this, see the Equal Opportunity Commission's fact sheet at `www.eeoc.gov/facts/jobapplicant.html`.)

If your symptoms are mild or moderate and you don't need special accommodations, what you tell your employer is up to you. Here are some good ground rules:

- **Be straightforward about symptoms that show.** Tell your boss about any problems he'll notice anyway. For instance, if you work in a building with armed security guards and the sight of someone wearing a gun makes you shivery and sweaty, casually mention, "I was injured a while back by an armed robber, and the sight of a gun still scares me, but don't worry if I get a little wonky when the security guard walks by — I'm getting over it."

- **Avoid TMI.** TMI stands for *too much information* — like when Great-Aunt Bertha tells you about her hemorrhoids. You want your new boss to view you as an asset, not a problem, so confine your explanations of your symptoms to a brief few sentences. Don't give her the history of your trauma and its aftermath or lots of other details. Your therapist wants to hear this information; your boss doesn't.

✔ **Explain your solutions.** If you need to tell your boss about a PTSD symptom, also note any solutions you have for handling this symptom. For instance, if your manager notices that you're hypersensitive to noises, you can note, "I found a great solution to this problem — I wear noise-cancelling headphones at my desk." Bosses like problem-solvers, so you can earn points with this approach.

Weighing your options if 9-to-5 isn't for you

If you're eager to get your career back in gear but you're not quite ready for the pressures of the full-time, on-site workday world, take heart: You may have other options. Depending on your skills and interests, these options can include

✔ **Telecommuting:** If your job involves working with a computer, your boss may be willing to let you work from home or combine on-site work with some telecommuting. This option can be great if you have trouble driving or handling office stress due to lingering PTSD symptoms.

✔ **Working part time:** If you can get by on a reduced salary, this choice is often a good one because it reduces the amount of workday pressure you need to handle. If you choose this option, make sure you understand how switching from full time to part time will affect your health insurance and other benefits.

✔ **Consulting:** Many people with PTSD find that their former employers are willing to hire them as consultants instead of requiring them to stay on as full-time employees. If you find this option attractive, remember that you'll need to make arrangements for health insurance. Depending on what field you're in, you may be able to sign on with a consulting firm that offers both job flexibility and benefits.

✔ **Working at home:** This option is excellent for many people whose PTSD symptoms make it hard to cope with interpersonal relationships or on-the-job pressures. Working at home gives you access to a wider range of relaxation and coping tools, and it can give you the flexibility to schedule your work for times when you're feeling up to par. On the other hand, it typically doesn't offer you the safety net of paid health insurance and other benefits. Working at home also requires self-discipline. Further, the lack of contact with other people may not be healthy if it causes you to sink into depression or loneliness.

Finding financial solutions if you can't return to work

For some people, returning to the workforce simply isn't an option because their PTSD symptoms are still too disabling. If you find yourself in this situation, finding a way to stay afloat financially is a huge concern.

In many cases, people with PTSD qualify for some form of disability benefits. The most common types of benefits include

- ✓ Workers' compensation if your PTSD is clearly linked to an on-the-job trauma

- ✓ Service-connected disability benefits if your PTSD stems from trauma experienced during military service (for more on this subject, see Chapter 5)

- ✓ Social Security benefits for people with disabilities — two different types of these benefits are available:

    - • Social Security Disability Insurance (SSDI), which pays benefits if your disability qualifies and if you paid Social Security taxes and worked long enough to be covered

    - • Supplemental Security Income (SSI), which pays benefits based on financial need if your disability qualifies you for coverage

- ✓ Private disability insurance coverage through an employer

You can't find a simple, one-size-fits-all answer as to whether you qualify for disability benefits because of your PTSD, but here are a few of the key factors that may play a role in determining whether you'll get coverage:

- ✓ Whether your PTSD is work-related or occurred outside work

- ✓ How severe and long-term your symptoms are

- ✓ Whether you have multiple disabilities

- ✓ How well you can document your symptoms and treatment

- ✓ How aggressive you're willing to be in pursuing your claim

 If you decide to seek disability benefits, be prepared for the fact that obtaining these benefits is often a chore and sometimes a battle. To weed out some bad apples, bureaucratic agencies put everyone through an inquisition — including the overwhelming majority of people who clearly need and deserve benefits. Here are some steps you can take to prepare for this challenging experience:

✔ **Gather your evidence.** Put together all the records you have to document your PTSD. If you don't have the records you need, ask your doctors or therapists for copies. (You may need to pay a small fee.)

✔ **Get legal help.** If you're not confident that your claim is ironclad, consider hiring an attorney who can help you prove your case. If you can't afford an attorney, ask your local Legal Aid Society about your options.

✔ **Brush up on your coping skills.** The agency you're approaching may appear obstructive, unsympathetic, or even hostile at times. Remind yourself that they're not really attacking you as a person; it's all part of the process, so don't take it personally.

✔ **Find out the facts.** Don't expect to master the fine points of disability law, which can give even lawyers a migraine headache. But if you bone up a little on general terms and broad laws, you should find it easier to understand the information you get from an agency or attorney. Most civilian claims involve the Social Security Administration (SSA). You can get information about the process at these Web sites:

- The SSA page "Benefits for People with Disabilities" at www.ssa.gov/disability

- The National Organization of Social Security Claimants' Representatives, www.nosscr.org, where you can find a wealth of information about the ins and outs of qualifying for Social Security benefits as a result of your disability

- Social Security Disability Secrets, www.disabilitysecrets.com, which contains materials written by a former disability claims examiner

If you're a veteran and you're pursuing a service-related disability, resources include

- Veterans Benefits Administration at www.vba.va.gov

- Iraq War Veterans Organization, Inc., at www.iraqwarveterans.org/disability_claim_info.htm

- Vietnam Veterans of America at www.vva.org/benefits/ptsd.htm

Recognizing the Positive Effects of Your Experience

There's an old story about a man who goes to his rabbi and complains, "Life is unbearable. There are nine of us living in one room. What can I do?" The rabbi replies, "Bring your goat into the room with you." The man stares at him, aghast, but the rabbi says, "Do it, and come back in a week."

The gift of perspective

Years ago, I saw two elderly women with arthritis in my psychotherapy practice on the same day. The first lady was very attractive and expensively dressed, and I didn't even realize that she had arthritis until she told me. Her mild case of the disease caused her very little pain, but she complained bitterly about how disfiguring her arthritis was and about how she needed to have her rings resized.

A few hours later, another elderly woman came into my office. She was hunched over and walked slowly across the room with the help of a cane. Her back and hands were deformed and twisted. Yet she also had one of the most radiant smiles I'd ever seen. Puzzled, I said, "I notice that you have severe arthritis and have difficulty walking, yet you have an amazing smile. I don't get it. How come?"

She looked at me and said, "I was just thinking how great this cane is going to look in a couple years, when I'm in a wheelchair."

This woman, at 75, had experienced loss, tragedy, illness, and all the other suffering that comes with living to a ripe old age. That suffering left scars and sadness — but it also gave her the perspective that allowed her (unlike my first patient) to treasure the good things in her life rather than take them for granted.

Like her, you'll carry some scars of your trauma for your entire life. But you'll also carry the gifts it gave you — if you're wise enough to see them.

Seven days later, the man comes back and says, "Life is even worse. The goat smells terrible, and we're even more crowded. Now what do we do?" The rabbi smiles and replies, "Put the goat back outside, and come back in a week."

Seven days after that, the man returns to the rabbi and says, "Life is beautiful! We're so happy that there's no goat — just the nine of us!"

What's the moral of the story? Often, whether you're happy or unhappy depends not on what's really happening in your life but on your perspective. That same perspective can help you as you recover from PTSD by allowing you to see that although you lost a great deal during your struggle, you also received some valuable gifts.

To help you identify those gifts, ask yourself the following questions. Remember that the goal is *not* to minimize the horrific ordeal you suffered or the intense pain you endured when PTSD took over your life but to help you become aware of the positive lessons you learned and the gains you experienced in going through this stage of your life. Recognizing the good changes in your life since PTSD struck can help put the bad changes in perspective and give greater meaning to your trauma and recovery.

✔ What new skills or inner strengths did you develop as a result of surviving your trauma and your PTSD?

- What new, positive relationships do you have as a result of this experience?

- How has your sense of empathy for other people changed as a result of what you went through?

- How has your sense of purpose in life changed as a result of overcoming your trauma and your PTSD?

- Do you feel a greater appreciation for the joys and blessings in your life?

- Do you have a better sense of who your true friends really are, based on how they came through in your time of need?

- Do you have a better sense of what's important in your life and what isn't?

Part IV
Healing and Rebuilding during and after Treatment

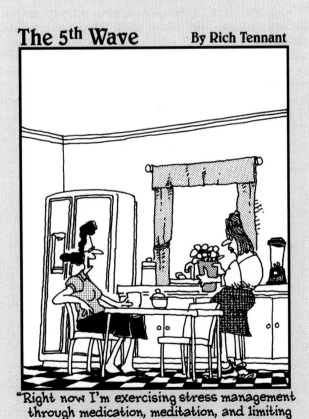

The 5th Wave   By Rich Tennant

"Right now I'm exercising stress management through medication, meditation, and limiting visits from my pain-in-the-butt neighbor."

In this part . . .

You're the quarterback of your PTSD recovery team, and in this part, I look at how you can make all the right moves. First, I talk about what you can expect in therapy and how you can maximize your results. I then describe the simple and highly effective steps you can take to heal both your mind and your body as you take control. I also talk about the effects of PTSD on your family and how you can strengthen family bonds frayed by PTSD. In addition, I offer advice on getting your life (both personal and professional) back in the groove as you recover.

Chapter 15

Getting Help for a Child with PTSD

In This Chapter

▶ Knowing when to seek professional help

▶ Understanding the different needs of children and adults with PTSD

▶ Weighing your therapy options

▶ Creating a game plan for helping your child at home

▶ Getting your child's school, friends, and family in the loop

Snakes and snails and puppy-dog tails. Sugar and spice and everything nice. That's what kids' lives are supposed to be made of.

All too often, however, fear and pain shatter a child's world. Frequently, the innocence of childhood ends abruptly when a parent dies, a natural disaster strikes, or a car accident occurs. In other cases, physical, sexual, or psychological abuse cuts the joy of childhood short.

Fortunately, the therapies that work with adults can also help children put the pieces of their lives back together again. In this chapter, I look at when to seek professional help for a child troubled by trauma; why treating kids is different from treating grownups; what kinds of therapy can help a child with PTSD; and how getting everyone on your child's team can speed up the healing process.

Recognizing the Nuances: Normal Childhood Behavior versus PTSD

Consider these scenarios:

> Davey refuses to go to summer camp.
>
> Seri, an honors student, stops doing her homework and gets a D in math.
>
> John gets into a fight at school and gets suspended.
>
> Darla clings to her mom's leg when it's time to go to school and screams, "No! Don't leave me!"

Maybe all these children are displaying symptoms of PTSD — or maybe they're all acting perfectly normally. As a parent trying to help a child come to terms with a trauma, how can you tell the difference between typical, healthy behavior and a serious problem?

The short answer: It isn't easy. In Chapter 3, I describe how to spot red flags for PTSD in children at different ages. Telling a normal childhood mood or behavior from a symptom can be difficult, however. In the end, you're likely to have to make a judgment call.

Here's why deciding whether a child's problems add up to PTSD is very hard for parents (and often even for doctors):

- ✔ Kids express the pain of PTSD differently from adults. In kids, anything from bedwetting to flunking an algebra test could be a reaction to trauma.

- ✔ Kids change from day to day, and telling normal changes from worrisome ones is hard — especially during the tumultuous teen years, when those scary hormones kick in.

- ✔ Children's PTSD symptoms often fluctuate over time. A child may be withdrawn and quiet for a month or two and then get jumpy or experience nightmares and flashbacks. These changing patterns can make it tough to identify the three core PTSD symptoms: intrusive thoughts, avoidance, and hyperarousal (for more on these subjects, see Chapter 3).

All these factors make deciding whether a child needs professional help a challenge, and that challenge usually falls squarely on the shoulders of Mom or Dad. In the next sections, I offer some guidelines that can help you answer this difficult question. If you're on the fence after reading these sections, err on the side of caution and consult your child's doctor.

Note: If your child's trauma occurred very recently (only a few weeks ago), he may be experiencing symptoms of acute stress disorder. See Chapters 2 and 4 for information about this problem and steps you can take to reduce the chances that the trauma will turn into PTSD.

Deciding Whether to Consult a Pediatrician

A strange rash or a hoarse cough is a clear sign that your child needs to visit the doctor. But PTSD is much harder to pin down, so you may have trouble knowing whether a consultation with the pediatrician is in order. Here are some guidelines that can help you decide whether your child's symptoms are serious enough that you should ask the doctor if it's PTSD.

Do the symptoms interfere with your child's life?

All children experience powerful feelings after a trauma, including fear, anxiety, irritability, confusion, anger, and sadness. For days or weeks after a life crisis, these emotions can get in the way of school and cause a child to avoid friends, lash out at family members, or simply curl into a ball in front of the TV and tune out the world.

All these reactions are perfectly normal, which is why doctors don't diagnose PTSD when people have short-term symptoms (see Chapter 2 for more on the differences between normal stress responses and PTSD). What *isn't* normal is when symptoms continue to interfere with a child's school, home, and social life for months or even years after trauma strikes. Here are some examples of the differences between typical and worrisome responses:

- ✔ It's normal for a child to have trouble concentrating on math or geography for a few weeks or months after a life crisis. But if a former A student seems to lose all motivation to study and her grades slide semester after semester, those changes are big warning signs.

- ✔ Kids overflow with conflicting emotions after a trauma, and those emotions can translate into crying jags, temper tantrums, or hostility. Again, all these responses are normal. But a child who continues to alienate good friends, cry at the drop of a hat, avoid social events, or get detention at school month after month is crying out for help.

Assessing overall changes in your child's lifestyle

To gain some clues about whether your child's symptoms add up to PTSD, you need to look at the big picture by analyzing his performance in different areas of life since the trauma. Remember that symptoms that are normal during the first few weeks after a trauma are cause for concern if they strongly affect his life for months or longer. Think about how he's doing in these areas:

- ✔ **School:** Did your child's grades drop dramatically after the trauma? Did he lose interest in getting good grades for college or stop caring about after-school activities he once loved (such as a sports team or drama) without replacing them with new, positive interests?

- ✔ **Friends:** Is your child breaking long-term bonds of friendship, hooking up with a bad crowd, or shrinking into a shell and avoiding contact with other people?

- ✔ **Family:** Is your child's relationship with you very different from the way it was before the trauma? Does he fail to find pleasure in family activities that he once loved or frequently lash out at family members, verbally or physically? If your child is young, does he have severe separation anxiety and scream or cry when you need to leave him?

✔ **Behavior:** Does your child act very differently from the way he did before the trauma? Does he now have a hair-trigger temper, jump at the least noise, or avoid places that remind him of the trauma? Do TV shows or movies upset him? Is he either too fearful (even of things not directly related to the trauma) or too quick to try dangerous activities? Does he suffer from frequent, intense nightmares? Does he seem abnormally numb and unable to experience normal feelings? Does he refuse to talk about the trauma at all — or conversely, seem to be unable to *stop* talking about it when the topic comes up? Is he wetting the bed or acting like a baby much of the time?

If you answer *yes* to any or all of these questions and if your child's trauma occurred one or more months ago, talking to your child's doctor is a good idea. On the other hand, if your child's symptoms are very mild and he's doing okay at school and at home, it's probably safe to assume that watchful waiting is fine for now. (See Chapter 4 for tips on ways to help your child recover if his symptoms are mild or if he's still in the early days after a trauma.)

Considering signs of depression

Many children with PTSD show signs of depression. Parents may miss these signs because they typically don't think of depression as a possibility unless a child is weepy or unhappy. But strange as it sounds, depressed kids don't always act sad (although sadness *is* a common symptom). Here are some of the other symptoms kids may show:

✔ Changes in eating (overeating, loss of appetite) or sleeping (insomnia, oversleeping, nightmares)

✔ A sense of hopelessness, worthlessness, or guilt

✔ Inability to express happiness or joy

✔ Loss of interest in favorite activities

✔ Fatigue, or periods of fatigue alternating with periods of overactivity (the latter may be symptomatic of bipolar disorder, also known as manic depression)

✔ Poor school performance and inability to concentrate on schoolwork

✔ Overreaction to minor failures or rejections

✔ Anger or hostility

✔ Isolation from friends or family members

✔ Headaches, stomachaches, or other chronic physical symptoms

✔ Suicidal thoughts or behavior

Many of these symptoms overlap with PTSD, so drawing a line between the two disorders is impossible. But from a parent's point of view, the distinction doesn't matter; both PTSD and depression require the urgent attention of a medical professional.

Could the symptoms endanger your child or others?

Just like adults, kids can react to a trauma by developing destructive behaviors. When they do, you need to act quickly before they can harm themselves or other people.

If your child exhibits any of these behaviors, seek professional help immediately:

- ✓ Violence toward family or friends — not the usual roughhousing or minor scuffling but serious acts that hurt or scare others
- ✓ Dangerous risk-taking, such as unsafe sexual behavior, speeding, or drunk driving
- ✓ Drug or alcohol abuse
- ✓ Depression (see the earlier section "Considering signs of depression" for symptoms)
- ✓ Eating disorders (see Chapter 3)
- ✓ Cutting or other self-injurious behaviors (see Chapter 3)
- ✓ Suicidal thoughts or behavior

In these situations, seeking help isn't an option — it's a necessity. To speed up the process, consider making an appointment directly with a child psychiatrist rather than starting with a pediatrician or general practitioner.

Are your child's symptoms getting better or worse?

The symptoms that stem from a trauma often follow a cyclical course but typically fade over time. If you're confident that your child's symptoms are decreasing, you can let nature take its course while you keep a watchful eye out for problems. But if your child's symptoms don't start improving by a month or so after the trauma — or if you think they're getting worse — you need to call for help.

One way to tell whether things are getting better, staying the same, or getting worse is to track your child's moods and behaviors. Stash a calendar in a drawer and note the days when your child is out of control, withdrawn, or otherwise troubled. Also note whether the behaviors are severe or mild so you can spot trends. If your child is a teenage girl, see whether her mood swings track with her periods; this information can help you decide whether you're facing PMS instead of PTSD. You may want to code your calendar (one parent wrote *water plants* every time her daughter went on a crying jag!) so your child doesn't get upset if she comes across it.

Among the things you can track on your timeline are

- ✔ How often your child has an emotional meltdown
- ✔ How often he has nightmares about the trauma
- ✔ How often she says *no* to activities she once enjoyed
- ✔ How often you feel alarmed or uneasy about his behavior (your gut feelings are a good indicator of whether things are getting better or worse)

Talk to your child. That's easier said than done with a teen, but even small clues can help you decide whether a behavior is worsening or whether your child is just going through a normal life issue. What strikes you as disturbing moodiness may turn out to be a typical reaction to getting the cold shoulder from a hot guy or losing a spot on the basketball team.

Enlisting the Help of a Doctor: The Order of Events

If you think your child's symptoms point to PTSD, share your concerns with a doctor. First, make an appointment to talk with the doctor alone. If she knows what to expect, she can be on the lookout for PTSD symptoms when you bring your child to the next appointment.

When you return to the doctor's office with your child, the doctor may ask both you and your child some questions that upset you. (For instance, if your child experienced a death in the family, the doctor may ask him questions such as, "Are you very angry about what happened?" or "Are you worried that other people in your family may die?") She needs to ask these questions to assess how troubling your child's symptoms are, so answer any questions openly and honestly and encourage your child to do the same. Kids are less likely to volunteer symptoms than adults are, so doctors need to do some poking around to fill in the blanks. Good doctors do this probing in a sensitive, age-appropriate way, but a few tears still may flow.

Most likely, your child's doctor will be able to form a preliminary opinion after one visit. If she suspects PTSD, she'll probably refer you to a psychological professional for an in-depth evaluation and therapy if the evaluation does indicate PTSD. (See Chapter 6 for info on the different types of professionals who specialize in treating PTSD.)

If you disagree with your doctor's conclusions, get a second opinion. Childhood PTSD is one of the hardest diagnoses for a doctor to make, and two doctors may come to very different conclusions because even the experts disagree on what PTSD looks like in young children and in teenagers.

Knowing Why and How Treating Children Differs from Treating Adults

If you and your child's doctor agree that your child shows signs of PTSD, try to find a therapist who's experienced in treating kids the same age as your child. Kids with PTSD are different from adults in several ways, and what works for a 40-year-old won't do the job for a 4-year-old or a 14-year-old.

In this section, I offer a quick look at the big differences between the PTSD treatments for grownups and kids, and I explain why therapists who treat children need to use approaches that differ from those used by therapists who treat adults.

Differences in language abilities and cognitive skills

Therapies for adults with PTSD typically involve a whole lot of talking. But a young child really doesn't have enough language to express his feelings and may not even be able to describe his trauma verbally. A therapist can address these limitations in several ways:

✔ By using words and concepts that a child can understand

✔ By using pictures or videos

✔ By using toys, dolls, puppets, clay, or crayons to help a child express what she can't say in words

In addition, a therapist who's trained in working with children understands the ways in which children think differently from adults and designs a therapy approach that takes these differences into account:

✔ Very young children often think that bad events stem from their own thoughts and actions. (Child development experts call this belief *magical thinking.*) Therapists who work with children are careful to reassure small patients that they aren't to blame for hurricanes, illnesses, or car accidents. This reassurance is crucial because guilt plays a big role in PTSD — for kids as well as adults.

✔ In different ways depending on their ages, children (and even teens) see their parents as omnipotent protective shields, so they feel betrayed and angry when Mom or Dad can't save them from a trauma. A therapist trained in helping children addresses this sensitive issue in a way that's appropriate to your child's developmental level.

✔ Teens often act out their PTSD in dangerous ways because at this age, they believe (to some degree) that they're invulnerable to death or serious injury. A therapist can help a teen take a hard look at the long-term consequences of risky behavior.

Differences in experience and coping skills

Life is full of big and little upsets, and weathering these storms gives you a wonderful gift called *perspective*. Perspective helps cushion the blows of life crises because you can look back at the past and say, "I overcame a problem like this before, so I know I can do it again."

To understand how this phenomenon works, think back to the first time you lost a pet or moved away from a best friend. At first, you thought you couldn't survive the pain. In a few weeks, however, you moved on with your life. The next time you suffered a similar loss, you instinctively knew that you'd get through it and feel better in time.

Kids, however, often have very little experience with the school of hard knocks. When a big trauma shakes their world, it can be even more shocking for them than it is for an adult because they can't call on experience as a guide. For this reason, a therapist may need to help a child develop the resilience and coping skills that an adult already possesses.

Another difference between kids and adults with PTSD involves the feelings of helplessness that often arise after a trauma. An adult often comes to terms with these feelings in therapy by realizing that he's not really helpless and that he has ways to cope if another crisis arises. An adult who develops PTSD after a natural disaster, for example, may recognize that he can protect himself in the future by buying better homeowner's or medical insurance, taking steps to make his home safer, or even moving to a less disaster-prone area.

The situation is not quite the same for kids because to a larger degree than adults, they *are* helpless, and they recognize this fact. A young child knows that she can't fend for herself if a hurricane, fire, or flood strikes. She can't drive, find shelter, or handle medical emergencies. Thus, her sense of helplessness following a disaster can be deeper than an adult's — especially if Mommy or Daddy couldn't be there to help her during the initial trauma.

Therapists who work with children can address this problem by helping even the youngest children identify what they *did* do to help take control of a situation (such as following the family's fire drill procedure during a home fire). In addition, the therapist can help a child come up with ways to feel a bit of control or take steps to help him regain his confidence that adults will do their best to protect him if another crisis occurs.

Understanding Common Treatments for Children and Teens with PTSD

Some aspects of medicine are so well studied that it's almost silly. (Do we *really* need another study saying that french fries are bad for you?) Other areas, however, are largely unexplored territory. Unfortunately, childhood PTSD falls into that category.

The research on what works and what doesn't for treating PTSD in kids is skimpier than it should be, but doctors and therapists can draw some good conclusions about the most common approaches. In the following sections, I discuss these approaches and explain what professionals know and don't know about their effectiveness.

Note: If your child's trauma is very recent and if a doctor or therapist recommends an intervention called *crisis intervention* or *psychological debriefing*, see Chapter 4 for a discussion of this approach. Because this therapy is used for at-risk children rather than those who already have PTSD, I don't discuss it in the following sections.

Cognitive behavioral therapy (CBT)

In Chapter 8, I talk about *cognitive behavioral therapy* (CBT), the most popular and well-validated approach for treating PTSD in adults. (This form of treatment is also referred to as *trauma-based CBT* because it asks patients to re-experience their trauma to overcome it.) Studies strongly indicate that CBT is also an excellent therapy for children.

Agreeing to let your child participate in CBT is a big step because this therapy requires your child to confront her trauma — though she'll do it in the safe setting of a therapy room. In the following sections, I look at how CBT therapists tailor their methods to children and why these methods are safe and effective even for young kids.

How CBT for kids differs from CBT for adults

Just like adult therapy, CBT for children starts by teaching children techniques for relaxation and stress management; then it helps them confront their trauma and make sense of what happened to them. CBT therapists who work with children, however, modify their techniques to take the following factors into account:

✔ **Age and developmental level:** CBT can work for children as young as 3 years old, but therapists often use techniques for children that differ from the ones they use for adults. A CBT therapist may ask a 6-year-old to act out the trauma with dolls or to draw pictures of his trauma, as well as describe the scene verbally. The therapist may also use role-playing to allow the child to understand the trauma from different people's points of view.

✔ **The role of parents:** Therapists who work with kids realize that parents are the most important people in a child's life and that they're crucial to the child's success in healing from PTSD. Thus, therapists include Mom, Dad, or both in many sessions.

CBT therapists who work with children use the same methods and have the same goals as those who work with adults, so to find out more about CBT in general, start with Chapter 8.

How CBT benefits kids and teens

Just thinking about letting a therapist ask your child to relive the terrifying event she suffered is likely to upset you. That reaction is natural because you want to protect her from any more pain. But in reality, she's in pain already — and the only way she can let go of the event that holds her in its grip is to revisit it in a safe setting and understand its effects.

As your child works through her trauma and figures out how to see it through new eyes, her initial fear and distress will fade, and she'll become more confident, happy, and ready to face the future. Her therapist can help her do this by zeroing in on these goals in particular:

✔ Helping her learn not to catastrophize events in his life so she won't be scared all the time; for instance, a therapist can help your child realize that

• If Daddy's feeling a little under the weather, it doesn't mean that he's having another heart attack.

• Cloudy skies usually don't mean that another tornado is on the way.

✔ Eliminating any misplaced guilt she feels as a result of the trauma

✔ Empowering her to feel strong and capable so that she's less fearful of potential future crises

Scientific support for CBT

Most research on the effects of CBT involves adults instead of children, but the number of pediatric studies is growing, and the results strongly support the effectiveness of this approach. Following are samples of recent findings:

✔ A 2006 study published by Ioanna Giannopoulou and colleagues in *Clinical Child Psychology and Psychiatry* followed 20 children who developed PTSD after a large earthquake in Athens, Greece. The researchers found that CBT resulted in a significant reduction in overall PTSD symptoms as well as symptoms of depression. Effects were long-lasting, with the children continuing to show positive effects four years after therapy.

✔ A 2006 study by Esther Deblinger and colleagues, published in the *Journal of the American Academy of Child and Adolescent Psychiatry*, involved 183 children who developed symptoms of PTSD after being sexually abused. The researchers compared CBT with a treatment called child-centered therapy (CCT), which doesn't specifically address the child's trauma. Their findings: Children treated with CBT had significantly fewer symptoms of PTSD and experienced less shame as a result of their trauma than the children who participated in CCT.

✔ A 2005 review in the journal *Depression and Anxiety* by Gili Adler-Nevo and Katharina Manassis compared three treatments for children with PTSD resulting from a single trauma; the report concluded that although all three therapies are effective, CBT has the best scientific support. (For info on the other two therapies, EMDR and play therapy, see the following sections.)

The National Center for Posttraumatic Stress Disorder recommends CBT for traumatized kids and teens, concluding that "this is the most effective approach for treating children." The Chadwick Center for Children and Families also highly recommended CBT in a comprehensive 2004 report on the best practices in the treatment of children traumatized by abuse.

Eye movement desensitization and reprocessing (EMDR) therapy

In Chapter 8, I explain how therapists use eye movement desensitization and reprocessing (EMDR) therapy to treat adults. This treatment is also growing in popularity for children because it's relatively quick and works well for children with limited verbal skills. In the following sections, I look at how pediatric therapists use EMDR and how effective it is.

Tackling inner-city PTSD

In some inner-city neighborhoods, crime or violence touches nearly every child's life at some point. A recent study of 6-year-olds at an inner-city pediatric clinic found that at one or more times in their lives,

- More than 40 percent saw another person being beaten up.

- More than one in eight witnessed someone being threatened with a knife.

- Seven percent saw someone being stabbed or shot.

These horrific statistics translate into sky-high numbers of inner-city children with PTSD.

Unfortunately, it's tough — if not impossible — for most families in these neighborhoods to find help for traumatized kids.

To address this problem, some therapists are offering school-based group sessions of CBT for inner-city students with PTSD symptoms. Research indicates that these interventions are highly effective in reducing PTSD symptoms, depression, and behavior problems in traumatized children. As a result, increasing numbers of inner-city schools are thinking about supplementing the three r's (reading, writing, and 'rithmetic) with a fourth r: recovery from trauma.

The basics of EMDR for children

EMDR is very similar to CBT (described earlier in this chapter and in Chapter 8) because it asks a participant to re-experience her trauma in the safety of a therapy setting. A patient participating in EMDR, however, recalls the trauma silently in short segments. At the same time, she uses her eyes to follow the therapist's finger as he moves it slowly and steadily from side to side.

Therapists use the same approach for children and adults when offering EMDR treatment, but they sometimes modify sessions in these ways:

- To hold a younger child's visual attention, the therapist may move an eye-catching finger puppet from side to side instead of moving a finger alone.

- Sessions tend to be shorter than those for adults. Sessions for children usually last about 45 minutes at most.

- Therapy for children often involves fewer sessions because children appear to react to the therapy more quickly than adults do.

The inside story on EMDR's effectiveness for kids

The scientific literature on EMDR for children is small but growing, and early results suggest that it's just as effective as CBT (which isn't surprising, because the two approaches are very similar). Here are some findings:

- In a 2002 study reported by Claude Chemtob and colleagues in the *Journal of Clinical Psychology,* researchers used EMDR to treat 32 children who still exhibited PTSD one year after a disaster. After treatment, the children showed significant improvements in PTSD symptoms, anxiety, and depression, and they continued to experience these positive changes at a six-month follow-up.

✔ A study by Guinevere Tufnell, published in *Clinical Child Psychology and Psychiatry* in 2005, followed four preteens treated with EMDR for PTSD symptoms. In all four cases, the children's symptoms were well-controlled within two to four sessions. A follow-up six months later showed that the children continued to do well.

EMDR has other advantages: It often works quickly, which can translate into faster healing as well as less expense for parents; and it's a good approach for very shy children or those with limited verbal skills because it asks children to recall their trauma silently rather than out loud.

Play therapy

Adults think of play as fun, but for kids, it's also a powerful tool for expressing love, rage, fear, and other very big emotions. For this reason, therapists often use play to explore what's going on in the mind of a child who's too young to describe his inner feelings in words.

In this section, I look at how professionals use play therapy to identify the psychic scars of children with PTSD and foster healing after a trauma, and I describe what professionals know about this therapy's usefulness.

The ABCs of play therapy

An adult knows about 50,000 words, but a child of 5 or 6 knows only about 5,000. What's more, an adult's vocabulary includes lots of expressions to describe emotions (such as "I was flabbergasted!" or "I was tense and on edge, like I was overcaffeinated"), whereas a young child's toolbox of words to describe his feelings is pretty limited. Because he has a small set of words to describe a big event, a young child can't always tell a parent or a therapist how he feels after a trauma changes his life.

Play therapy gets around the language problem by giving a child other outlets for expressing himself, including dolls, puppets, stuffed animals, toy houses and cars, sand, water, paint, clay, and crayons. Watching a child's play, a therapist can gently guide him to air his feelings. Here's an example of how this approach works:

✔ If the child repeatedly crashes two toy cars together, a therapist may ask, "How do the people in those cars feel when they crash together?"

✔ If the child draws a picture of a person screaming, the therapist may ask, "What is happening that's scaring that person?"

Gradually, a therapist can get a child to open up more and more about the trauma he experienced. The therapist has two goals in this process: to understand the child's thoughts and feelings and to use play to guide him to explore new ways of thinking and feeling.

A child traumatized by a dog attack, for example, may spontaneously reenact the trauma by using a toy dog to attack a doll named Charlie over and over. The therapist may respond in these ways:

✔ First, she may ask how the doll feels when the attack occurs. ("Is Charlie scared when the dog bites him on the foot?")

✔ Next, she may ask how the doll feels after the trauma occurs. ("What happens later, when a dog comes up to Charlie in the park?")

✔ Eventually, she may have the child experiment with different ways the doll could feel and act now. ("Here's a little friendly dog that's very different from that big mean one. This dog is very kind and gentle, and he's on a leash, so he can't run up and jump on Charlie. This dog really likes Charlie and wants to be his friend. Do you think that Charlie will be able to pet him?")

Play therapy can also be effective for older children who have trouble opening up verbally about their trauma. Doctors sometimes recommend this approach for children as old as 12.

The bottom line on play therapy

Play therapy is one of the oldest treatments for traumatized children, but judging its overall effectiveness is hard because most studies of this approach involve only one or two children. These small case studies don't offer much insight into how useful this approach is for kids in general.

In general, play therapy appears to be less effective than trauma-based CBT or EMDR, both discussed earlier in this chapter. It's an excellent choice, however, for children who are too young or frightened to benefit from CBT or EMDR and for kids with very limited verbal skills. It's also a gentle and non-threatening approach for many children with developmental disabilities.

In individual cases, the effects of play therapy can be very dramatic. Recently, WBHM, a National Public Radio affiliate in Birmingham, Alabama, reported on the effects of play therapy on a 4-year-old girl who had lost both kidneys to cancer. Before therapy, the child refused to speak to people in lab coats, regressed to baby talk, and covered herself with her sheets if a doctor entered the room. Now, after therapy, the little girl actively seeks out her doctors — and she doesn't hesitate to give them an earful about whatever's worrying her!

Play therapy is very safe and unlikely to cause any problems for your child, but one caution is in order: If your child is involved in legal proceedings stemming from a trauma (if he'll need to testify about an assault, for example), you should consult your therapist and your child's lawyer about the impact this therapy could have on the validity of his testimony. This consultation is important because without meaning to, a play therapist may alter a child's recollection of a trauma.

If you choose play therapy as the best option for your child, be sure your therapist is certified as either a Registered Play Therapist (RPT) or a Registered Play Therapist Supervisor (RPT-S).

Medications

Just like adults, children with PTSD sometimes benefit greatly from medications. For a child who's out of control, the right medication sometimes puts on the brakes long enough for psychological therapies to take hold. Drugs can have some serious adverse effects, however, so do your homework before you agree to any prescription for your child. Chapter 9 outlines the primary drugs used to treat PTSD, along with their benefits and dangers.

Doctors prescribe many of the same medications for children and teens, but these drugs can be far riskier for the younger set than for adults. Here's why:

- ✔ Researchers tend to study the effects of psychiatric drugs on adults more thoroughly than they study these drugs' effects on children. As a result, proof that a drug is relatively safe for an adult doesn't necessarily translate into proof that it's safe for a kid.

- ✔ Kids aren't just little grownups when it comes to medications. Because children are growing and changing, their metabolism and brain function can be very different — which means that drugs can affect them differently than they affect adults.

As a result, psychiatric drugs can have serious and sometimes surprising effects in kids, especially when a doctor combines two or more of these medications. I recommend using them only if a compelling reason for using them exists.

In particular, be extremely cautious if your child's doctor recommends antidepressants. Some of these drugs now carry "black box" warnings — the strongest warnings that the U.S. Food and Drug Administration can require — cautioning that the drugs may cause suicidal thoughts or behavior in children. Doctors are still debating whether antidepressants actually increase or decrease the overall risk of suicide in young people, but be aware that this is a potential concern.

If your doctor does recommend a medication for your child, here are some suggestions:

- ✔ If the doctor who recommends the medication is a family practitioner, ask for a referral to a child psychiatrist before accepting the prescription. Child psychiatrists are more likely to be up-to-date on the good and bad effects of psychiatric drugs on children than general practitioners are.

- ✔ Get a second opinion before you say *yes* to a medication, even if a child psychiatrist recommends it.

If you decide that medication is a good option, be sure that your child receives regular medical monitoring. Frequent tests can help prevent side effects or catch them at an early stage.

Also, realize that medications — even when they work wonders — should supplement psychological interventions instead of being a primary or sole treatment. See Chapter 9 for more on this important point.

Seeking Out a Therapist and Starting Therapy

Therapy can work wonders for a child with PTSD, especially when you find a sensitive and knowledgeable therapist who's able to develop a good rapport with your youngster. In this section, I offer advice on how to find the therapist who best suits both your child's needs and yours. In addition, I offer tips on getting your child to agree to go to therapy sessions, and I tell you a little about what to expect when you get to the therapist's office.

Finding a good therapist for your child

In Chapter 6, I list a variety of ways to locate a therapist. In addition to following the leads I suggest in that chapter, you may want to check with your child's school counselor for recommendations (but be discreet). Your pediatrician may also be able to make a referral.

If possible, get referrals for at least two or three therapists. Call each one and ask for a brief interview, either in person or over the phone. (If you meet in person, leave your child at home for the interview so you can talk frankly with the therapist.) Here are good questions to ask:

- ✔ Do you have specific training in working with children who are the same age as my child?

- ✔ How many years have you worked with children?

✔ What type of approach do you use?

✔ What credentials do you have?

✔ What's your philosophy about involving the child's family in treatment?

✔ Are you willing to collaborate with a child's school or doctor to address problems?

✔ What's your philosophy about using medications?

In general, you want a therapist who's licensed and has several years of experience in treating children with PTSD. Beyond that, look for a therapist whose ideas on issues such as medication use or family involvement in therapy jibe with your own. Also, use your instincts to decide whether the therapist seems like someone who can make your child feel comfortable.

For information on the different types of professionals who offer therapy for PTSD, as well as the financial aspects of therapy, see Chapter 6.

Getting your child to go

In most cases, adults seek therapy for PTSD because they accept the fact that they need help. They may come to this decision slowly, and friends or family members may need to help them overcome their denial, but in the end, the choice is generally theirs.

The situation is different for kids because usually parents — not the children themselves — decide that therapy is necessary. This arrangement typically isn't a problem with younger kids, who tend to go along with what their parents say. But a preteen or teenager may say, "I'm not going," or "You can drag me there, but you can't make me talk when I get there."

If your child objects to therapy, realize that kids (just like adults) often fight the idea of getting help because they're frightened or in denial. Also, your child may be scared that her friends will think she's "crazy" if they find out she's seeing a therapist. Here are some ways to win her cooperation:

✔ **Reassure her.** Let her know that getting therapy is like getting medical treatment for a sore arm or a headache and is nothing to be embarrassed about. But also agree that you won't talk to her friends (or yours) about her therapy if privacy makes her feel more comfortable.

✔ **Negotiate.** Make a deal that she needs to go to only a half-dozen sessions or so; then you'll evaluate how therapy is going. If you can get her foot in the door, she's likely to find that talking about her feelings with a caring therapist is easier and more rewarding than she expected.

✔ **Let her be part of the decision process.** Explain the different types of therapy to her, and get her input on what sounds best. Giving her some control of the situation may improve her attitude.

> ✔ **Offer a bribe.** Under normal circumstances, bribing your kid isn't the greatest idea — but if your child has PTSD, the circumstances aren't normal. So consider telling a reluctant child that you'll upgrade her computer, give her more cellphone minutes, or let her slide on her chores for a couple of months in exchange for her promise to participate willingly in therapy.

Picking your place: Therapy room or waiting room

Studies show that a parent's positive attitude and willingness to participate in therapy have a powerful effect on a child's ability to heal from PTSD. In addition, a parent's involvement in therapy can reduce a child's behavioral problems and symptoms of depression.

Parents often wonder whether they should participate in every therapy session with their children. The answer depends on your child's age. If your child is very young — say, 3 or 4 years old — a therapist may want you to participate in every session. If your child's older, however, the therapist may want to talk to him alone some or most of the time. Here's why:

> ✔ Your child may be embarrassed or ashamed about some aspects of the trauma and may be unwilling to discuss them with you in the room.

> ✔ Your child may want to avoid upsetting you and will hold back — an act that can reduce the effectiveness of therapy.

> ✔ If your child is a teen who's full of attitude — and what teen isn't? — he may spend less time being hostile or defensive if his favorite target (you) is out of the room.

If the therapist asks you to be involved in the sessions, give these sessions top priority in your life, no matter how many other work and home responsibilities you have. But bring a good book along to therapy sessions in case the therapist asks you to sit in the waiting room — and don't feel slighted if she does. Being asked to wait outside doesn't mean the therapist doesn't like you; it means that sometimes, three really is a crowd.

If you're very uncomfortable leaving your child alone with a therapist, look for a professional whose therapy room includes a one-way mirror so you can view your child's session without participating.

When you do take part in therapy sessions, resist the urge to be defensive if the therapist suggests ways to alter your own actions in order to foster your child's healing. (For instance, a therapist may suggest being firmer in handling some of your child's behaviors or, conversely, cutting your child more slack in some areas.) The therapist may seem to be challenging your skills as a parent if he offers you advice, but he's not. He just has a good feel for the ways in which PTSD can change family dynamics — something that's true in every family dealing with PTSD, not just yours — and he knows tricks for tweaking those dynamics in positive ways.

Also, help and support your child with any homework the therapist recommends. If the therapist asks your child to write in a journal each night, for example, schedule your child's chores so that they don't interfere, and make sure she has some quiet, uninterrupted time for this important task.

Helping Your Child Heal outside the Therapist's Office

When a trauma leads to PTSD, your child needs a whole team of people in his corner, including a therapist, a doctor, and a supportive school staff. Most importantly, he needs *you,* because you're the most important person in his life.

In the following sections, I talk about some simple steps you can take to assist your child in healing after a traumatic event. These steps can help both children at risk of developing PTSD and those already diagnosed with the disorder, so you don't need to wait for an official diagnosis to put these pieces in place.

Get on the same page as your partner

If you have a partner who's very involved in your child's life, talk together about what you can do to help your child. Have this conversation when your child isn't home so you can be frank and iron out disagreements.

Here are some issues you should resolve to make sure you're a solid team:

- ✔ **Do you both agree that your child's problems are significant?** If not, talk to a doctor or therapist together and see whether you can resolve this crucial question.

- ✔ **Do you agree on what type of therapy is appropriate?** If not, do some extra reading on the topic or interview additional therapists until you find an approach you both can accept.

- ✔ **What other steps can you take to aid in your child's healing?** Can either of you spend more time with her? Can you come up with a consistent plan for dealing with her emotional outbursts?

Don't be too upset with yourselves if you occasionally squabble about issues related to your child's PTSD; you're both experiencing some powerful emotions as well. But do try to present a united front and to keep your personal issues from affecting your child during this tough time in his life.

Understand your own feelings so you can foster your child's healing

When your child suffers a trauma, you suffer right along with him. In addition, you feel some very complex emotions because of your special relationship with your child. Here are some of the feelings you're likely to experience:

- ✔ **Guilt:** As a parent, you see yourself as your child's protector, and right now, you feel like you let him down. You're probably second-guessing every move you made before the trauma ("If only we'd sent him to a different school . . . forbidden him to go to that party . . . gotten him a safer car . . .").

- ✔ **Anger:** After a trauma hurts your child, you're angry, and you don't always direct that anger at the right targets. You may find yourself blowing up at a partner, your child's teacher, or anyone else in your path, even if that person had little or nothing to do with the situation. If you have a partner, the two of you may also argue about how serious your child's symptoms are and whether she needs help (see the preceding section for advice on resolving such issues). At times, you may even feel angry at your child if her symptoms cause her to say or do hurtful things.

- ✔ **A sense of rejection:** If you didn't experience the trauma with your child, he may say, "You can't understand; you weren't there." He may turn away from you at times and seek out the company of other people who lived through the trauma, making you feel like you're out in the cold.

- ✔ **Grief:** When your child experiences a trauma, your world changes, too. While you're busy trying to help your child cope, you're also coming to terms with your own grief about her pain and lost innocence.

All these emotions are normal. If they get in the way of both your healing and your child's, however, seek therapy for yourself. A support group (see Chapter 4) can also help you work through your feelings in a constructive way.

Keep life as calm as possible

When a trauma turns your child's world upside down, he needs to regain a sense of security, especially when PTSD enters the picture. One of the most powerful ways you can help your child re-anchor himself in the present is to keep his life as normal as possible. Here are some ways to reestablish routines after a life shakeup:

- ✔ If a natural disaster displaced you from your home and neighborhood, see whether your child can still get together with his friends. If possible, keep him in the same school and find ways for him to participate in activities he's used to, such as sports teams.

- ✔ If you can, keep mealtimes and bedtimes consistent and try to continue family rituals such as pizza nights or weekend bike rides. Mundane routines can be incredibly calming when the world seems off-kilter.

- ✔ If your child's favorite book, toy, or video was lost or destroyed in an accident or disaster, replace it as quickly as possible. A beloved possession, no matter how small, can serve as a link to reality and routine in a time of turmoil.

- ✔ If possible, keep familiar faces around: your child's usual babysitter, well-known relatives, familiar neighbors, and friends.

- ✔ Talk about the future to help your child understand that life will get back on track. For instance, if a fire temporarily displaces you, say, "By your next birthday, we'll be back in our house again — and I'll be making that chocolate cake you love." Conversations like this can help your child see his life crisis as a temporary disruption rather than the end of the world.

Encourage relaxing activities

A peaceful environment can help soothe a troubled soul, so keep your child's physical surroundings as calm and relaxing as possible. Here are some ways to accomplish this goal:

- ✔ Play relaxing or cheerful music that your child likes.

- ✔ If your child is a reader, get her a big stash of books by her favorite authors. If possible, look for books with calm plots (though books in which heroes overcome adversity can be inspiring, too, so don't say no to hobbits or Harry Potter).

- ✔ Follow holiday traditions, but tone them down if necessary. Focus on rituals that your child loves instead of overwhelming him with company or parties.

- ✔ If you have a budding chef at home, plan some cooking projects. A little thing like the smell of cookies baking can help a child relax and enjoy the moment.

✔ Encourage a good night's sleep with soft bedtime music and calming stories. If your child can't fall asleep on his own, it's okay to let him sleep in your bed (or in a sleeping bag in your room) for a few weeks.

Focus on your child's resilience

For decades, therapy for both children and adults focused almost exclusively on problems and psychic wounds. Now, however, experts know that focusing on a person's strengths is equally important — if not more important. Most people who survive a trauma are resilient and capable of healing. Therefore, sending the message "You're a survivor" is much more effective than sending the message "You're a victim."

Have faith in your child. She may always carry some scars from her ordeal, but she needs to know that you think she's strong and has the power to recover. Your actions and conversations should convey the message that you have confidence both in her and in her future.

Conversely, don't belittle what happened to your child. Acknowledge the depth of the trauma he suffered, as well as the fact that he suffered wounds and needs time to heal. Don't expect him to just get over it. Do expect some fallout from his ordeal to linger for months or possibly years.

Take charge of the remote

The magic of TV lies in its power to connect you to people, places, and events around the world. But that magic can turn dark when a trauma strikes your child because nonstop coverage of a crisis can overwhelm a traumatized child who can't come to grips with what she's seeing.

If the trauma that affected your child makes the nightly news, do your best to minimize the amount of coverage he sees. Watch TV when it's necessary (if your family survived a natural disaster, for example, and you need info on where to go and what to do), but try to avoid sensationalistic coverage or specials that air on the anniversary of a traumatic event. This advice applies both to children who already have PTSD and those who are at risk.

Understand symptoms (but don't dismiss everything as a symptom)

If you're the parent of a child with PTSD, you need the wisdom of Solomon and the patience of a saint, especially when your child acts up and you're left wondering, "Why is she doing this?"

It's important to acknowledge your child's symptoms while still expecting her to behave in ways that don't harm herself or others. Here are a few ground rules to help you walk this fine line:

- **Call on the pros.** When alarming behaviors arise, consult your child's therapist for ideas on how to handle them. If you don't have a therapist, your family doctor or a pastoral counselor (see Chapter 6) may be able to help.

- **Spot the connections.** Be sensitive to behaviors that probably stem from your child's trauma. Cut your child some slack if he's weepy, whiny, or irritable on anniversaries of his trauma, and don't make him attend holiday parties if they trigger emotional outbursts.

- **Draw the line.** No matter how much your child's hurting, you need to say a firm *no* to destructive or hurtful behavior. If your daughter slaps her sister, for example, say something like this: "I understand that you're in pain because of what happened to you and that it's going to take time to work through all your emotions. We're here to support you every step of the way. But it's never acceptable to hurt Janey or us. First, you need to apologize to Janey — and then you're going to do all her chores for the next month. Now let's talk about things you can do when you feel these overwhelming emotions and ways we can help you get control over them."

When your child's out of control, it's tempting to let him off the hook because your heart's aching for him and you don't want to add to his pain. But in reality, a child who can't rely on himself to set limits desperately needs you to set them for him. Be loving but firm.

Consider a support group

Face it — as much as you love your child, you can't really understand her a lot of the time (and vice versa). No matter how hard you work to bridge the generation gap, sometimes it's easier for a child or teen to open up to people her own age. For that reason, you may want to ask your child's therapist or your family doctor whether your child could benefit from attending a support group.

Also, think about joining a support group for parents of kids with PTSD if one exists in your area. Helping a child with PTSD is a huge challenge, and that burden can seem a little lighter if you share it with understanding people.

For information on how to locate support groups and for the benefits and possible drawbacks of these groups, see Chapter 4.

Getting School, Family, and Friends in the Treatment Loop

When your child is hurting, you need all the help you can get to make things right. For a child with PTSD, that help comes mostly from parents and therapists. But teachers, school counselors, friends, and relatives can aid in the healing process. In this section, I talk about how you can put these people to work for you and make sure that they do good rather than harm.

How teachers and other school staff can help

When PTSD enters the picture, you need to get your child's school in the loop. Here are some ways to get your child's teachers and other school personnel on your team (and the big advantages of doing so):

- **Talk to your child's teacher(s).** Ask for an appointment before or after school so you can speak privately. If your child has significant symptoms that interfere with schoolwork or socializing, describe these symptoms to the teacher and explain the best ways of handling them. Also offer the teacher some basic information on PTSD to help him understand the disorder and how it affects your child. You may also want to put the teacher in touch with your child's therapist so they can work together to solve school problems.

  If your child's schoolwork takes a hit, a teacher who's in the loop is more likely to find constructive ways to deal with the problem, such as letting your child make up for a failed test by doing an extra-credit project at home. A teacher who's on your team is also more understanding about PTSD-related behavior problems in the classroom or on the playground.

- **Meet with the principal if necessary.** If PTSD causes your child to act out, a principal who's aware of your child's issues will be in a better position to handle behavior problems in a positive way. Provide the principal with the same material you offer your child's teacher, and ask her to let you know if she spots problems the two of you can address together in a positive way.

- **Consult with the nurse.** Scheduling a meeting with the school nurse is a good idea if your child has significant symptoms such as panic attacks. A nurse who's part of your backup squad may be able to offer a safe haven to your child if he occasionally needs a place to hide out until he can get his symptoms under control. Also, make sure you update your child's medical information at school to reflect any medications being prescribed for his PTSD.

✔ **Chat with the school counselor.** If your child's symptoms affect her schoolwork or behavior, schedule a talk with the school counselor to inform him about the situation. A counselor who has the full picture may be able to offer good suggestions for handling these problems. In addition, he may be able to steer you to many community resources for both you and your child.

The key to getting your child's school on your side is *sensitivity*. Your daughter probably doesn't want to broadcast her PTSD to everyone on campus, so keep your conversations confidential. Discuss your concerns on the phone with teachers or other school staff members, or make an appointment to come in before or after school (and have a ready excuse for your visit handy if you spot any of your child's friends). PTSD is nothing to be ashamed of, but kids can be cruel, and your child needs to share her situation with friends in her own way.

How to bring friends and family into the picture

In Chapter 16, I outline a host of ways in which friends and family members can lend a hand in the recovery process. These methods are one-size-fits-all approaches because they work just as well for kids as they do for adults.

There's one difference, however: Deciding which people to tell about your child's PTSD, and exactly what to tell them, can be even trickier than it is for an adult with this disorder. Here are some suggestions:

✔ **Tell your child before you spread the news.** You don't want a sensitive child to be blindsided by Uncle Roy ("So I hear you have PTSD. How's the therapy going?"). If you decide to discuss your child's PTSD with other relatives, let your child know ahead of time and make sure he's comfortable with the information you're giving out.

✔ **Keep your explanations to friends and family upbeat and matter-of-fact.** You can tell Grandma, "We're very pleased that we've found an excellent doctor who's helping Alison with some of the symptoms she's experiencing as a result of the hurricane." Another helpful method is to talk about symptoms that friends and family are likely to witness ("Loud noises bother Mike, so we'll probably skip the Fourth of July party this year") — but unless people are very close and trusted, don't go overboard on the details.

✔ **If your child is young, let her best friends' parents know a little about the situation.** That way, they'll be more understanding if your child has an emotional meltdown or acts in hurtful ways. Describe the behaviors your child may exhibit and good ways to respond to them, and encourage them to talk with you if they have any questions or concerns.

✔ **Be matter-of-fact with a young child's friends.** Your child's buddies don't need a lecture on PTSD, but a little basic info can help keep friendships strong. For instance, you may say, "Right now, Heather feels sad and upset because she's remembering her mommy and missing her. That's why she sometimes doesn't feel like playing or talking. But you're still her best friend, even if she can't always show it right now."

✔ **If your child is a teen, let him choose how to handle the situation.** He'll probably have two words of advice for you: Butt out! If so, honor his wishes and let him tell his friends as much (or as little) as he wants about his PTSD.

One exception: If he says or does hurtful things, you may want to take his friends or their parents aside and give them a quiet heads-up. If you're discreet, you can respect your child's privacy while keeping his friends and their families on his side, which can play a big role in his recovery.

Chapter 16

Supporting a Loved
One with PTSD

*I*f you're trying to help a loved one with PTSD, you have my sincere respect, because supporting someone who's scarred by the deep, invisible wounds of trauma is a tough job. PTSD can make a person act cold and uncaring, push others away, or lash out cruelly. Trying to respond to these behaviors with love and loyalty is a huge task, and you deserve all the credit in the world for accepting this challenge.

To make your path a little easier, this chapter offers advice about the best ways to help a person with PTSD, as well as some common missteps to avoid. The chapter as a whole offers info for anyone who's trying to help — no matter what the connection to a person with PTSD — so you can find valuable advice in every section. However, because different people have different relationships with a person battling PTSD — parents, partners, extended family, or friends — I also offer sections tailored to the specifics of each relationship.

I begin by taking a look at the special role a partner or parent plays in the healing process. Next, I talk about how other family members and friends can show their love and support. In addition, I talk about the importance of watching out for your own health and well-being as you reach out to your loved one with PTSD.

The Biggest Struggle: Coping Strategies for Caregivers

If you're the partner or parent of someone with PTSD, you're the most important player on your loved one's support team. You may not feel like it, however, because right now, the person you care about isn't doing a good job of caring about *you*. In fact, you may often feel ignored, unloved, neglected, and ill-treated. (See Chapter 13 for more on the problems that PTSD causes in a partner's or parent's life.) But if you're reading this book, most likely you're committed to toughing it out and helping your loved one heal, no matter how rocky the road gets.

The tips I offer throughout this chapter can aid you in that mission. In this section, however, I offer advice that's tailored specifically to partners or parents — typically the unsung heroes in a person's battle against PTSD. Here are the best ways to help your loved one while keeping your own sanity.

Call for backup!

Living with a person with PTSD is stressful and often unsatisfying because your loved one can't meet all your needs when she's trapped in her own nightmare. Burning out is easy if you don't have someone to help you carry your load. In fact, social support is one of the biggest keys to keeping families together when they're battling PTSD. Getting this support isn't important just for you — it's vital to your loved one with PTSD as well.

 One place to turn for help is your extended family — aunts, uncles, in-laws, siblings, and grandparents. When these family members can't help enough — or when they're part of the problem — you need to tap other sources. The best idea is to visit a therapist, either with your loved one or by yourself (see Chapter 13).

 Another excellent option is to find other families dealing with PTSD who are facing the same challenges. These folks know just how it feels to live with a hubby with a hair-trigger temper, a wife who can't bear to be touched, or an adult son or daughter who drinks or uses drugs to mask the pain. They're happy to share their wisdom and experience or simply to offer moral support.

Here are two ways to team up with other people who are in the same boat as you:

> ✔ **Attend support groups.** If your loved one has drug or alcohol problems, look into groups that focus on these issues. Al-Anon and Families Anonymous are two of the best-known groups for family members of people with substance abuse problems. (See Chapter 4 for good ways to locate a support group in your area.)

✔ **Join a virtual community.** Online discussion forums can be outstanding sources of support and practical advice. (Be careful, however, not to give away too much personal info in these forums — something that's easy to do when you're having heart-to-heart conversations.) Dozens of discussion groups are available for partners or parents of people with PTSD, including this sampling:

- **General forum for loved ones of people with PTSD:** `www.ptsd-forum.org` (click the *Chat – Carers* link)

- **For partners of combat veterans:**
  `forums.grunt.com/forums/123.aspx`

  `groups.msn.com/AftermathofwarcopingwithPTSDtoo`

  `groups.msn.com/LivingwithPTSDVietnamWives` (this group also includes a forum for wives of veterans of other wars)

- **For partners of people overcoming sexual or physical abuse:** `www.thelighthousesanctuary.com/forum`

Even people who don't know much about PTSD can help if you give them a chance. Friends, neighbors, church members, and others may be willing to lend moral support or practical assistance. Be patient if they don't always say or do the right things (especially at first). Offer them books or articles, or steer them to Web sites that can help them understand PTSD (I provide a list of my favorites in the Appendix).

Know what you can and can't do

When you love a person with PTSD, you want more than anything to make that person feel better. But here's the hard part: Much of the time, you can't. The most important thing you need to know to help your loved one is this: *You didn't cause his PTSD, and you can't fix it.*

Drawing boundary lines between what you can and can't do maximizes your power to help and minimizes your risk of frustration and burnout. Here are some of the things you *can* do:

✔ **Be a sounding board.** Learn to listen without feeling that you need to solve every problem yourself. You can't solve all the problems, anyway, because your loved one has to find solutions on his own. Instead, offer a sympathetic ear and resist the urge to say, "I know just how you can handle that."

✔ **Recognize that your loved one's pain is real.** A person with PTSD has deep, unhealed wounds, and she lashes out because she's in agony. Acknowledging the reality of PTSD is the only way to understand why she does hurtful, self-destructive, or off-the-wall things. Do *not* let anyone tell you that her problem is "all in her head" or that she can "just get over it." (See Chapter 2 for more on the biochemical and physical realities of PTSD.)

✔ **Be patient.** Healing from PTSD takes a long time — sometimes a lifetime — and recovery often follows an ebb-and-flow pattern. Here are two corny but very true thoughts that many people find helpful in coping with day-to-day crises:

- **"This, too, shall pass."** Change is a fact of life, and your circumstances may be very different in a year or two. If your loved one is in therapy, you may see big changes for the better — but these changes rarely happen overnight.

- **"One day at a time."** Confronting all your problems at once can overwhelm you. A smarter plan, if you're overwhelmed by your responsibilities as a caregiver for a person with PTSD, is to focus solely on the issues you can deal with today. When you feel like you're drowning in crises, pick one you can handle — even if it's something small, such as a broken doorknob or a stack of paperwork that's piling up — and tackle it.

✔ **Keep up routines.** The familiar patterns of life can help anchor a troubled person to reality. Conversely, breaks in routine sometimes cause distress all by themselves, even for people who don't have PTSD. In fact, breaking regular routines can create withdrawal symptoms very similar to those in people withdrawing from drugs or alcohol! So keep up comfortable routines such as Friday-night pizza or weekend bike rides, and be sensitive to issues that arise if you need to alter those routines.

✔ **Have realistic expectations on big days.** Festive occasions like Thanksgiving and Christmas can be brutal for a person with PTSD because everyone's expected to be joyous and loving — something your loved one may not be able to do. Play it by ear on holidays, birthdays, and anniversaries, and let your loved one retreat to a quiet place if necessary. Be especially sensitive about holidays linked to the trauma in some way, such as a birthday that falls right before or after the anniversary of the trauma. Remember that a *reasonable* expectation (what you'd have every right to expect, under normal circumstances) isn't the same as a *realistic* expectation (what's likely to happen) — and plan for the latter.

✔ **Take care of your health.** Right now, you're the Rock of Gibraltar for your loved one, and you can't be there for him if you fall apart yourself. So do your best to exercise, eat well, and get sleep. If you have your own issues with drugs or alcohol, seek help. Take care of your mental and emotional health as well (see the section "Make sure you don't get lost in the mix," later in this chapter, for advice).

✔ **Recognize and accept that both of you are scared.** You're both frightened by the alarming symptoms and unpredictable course of PTSD. If the person with PTSD is your partner, you may also be scared that therapy will change your relationship — and scared that it won't. In addition, you may also be afraid that if your loved one heals, she won't love or need you as much. When you spot these fears and face them honestly, getting past them and tackling the hard work of recovery is easier.

Now here are some of the things you can't do and the burdens you shouldn't try to shoulder:

✔ **You can't handle your loved one's troubles alone.** Often, families coping with PTSD try to hide their problems from the world and tough it out on their own. But when you mix PTSD with denial and secrecy, you create a toxic cocktail that's bound to poison your relationship. Worse, this situation leaves you as your family member's therapist, caretaker, and problem-solver — a burden that causes resentment and sky-high stress levels (see more on this in Chapter 13). If your loved one refuses to seek help, seek it for yourself.

✔ **You can't turn your family into the Brady Bunch.** The household of a person who's suffering from PTSD can easily become a battleground. That's especially true if

- Your loved one's PTSD includes serious problems with anger or other emotional meltdowns.

- Your family includes kids — especially if you have one or more teenagers with big attitude.

- You're a parent whose adult child has moved back home after you and your spouse have gotten used to having your home to yourself — and you're discovering that three's a crowd.

You can easily tie yourself in knots trying to keep the peace in your household, but you probably won't succeed. Instead, if things get out of control, seek out a therapist and ask for ideas on handling stressful situations. If your partner or child with PTSD says no to family therapy, go yourself — and if you have kids, bring them along too. That way, the therapist — not you! — can shoulder responsibility for helping everyone sort out the mess. Or if the budget's tight, check out support groups for families dealing with PTSD. (For help in finding these groups, see Chapter 4.)

✔ **You can't always be Pollyanna.** PTSD shattered many of your dreams, so feeling resentful or angry is natural — especially if you're dealing with a loved one's alcohol or drug problems or if you're struggling financially because of your family member's disability. Don't feel guilty if you let your happy mask slip once in a while. You don't need to be a saint to help your loved one; in fact, sainthood can irk the heck out of a family member with PTSD who's feeling pretty imperfect himself.

Make sure you don't get lost in the mix

Fran, a patient I saw years ago, coined the phrase "Cheshire Cat Syndrome" — a concept that may ring a bell with many family members of people with PTSD. Fran spent her life trying to please her parents, lovers, friends, and co-workers while ignoring her own needs. As a result, she felt like the Cheshire Cat in *Alice in Wonderland,* fading out of the picture, leaving nothing but a perky smile behind. "I'm afraid I'm going to disappear altogether," she told me.

It's not hard to spot a Cheshire Cat in a family dealing with PTSD. Cheshire Cats watch only the TV shows that their loved ones like. They never express political opinions that could make their family members angry. They don't travel if their loved ones can't handle trips. They avoid friends and family members whom their family members don't like. They spend their days trying to figure out what makes Bob or Jane happy — and as time goes on, they forget to ask, "What makes *me* happy?" In the following sections, I explain why falling into this self-denying pattern is unhealthy, how you can tell if you're doing it, and how to get back to a healthy relationship.

Seeing the importance of a healthy balance

In Chapter 13, I talk about what to do if you're in a *codependent* relationship — a problem that occurs when one person, in order to keep the peace and prevent confrontations, lets another person fall into a pattern of selfish and self-destructive behavior. There are effective ways to turn around a codependent relationship, but it's far better to avoid falling into one in the first place.

If you're showing signs of Cheshire Cat Syndrome (see the section intro), that's a big warning sign that you're becoming codependent because you're starting to neglect your own needs in order to avoid arguments or other emotional upsets. Now's the time to change your behavior, and in turn, your loved one's.

This change is important because denying your own needs hurts both you and the person with PTSD. Over time, it makes you resentful and frustrated — and it makes you less an ally than a hostage to your loved one. It harms your loved one, too, because it allows her to fall deeper into maladaptive behavior patterns that reinforce her PTSD instead of helping her conquer it.

Determining whether your scales are tipped

If you suspect that caring for a person with PTSD is causing you to sacrifice your own needs (and make your loved one overly dependent in the process), here's a quick quiz. Ask yourself the following two questions, rating your answers on a scale of 0 to 10, with 0 representing *none* and 10 representing *all:*

- How much of your energy do you devote to pleasing, comforting, protecting, or caring for your loved one with PTSD?

- How much of your energy do you devote to pleasing, comforting, protecting, or caring for yourself?

If your two scores are the same or close together — say, 6 and 4 or 5 and 5 — that's healthy. If you answer 7 to the question about your loved one and 3 to the question about yourself, you're veering into Cheshire Cat territory. And if you say 9 and 1, you're sitting right in his tree.

Balancing your needs (and wants) with your loved one's

The solution to balancing your needs — not easy, but doable — is to start focusing more on your own needs and less on the other person's. Here are three ways to do that:

- Once a week, stop and ask yourself, "What can I do today to make myself feel better?" Whether it's a soak in the tub with a good book, a round of golf, or a phone call to a friend, do it. When you get into the habit, take this step at least once every day.

- Make a list of five things you used to enjoy doing but don't do now because of your loved one's PTSD. Then ask yourself, "Is there a way I can still do these things?" If your family member can't face traveling, for example, maybe you and a friend can take short out-of-town hops. If she refuses to let your relatives visit, maybe you can put them up in a hotel and spend time with them away from your home. Instead of giving up the things you love, find creative ways to work them into your life.

- Here's the biggie: Start letting the person with PTSD solve his own problems. This step is very, very difficult if you're a kind-hearted person who's fallen into the trap of letting your family member shove his responsibilities onto you. It's also hard if you're trying to keep your house safe and sane for children. A therapist can help you discover ways to avoid the co-dependency trap and point you in a healthier direction (see Chapter 13).

Recognize that you're not the problem

Your self-esteem may take a nosedive when you're the primary caregiver for a person with PTSD. Even after getting a diagnosis, your loved one may still turn denial into an art form by blaming you for problems that really stem from PTSD. Here are the types of accusations you may hear:

- **From a person with anger issues:** "Of course I'm mad all the time. It's because you let the kids make so much X#$% noise!"

- **From a loved one with avoidance issues:** "I wouldn't hide out in the den if you'd stop inviting those annoying friends of yours over."

> ✔ **From someone who's hypervigilant:** "No, I'm not relaxed. Nobody can relax with that stupid TV on. Do you have to watch that show every week?"
>
> ✔ **From a person who's linking to an earlier betrayal:** "Yes, I'm crying. It's the biggest holiday of the year, and you got me a dumb ring I don't like."

If you fall for these lines, you can wind up thinking you're inadequate, unlovable, or guilty of causing your loved one's troubles — or you can wind up yelling back and saying hurtful things in return ("Maybe I'm not the greatest wife in the world, but hey, buddy, you're not exactly a prize yourself!").

Identifying your loved one's hurtful words as symptoms of PTSD, on the other hand, can help you get a handle on them. Once again (am I starting to sound like a broken record?), a therapist can help by showing you how to sort the wheat of real family issues from the chaff of PTSD.

Special Guidance for Partners of People with PTSD

If your partner has PTSD, you have two extra issues to consider. One of these issues, of course, is sexuality: How can you cope if PTSD is dousing the flames of romance? Another is the $64,000 question: Should you stay in your relationship if PTSD is making your life a wreck? In this section, I help you get a handle on both of these questions.

Coping when love turns to neglect

When Audrey's husband Chuck came home from the war, she anticipated romantic evenings and lots of hugs and cuddles. What she got, instead, was excuses: "I really don't feel good," "Maybe tomorrow night," and "I just need some sleep." She was devastated and felt unattractive and inadequate. She didn't realize that Chuck's responses had nothing to do with her and everything to do with PTSD. (See Chapter 3 for info on how PTSD can make a person feel distant or unromantic.)

The key to coping with this problem is to understand that you can't make your partner desire you. If candlelight, soft music, and a come-hither look do nothing to stir romance in your partner's soul, don't feel like a failure. Loss of sexual desire is a primary symptom of PTSD, especially if your partner experienced a sexual assault. Only time and therapy can solve this problem, so don't think it's your responsibility to seduce an iceberg. Be patient — and if your partner is afraid of physical contact or intimacy, point him to the suggestions in Chapter 12 for overcoming this problem.

Deciding whether to stay or leave

Dana said, "It was awful at first. He said he didn't love me anymore and he wanted to leave. When I tried to get close, he pushed me away. For a while, he even moved out and lived on his own. But once he got therapy, things got better. We still take it one day at a time, but I'm glad I stayed."

That story is a common one in PTSD families. Often, a person with PTSD will shove you away just when she needs you most desperately. If you firmly believe that she's the person you want to spend your life with, try to stay connected even if she's acting distant or cold. In some cases, you may want to try a separation rather than file for divorce — or live in different houses for a time while you sort things out.

You're the only one who can know whether a relationship is worth the pain that PTSD puts you through. If not, cutting ties is the right move. But if you sense that you and your partner have something worth fighting for, stay strong and give therapy a chance — and then another chance. Even if your loved one walks out on you, keep the lines of communication open through phone calls, letters, or e-mails.

Be aware of one big exception: Never, *never* stay with a partner who's physically dangerous or so emotionally abusive that you or your children are at risk. No one benefits, and everyone suffers, if you allow your partner to abuse you or your kids. What's more, walking out the door can be the best gift you can give a person with PTSD if it jolts him into getting help for his destructive behavior. If you stay, on the other hand, you give your partner permission to continue on a downward spiral. Worse, you run the risk that you or your children will develop PTSD as a result of his abuse.

Also be aware that no matter how hard you try to keep your relationship on track, overcoming the obstacles may be impossible. PTSD breaks up many wonderful, loving couples. For example, the National Vietnam Readjustment Study (1990) indicates that Vietnam vets with PTSD divorce twice as often as those without PTSD and are three times more likely to have multiple divorces. If you give your relationship your best shot and it doesn't work out, don't sit around wondering whether you could've done something different to save your relationship. Almost assuredly, the answer is *no*.

REAL-LIFE STORY

A tale of two couples

It was love at first sight for David and Lucy. Six months after they met, he proposed to her on the beach and gave her a ring hidden in a seashell. Everything was hearts and flowers — until the night she went out for a quick jog and an attacker raped her at knifepoint.

For two years afterward, Lucy couldn't bear a man's touch. David went to group therapy with her, gave her space to heal, and agreed to postpone the wedding — twice. "I kept backing off," Lucy said, "but he kept saying, 'I'll wait.'"

David did wait, and as Lucy gained control over her PTSD, she got brave enough to commit. Three years later, the couple was expecting their first child.

Rita was just as supportive when her husband, Ed, returned from Iraq. She was the first to recognize the warning signs of PTSD, even before Ed did. She encouraged Ed to seek therapy and took a second job to pay the bills when his symptoms kept him from getting work in the civilian world.

"We both tried so hard," she said. "But Ed just couldn't take the pressure of being in a relationship anymore. We tried a separation, but it was too painful to keep getting together and splitting up, so we finally divorced. But he's still my best friend, and I love him dearly."

David and Rita both did everything humanly possible when it came to holding their relationships together, but only one of them lucked out. The moral of their stories is that "happily ever after" is possible when a partner has PTSD, but there are no guarantees.

Special Guidance for Parents of Adults with PTSD

In helping a loved one with PTSD, parents are often the brave souls on the front lines. What's more, moms and dads can often help in ways that no one else can (for instance, by spotting behavior changes that other relatives overlook — after all, nobody knows a kid like Mom or Dad does.) Sometimes however, it's hard to know where to draw the line when you're aiding a grown child with PTSD. (For info on helping a young child or teen, see Chapter 15). Here's some helpful guidance on parenting an adult child who's battling this disorder.

Handle family disagreements wisely

One problem that often arises when an adult child with PTSD lives with her folks is that Mom and Dad disagree over how much to help her. For instance, Dad may say, "Letting her live here rent-free isn't helping her to recover — it's just letting her avoid real life." Mom, on the other hand, may argue, "She needs a safe place while she's healing — and she doesn't need financial burdens right now." If disagreements like these arise, here are some smart ways to handle them:

✔ Agree to discuss your issues at a time when your son or daughter isn't around. That way, you can air your differences openly, without adding to your child's stress. With luck, you'll be able to compromise on a plan you can both accept.

✔ If you can't agree on what actions you should take, schedule a session with a family therapist who can help you sort through your differences. If that's not in your budget, a member of the clergy may be able to help.

✔ If your child gives you permission, talk with her therapist. This professional has a good handle on what your child needs right now and can help you both understand the actions you should or shouldn't take.

A different situation arises if your adult child is married and you disagree with your child's partner about PTSD-related issues — for example, what kind of therapy your child should try. In this case, the smartest course is to offer your suggestions tactfully but also respect and support the decisions your child and his partner make. One exception: If you firmly believe your child's behavior is endangering his life or other people's (for example, if he appears suicidal or has bouts of violent anger that endanger his children), then argue forcefully for intervention even if you risk straining the bonds with your child's partner.

Make your help as temporary as possible

Sometimes letting a young adult child fly from the nest is difficult, and that's especially true when your child has PTSD. But adult children need to spread their wings in order to grow and mature — so let your child stay at home and mend while it's necessary, but also facilitate independence.

Here are some questions that can help you determine whether you're providing necessary support or merely babying an adult child with PTSD and preventing your son or daughter from becoming independent:

✔ **Does your child help out around the house and chip in financially to the extent that she can? Or does she treat you like an unpaid maid and your house like a hotel?** If you spot the latter pattern, you're slipping into codependency (see Chapter 13). Look for areas in which your child is capable of lending a hand and expect her to do so instead of letting her act like a permanent guest.

✔ **Does your child talk about being independent in the future?** If not, gently bring up the topic yourself. You don't need to set a firm deadline, especially if he's battling serious PTSD symptoms right now, but do talk about "when you're back at work" or "when you have your own place" so he knows he needs to face adult responsibilities again when he's better.

✔ **Is your child actively seeking help for his PTSD or related problems such as substance abuse?** If not, make it crystal clear that you expect her to take steps to promote her own recovery. You can't force an adult child to get help, but you can strongly encourage her.

As your child heals from PTSD, taper the amount of support you offer and let him start standing on his own two legs again. Let him know that you're always there to offer emotional support but that you trust him to take charge of his own life. For instance, if he gets a job, you can say, "That's great that you're getting back on your feet. And after you get your own bills paid off, you can start pitching in on our phone and electricity bills. We'll really appreciate the help!" That's not being mean — it's acknowledging your child's healing and promoting his growing independence.

When the Sufferer Is Your Friend or a Member of Your Extended Family

Think of family and friends, and you picture holiday get-togethers, backyard barbecues, and weddings. If your friend or relative has PTSD, however, life's not all sunshine and laughter.

If you know that fact and you're still sticking by a person with PTSD, you're a true-blue friend, and your friendship can be powerful medicine for someone who's battling this monster. In this section, I give you tips on how you can help and a few cautions about mistakes to avoid.

Be there

Loneliness is a heavy burden for someone with PTSD. Your friend is suffering, and she needs to talk about her pain with people she trusts, but right now she's probably afraid to open up to you because she thinks you won't understand.

In a sense, she's right: If you don't have PTSD, you can't really picture the depth of the suffering it causes. You don't *need* to understand everything your friend is going through, however. All you need to do is be there and be supportive. Here are the best ways to do that:

- **Be honest.** It's human nature to comfort traumatized people by saying, "Don't worry; it'll be okay," or "Just get your mind off it, and you'll feel better." But PTSD is real, and it's serious. Accept this fact. Don't try to pretend that everything's just dandy when it's not.

- **Let your friend talk.** Listening to the details of a rape, a bombing, or a car wreck is painful and upsetting. But your friend needs to talk openly to someone who won't shut him out, so do your best to hear him out. Equally important, respect his wishes if he asks you not to share secrets he tells you in confidence. (See "Know when to nix confidentiality," later in this chapter, for an exception to this rule.)

- **Offer practical help.** Sometimes, an extra pair of hands is as useful as a shoulder to cry on. If you know that your friend doesn't have a car right now, offer to drive her to therapy. If her family is going through a rough patch, invite her kids to stay with yours for a weekend so that everyone can cool off.

- **Inject some fun into tough times.** Because you're close to your friend, you know what makes him smile. So watch a silly movie with him, toss a baseball together, or hit the computer store and pick up some new video games. If your friend vetoes one plan, realize that it may be too threatening because of his triggers, and suggest another option.

- **Encourage healthy habits.** Now's not the time to nag your friend about smoking or a junk-food diet. But if you can think of positive ways to get her into a healthy groove, you'll do her a big favor. Take nightly walks together, for example, or go for hikes or bike rides.

- **Know when to butt out.** Your friend needs support, not advice or lectures. Share with him your thoughts about how PTSD affects his life, but let him find his own answers. It's okay to say something like, "I found an interesting book on PTSD," but resist the urge to say something like, "You really need to read this book." Also, be sensitive to the fact that his partner, parents, or very close family members should play the primary role in helping him make decisions, with you serving as the supporting bench.

- **Offer validation.** The trauma your friend suffered shook her world, and she's not sure who she is anymore. You can help her by reminding her of all the things that make her special. If she says, "I just feel so stupid," remind her by saying something like this: "You're not stupid. You're the one who got me through algebra, remember? You're just hurting right now. You are strong and wonderful and smart, and you will get through this. And I'll be here to help you."

Be informed

You can't walk a mile in your friend's shoes — and you wouldn't want to — but books, articles, and Internet sites can give you a basic idea of what PTSD is all about. This knowledge can help you put brush-offs or outbursts into perspective so that you know when to think, "He's a jerk," and when to think, "He's really hurting, so I'm not going to get angry."

This book, of course, is a good start. You can also find valuable info at these sites:

- The U.S. Department of Veterans Affairs' National Center for PTSD site, www.ncptsd.va.gov

- The Sidran Institute, www.sidran.org

- The National Child Traumatic Stress Network, nctsnet.org

- The National Institute of Mental Health's PTSD site, www.nimh.nih.gov/healthinformation/ptsdmenu.cfm

Here are two other ways you can help a friend in need:

- **Do some detective work.** If your friend doesn't have the medical care or social support she needs, see whether you can find resources in your area. Check out Chapter 4 for ideas on locating support groups and Chapter 6 for ways to find free or low-cost therapy if money is an issue. But don't be surprised if your friend doesn't follow up on your leads right away. Often, people with PTSD are in denial, and it takes time for them to realize that they need help. Offer information, but don't push.

- **Surf the Net.** To get an insider's view of your friend's battle with PTSD, visit Internet forums. Some useful ones include

  - PTSD Forum at www.ptsdforum.org

  - The Broken Spirits Network at www.brokenspirits.com

  - Trauma Anonymous at www.bein.com/trauma

People in these forums — both survivors and their loved ones — appreciate the fact that you're trying to help a friend, and they can often offer insight or advice. Just remember that no two people are alike, so what works for another person may or may not work for you.

Be realistic

The biggest fact you need to face is that your friend is different now, and he probably always will be. A big dividing line in his mind separates *before the trauma* from *after the trauma*. Even if you knew him inside-and-out before he developed PTSD, you may never fully grasp the changes your friend went through when trauma turned his life inside out. Those changes can include

- ✔ A loss of beliefs your friend once shared with you, such as religious convictions or opinions about fairness and justice
- ✔ A loss of trust in other people
- ✔ A loss of confidence in the future
- ✔ A loss of innocence and lack of interest in innocent pleasures you once shared
- ✔ A new fear of getting too close to someone who may leave or die

When you recognize and accept these changes, you find it easier to let go of what *was* and accept what *is*. Maybe your friend doesn't want to go clubbing anymore. Maybe she's no longer the happy, carefree person you used to hang out with. Maybe he wants to keep you at arm's length instead of treating you like a brother. But you can start from where you both are now and build a new, different relationship that works for both of you.

Be realistic, too, about the up-and-down pattern of PTSD. Because this condition is a wild roller-coaster ride, your friend may be smart, funny, and warm one day and a blank-eyed stranger the next. She also may take some deep slides into anger, despair, or self-harm. If you get to the point where you can't stand to watch your friend's hurtful or self-destructive acts, keep your distance for a while — but always let her know that the door's open when she's ready to return your friendship.

Know when to nix confidentiality

Keep your heart-to-heart talks confidential unless you have your friend's permission to share them. That advice is almost always good, but be aware of one exception: If you pick up clues that your friend is suicidal, you need to act. Taking action is especially important if your friend

- ✔ Says he's actively thinking about ways to kill himself
- ✔ Asks you to take care of the people he loves if he's not around any longer
- ✔ Was very depressed and suddenly seems very agitated

If you spot these red flags, tell your friend's partner, other relatives, or anyone else you can trust (such as a pastor or doctor). In doing so, you may destroy trust and lose a friendship — but that's better than risking your friend's life.

If you're not sure whether your friend is suicidal, call your local suicide-prevention line and tell someone about your concerns. Whoever takes the call can help you decide what steps to take.

Part V

Stepping In: When You're Not the One Who's Suffering

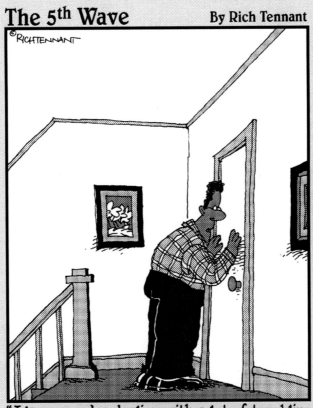

"I know you're dealing with a lot of troubling issues from your past, but if you need to talk, remember, I got straight A's in history, so I'm very good with things that happened a long time ago."

In this part . . .

If you're a relative or friend of someone who's hurting because of PTSD, you want to help — and in this part, you find out how. First, I talk about how you can identify signs of PTSD in a child or teen and what treatments work best for the younger set. I also describe the key role you can play in a friend's or relative's healing, and I offer a list of important do's and don'ts that can help you provide support and inspiration while avoiding a false step.

Chapter 17

The Ten Most Common Myths about PTSD

In This Chapter

▶ The myths that other people believe

▶ The myths you may buy into

▶ The myths that can stand in the way of treatment

Winston Churchill once said that "a lie gets halfway around the world before the truth has a chance to get its pants on." That goes for errors, half-truths, and downright silly ideas, too — and if you have PTSD, you'll hear lots of them.

If your friends and family inflict foolish advice on you, don't hold it against them, because they probably mean well. Just be ready with the facts so you can do your part to dispel the tall tales that many people believe. Here are ten of the biggest whoppers you're likely to hear (and even a few you may tell yourself), along with the facts to counter them.

PTSD Isn't Real

Wouldn't it be nice if PTSD were merely a figment of your imagination, like unicorns or leprechauns? Unfortunately, that's not the case. The symptoms of PTSD stem from biochemical and physiological changes, and those changes affect everything from your blood pressure to your digestive system. They're as real as the symptoms of pneumonia or bunions — so don't let anyone tell you otherwise.

In one way, of course, PTSD is largely "in your head." That's because PTSD changes the chemistry of your brain (and apparently its structure and wiring as well). Experts can actually see evidence of some of those changes in laboratory tests and brain scans, which means that they're far from imaginary.

Only Soldiers Get PTSD

The idea that PTSD is a "soldier's problem" that stems only from combat is a common misconception. In part, that's because the first insights about PTSD came from combat vets. Also, war is indeed one of the biggest risk factors for PTSD. (One study of Vietnam combat vets, conducted in 1992, found that they were six times more likely to have PTSD than men who never saw combat.)

But in truth, anyone from a kindergartener to a corporate CEO can develop severe symptoms following a trauma. What's more, as I explain in Chapter 2, *any* horrifying situation — not just battle — has the potential to cause PTSD.

People with PTSD Are Weak

Movies and TV shows send the message that heroes can withstand terrible abuse and bounce right back. For instance, spaceship captains are attacked by hideous aliens, sucked into time warps, shot at, swallowed by slime monsters, you name it — and the next week, they're right back at the helm, just as perky as ever.

In real life, however, trauma takes a toll on everyone, and brave people don't have any special powers that make them immune from developing long-term symptoms. In fact, the braver you are, the more likely you are to get in a situation that can provoke PTSD. That's why the people at highest risk for PTSD include those who willingly take on dangerous jobs: firefighters, police officers, and soldiers. These people ain't sissies — and neither are you.

Time Heals All Wounds

People with good intentions often say, "Give it time — you'll get over it." If you have PTSD, don't take this advice. If you're a friend or relative, don't give it. In reality, PTSD is like an infected wound: It's not likely to heal on its own, and without special treatment, it's likely to fester. That's why therapy, not time, is the best medicine.

Waiting for time to heal your PTSD can backfire in a big way because PTSD alters your thinking and behavior in ways that create secondary problems — drug or alcohol issues, financial problems, broken relationships. After PTSD messes with how you live your life, causing you to develop bad habits (*bad* = they make things worse for you), recovery can be further complicated by the need to unlearn *those* habits before you can replace them with good habits. Thus, the best time to treat PTSD is *before* it complicates your life any further.

Therapy Will Dissolve All Your Troubles

Here's the truth: *Lots* of your troubles probably stem from PTSD. But if you didn't have PTSD, you'd still have troubles. Remembering this point as you go through therapy is important so you don't expect the impossible. Therapy can make your life better, but it won't make it perfect. Instead, with luck, it'll give you the energy, strength, and confidence to handle your remaining problems after the weight of PTSD lifts.

Blocking Traumatic Memories Is Easier than Facing Them

Here's a quick exercise: Try *not* to think about a pig in a pink tutu. Now, try again *not* to think about a pig in a pink tutu. Now, try again . . .

Okay, you get the picture. Several seconds ago, you didn't have the least urge to think about a pig in a pink tutu. Now, however, you have to work hard to avoid conjuring up this picture (and you're probably not succeeding). What's more, the pig ballerina in this exercise isn't "loaded" — that is, it's not a memory etched into your brain by trauma and kept captive by brain chemicals that refuse to let it go.

What's the point? That the memories that grab onto you in PTSD don't just politely disappear if you try to shove them away. Ironically, the more energy you devote to ignoring bad feelings, the more you feed them. Why? Because those feelings *need* you to hear them out — they're there for a reason! So until you listen to them, explore them, and let yourself start working with them, they'll continue to intrude, and your efforts to clamp a lid on them will exhaust you. To do that, you need to team up with a therapist.

It Can't Be PTSD — It's Been Too Long

PTSD doesn't always show up right on schedule after a terrible event. Sometimes, especially if you suffered abuse as a child, it can rear its head years or even decades after a trauma is over. (See Chapter 2 for details.)

One common scenario occurs when a second trauma, often but not always related to the first one, dredges up long-submerged memories of the original event. For instance,

- A veteran of a long-ago war may come through his own combat traumas without experiencing PTSD, only to have symptoms develop many years later when his own child goes off to fight another war.

- A woman who had an extremely difficult labor and delivery may do fine but then develop PTSD following a second difficult birth.

- A person injured in a serious car wreck may come through seemingly unscathed but then experience a meltdown years later when she goes on an amusement park ride that makes her re-experience the same feelings of danger and loss of control.

If you experience delayed PTSD, the event that led to your PTSD was so horrible that you did whatever you could at the time to just survive it. You got past it, but you never got completely over it. It created a deep crack in your psyche and well-being that you hid from yourself and everyone else — like turning a crack in a vase to the back, where nobody (including you) could see it. But because that crack never healed completely, it left you with a vulnerability that could be reopened years later by even a small triggering incident.

Speaking of backs, many people have lower back pain problems from an injury but manage to get by for years with only a few twinges. Then one day they reach for something small in the wrong way and *bang!* — they're flat on their backs for a week. Delayed PTSD can lay you low in much the same way.

PTSD Causes Violence

Only a small percentage of people with PTSD commit serious acts of violence; it just seems like a common occurrence because the media blows these cases out of proportion. (Did you ever see a movie about the hundreds of thousands of Vietnam veterans who *didn't* commit violent acts? Probably not.) In reality, people with PTSD are far, far more likely to commit acts of violence against themselves in the form of alcoholism, drug abuse, self-injury, or eating disorders. True, people with complex PTSD for instance, combat veterans or people who were chronically abused as children — are at higher-than-normal risk for episodes of violence, but only a minority of people with complex PTSD has this problem.

That said, you need to take violent thoughts or urges very seriously and have them immediately addressed by a professional. The same is true for suicidal thoughts or urges. And if you find yourself abusing a partner or child, get help right away (see the emergency numbers listed in the Appendix).

You Deserve to Feel Bad for Making Mistakes When Your Trauma Happened

Guilt is often a healthy thing. Like a stern schoolteacher, it can make you see the error of your ways and prevent you from making the same mistakes over and over.

At other times, however, guilt is simply a sadistic thug. Often, it blames you for things you didn't do or makes you feel terrible for reacting in perfectly normal, logical, and human ways. For instance, someone who survived the World Trade Center attack may feel guilty if she ran away instead of helping others — even though running away was a smart and logical thing to do, and staying probably would've gotten her killed.

If you're using guilt to avoid therapy — if you're saying to yourself, "I deserve this punishment because I survived and other people didn't" — then recognize this as an excuse. Unless you're a robber, rapist, or Mother Nature, you didn't knowingly and willingly do anything to cause your trauma. What's more, when it happened, you did the best you could to get through it. So you don't deserve the pain you're living with, and both you and your loved ones will be happier as soon as you let go of your guilt and start on the road to healing.

You Don't Have the Time or Money for Therapy

In Chapter 6, I describe some low-cost or inexpensive ways to get therapy, such as community clinics, support groups, and pastoral counseling through a church — so no excuses there! Also, therapy takes only a few hours of your life each week, and it doesn't last any longer than you need it to. PTSD, on the other hand, is an uninvited guest that plans on staying *forever,* unless you chase it off. That definitely makes confronting your PTSD the better choice.

Chapter 18

Ten Ways to Recognize that You're Getting Better

Sometimes, events announce themselves with a big fanfare — the first squawk of a newborn, for example, or fireworks on the Fourth of July. At other times, the signs are subtle, such as the nip in the air that tells you Halloween's approaching or (ugh) the first gray hair that signals that you're *really* a grownup now.

As you heal from PTSD, you can see both clear and subtle signs of recovery. Spotting these signs can give you renewed motivation to keep moving forward, even if you still have some big hills to climb. Here's a sampling of clues, both large and small, that you're on the mend.

You Avoid a Blowup or Meltdown

PTSD can short-circuit your control over your emotions, causing your feelings to explode like champagne from a shaken bottle. No matter how hard you try, keeping your tears, anger, or fear from boiling over may be impossible sometimes.

As you heal, you start getting a handle on your emotions. Tense situations start to have less effect on you, and you stay calm (or even find something to laugh about) when problems pop up. You know you're making progress on this front if you keep your cool during an argument with your partner, a spat with your kids, or a tension-packed meeting at work — or even if you handle a frustrating encounter with your cable company without using any four-letter words.

You Become an Optimist

If you ever saw the musical *Annie,* you probably remember Little Orphan Annie's famous lyric "The sun'll come out tomorrow." When you have PTSD, you feel just the opposite way: You're pretty sure that even if today's going okay, the skies will cloud up and lightning will strike you the next day. You may think, "It's great to get this job, but I don't expect it to last," or "It's no use saying yes to this date because it's just going to be another bad experience."

When PTSD's grip starts to loosen, your inner Annie peeks out again. Instead of expecting the worst, you start to think that maybe — just *maybe* — tomorrow will be a good day. You may catch yourself saying, "I'm going to the picnic tomorrow because it might be really fun," or "I should interview for that position; I probably have a shot at it." These thoughts are big signs of healing because they mean you're ready to seek out happiness instead of spending all your time fearing misery.

You Turn "I Can't" into "I Can"

In a thousand different ways, PTSD limits your life by telling you that you can't do the things you want to do: take a cab, go to the store, board a plane, trust a loyal friend, or maybe even walk to your mailbox. And with each *can't,* your world shrinks a little bit more.

The first time you conquer one of these *I can't* thoughts and instead say, "I can" — a step you can take safely in therapy (see Chapters 8 and 10) — you feel your horizons expanding. Each *I can* gets easier than the last one, so no matter how large or small that first *I can* is, chalk it up as a major victory.

You Widen Your Circle of Friends

People with PTSD often shed friends like a duck sheds water, for reasons I talk about in Chapters 14 and 16. As a result, you can wind up feeling very much alone. As you recover from PTSD, you eventually spot this big hole in your life and start getting the urge to call up old buddies, make new friends, or patch up problems with the people you hurt when PTSD made you act in destructive ways. That itch to reconnect with people, like the itchy scab over a skinned knee, is a powerful sign of healing.

You Feel Another Person's Pain or Joy

If you have PTSD, your mind tries to protect you from excruciating emotions by making you feel numb to *all* emotions. Often, it does such a good job of wallpapering over your feelings that you have trouble feeling empathy even for the people closest to you. When that iceberg starts to thaw, you once again begin to care about the people around you. You see the first signs of this progress in little ways: a surge of sympathy for a co-worker who's divorcing, a thrill of pride when your child brings home a good report card, or a rush of love for a parent or partner who stood by you in your battle against PTSD.

You Say, "I Like You" — to Yourself

PTSD reminds me of the little devil sitting on a cartoon character's shoulder. At every turn (and especially when you're facing a challenge), it whispers destructive remarks like, "You can't do this," "You're weak," "Nothing ever turns out right for you," and "You're a loser."

Healing teaches you that all these lines are bogus. Instead, you learn to recognize your strengths — including the strength that helped you survive your trauma and start on the path to healing. You know you're making this change for the better when you catch yourself thinking things like, "I'm proud of myself," "I'm strong enough to deal with this problem," and "I deserve this happy relationship."

You Take a Leap of Faith

For a long time, PTSD kept you from trusting other people. You built a brick wall between yourself and the world and added an extra strand of barbed wire on the top each time you spotted somebody trying to climb over that wall.

Therapy can help you identify the reasons for this distrust and overcome them. You know you're starting to trust again if you hear yourself saying, "Sure, I'd like to go to out with you," or "Yes, I'd like to be your friend." Or if you're already in a relationship, you may even startle a longtime partner by making a big commitment, saying something like, "Let's get married," or "Maybe it *is* time to start a family."

You Enjoy Skipping Down Memory Lane

For people with PTSD, snapshots or videos from the time before trauma struck can be powerful reminders of lost innocence, hope, love, and happiness. As a result, trauma survivors often feel pain instead of pleasure when they flip through the pages of a family album or pop in a video from earlier days.

As you come to terms with your trauma, old memories can take their rightful place in your life, especially when you start to look forward to your future. You may find yourself smiling at the same home movies that used to upset you or feeling warm and fuzzy rather than bereft and abandoned when you come across a picture of a lost loved one.

You Wake Up with the Sun

People who don't have PTSD can't know how hard it is to face each new day. Getting started in the morning is especially hard if you're battling both PTSD and depression, a tag team that leaves you feeling so low that just putting your feet into your slippers is an act of courage.

In therapy, you discover that the rest of your life *doesn't* have to revolve around PTSD. In fact, you find that each new day can bring good surprises and happy times. In addition, you get a handle on your bad dreams and spend less time lying awake in the dark. You may find yourself throwing back the covers and greeting each morning with anticipation rather than the usual sense of dread — a clear sign that life is getting better.

You Get Back into the Swing of Things

What lit up your life before trauma struck? Maybe you cared deeply about politics or donated your time to charity work. You may have lived for major-league baseball or opera, collected salt shakers, worked in macramé, or raised potbellied pigs.

Whatever your passions, you probably abandoned many of them when PTSD focused all your attention on your internal demons. As you chase those demons away, you find yourself rekindling old interests or taking up new hobbies — a very healthy sign. So if you drag your easel out of the closet, start your own blog, or dust off your old piano books and try tickling the ivories, congratulate yourself. You're healing!

Part VI
The Part of Tens

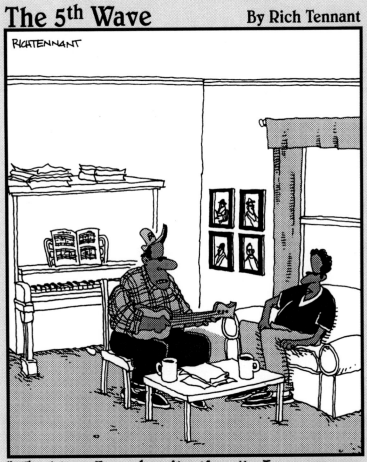

The 5th Wave — By Rich Tennant

"The blues I can handle. Usually I can express it with a simple 12-bar guitar lick. PTSD, on the other hand, takes a 3-act opera."

In this part . . .

In this part, I mix some practical information with a little bit of fun. I start by debunking ten myths about PTSD and offering some facts in their place. Then I offer ten signs — big and small — that you're on the road to healing.

Appendix

PTSD Resources

‸ ‸

*L*ooking for additional information to help in your healing or that of some-one you love? If so, this appendix provides a wealth of Web sites and other resources to aid you in understanding PTSD and in taking control of it if you're the one caught in its grip.

Emergency Phone Numbers

These numbers can be lifesavers if conditions get really tough. Keep them handy if you have any suicidal thoughts or if you're living in a dangerous situation.

✔ **National Suicide Prevention Lifeline,** 800-273-TALK (800-273-8255)

✔ **National Domestic Violence Hotline,** 800-799-SAFE (800-799-7233)

✔ **National Child Abuse Hotline,** 800-4-ACHILD (800-422-4453), for help if you're being abused or are committing abuse and know you need help

Web Sites

If you have access to the Internet, you can locate anything from basic info about PTSD to discussion forums and organizations offering practical sup-port. This section lists some good sites to check out.

General information

The Internet is full of facts (and nonfacts) about PTSD, so knowing where to begin if you're looking for information online can be hard. I recommend these sites as good starting points. The first two in particular are outstanding.

✔ **National Center for Posttraumatic Stress Disorder** (www.ncptsd.va.gov)

This site, created primarily for veterans and their families and for care providers, also provides excellent info for civilians dealing with PTSD. The site is a must-see if you're seeking basic information, whether you're a person with PTSD, a family member or friend, or a healthcare professional. It provides both basic information and loads of links to other sites, including excellent sites with info on helping children with PTSD. Another great feature: the PILOTS database, an electronic index to the worldwide literature on PTSD.

✔ **Sidran Institute** (www.sidran.org)

This site is a top source of information about all aspects of PTSD. It offers a help desk providing information on finding therapists, treatment centers, and support groups, as well as recommendations regarding books, videos, newsletters, and journals about PTSD. Highly recommended!

✔ **National Institute of Mental Health** (www.nimh.nih.gov/healthinformation/ptsdmenu.cfm)

This site offers basic information about PTSD, links to breaking news stories about the disorder and its treatment, downloadable publications and resource materials, and a link to a list of clinical trials of new PTSD treatments.

✔ **Association for Behavioral and Cognitive Therapies** (www.aabt.org/public)

Formerly the Association for Advancement of Behavior Therapy (hence the Web address), this organization's public site offers both information and a search tool you can use to find a local therapist who offers cognitive behavioral therapy, or CBT (see Chapter 8).

✔ **PubMed** (www.pubmed.gov)

This free site, which offers abstracts from medical journals, can help you keep up-to-date on new treatments.

Discussion groups or support groups

If you're looking for other people who understand the pain of PTSD and who can offer both moral support and practical advice, the Internet is a great place to find them. Here are good sites that can get you started:

✔ **PTSD Forum** (www.ptsdforum.org) is one of the best of the online discussion groups about PTSD.

✔ **American Self-Help Group Clearinghouse** (mentalhelp.net/selfhelp) can help you find PTSD support groups in your area, whether you're battling PTSD yourself or you're a family member seeking ways to cope.

PTSD-related issues

If you're battling PTSD, related problems such as substance abuse or mental health disorders may come along for the ride. The following Web sites can be a big help if you're facing several of these challenges at once.

✔ **National Council on Alcoholism and Drug Dependence** (www.ncadd.org) offers links to dozens of programs that can help if you're dealing with a substance abuse problem.

✔ **National Eating Disorders Association** (www.edap.org) includes advice and referrals for people who develop eating disorders as a result of PTSD.

✔ **S.A.F.E. Alternatives** (www.selfinjury.com) offers information and a therapist referral list for people with trauma-related issues involving self-injury (see Chapter 3).

✔ **Agoraphobics Building Independent Lives** (ABIL) (www.anxiety support.org/b001menu.htm) is a support group that can help you if your trauma caused severe anxiety that makes it difficult for you to be in public places.

✔ **PDRhealth** (www.pdrhealth.com) is helpful if you want more information on a drug your doctor prescribes for PTSD. Just go to the index (www.pdrhealth.com/drug_info/index.html) and type the drug's name.

For soldiers and vets

If you're serving your country right now or you wore a uniform in the past, check out these sites for information on the services available to you — and for moral support and practical advice from people who know the PTSD drill.

- ✔ **Military OneSource** (www.militaryonesource.com) offers assistance in finding help for PTSD, for drug or alcohol problems, and for a wide range of other issues.

- ✔ **The Veterans Coalition** (www.theveteranscoalition.org) offers support and advice for people coping with PTSD and other post-combat issues.

Also see "General information," earlier in this appendix, for info on the National Center for Posttraumatic Stress Disorder, which focuses much of its efforts on helping vets and their families.

For people caring for children with PTSD

As I explain in Chapter 15, kids react differently than adults do to a traumatic experience. If you're caring for a child or teen who is at risk for or was diagnosed with PTSD, the following resources and articles can help you understand what he's going through and how you can help.

- ✔ **National Child Traumatic Stress Network,** www.nctsnet.org

  This site contains excellent information for both parents and professionals. Professionals dealing with children who've experienced a traumatic experience can also find an excellent downloadable publication titled "Psychological First Aid" at this location on the site: www.nctsnet.org/nccts/nav.do?pid=typ_terr_resources_pfa.

- ✔ **"Stress, Trauma, and Post-traumatic Stress Disorders in Children,"** **ChildTrauma Academy,** www.childtrauma.org/ctamaterials/ptsd_interdisc.asp

- ✔ **"PTSD in Children and Adolescents,"** National Center for Posttraumatic Stress Disorder, www.ncptsd.va.gov/ncmain/ncdocs/fact_shts/fs_children.html

- ✔ **"Helping Young Children Cope with Trauma,"** American Red Cross, www.redcross.org/services/disaster/keepsafe/childtrauma.html

- ✔ **"Children, Stress, and Natural Disasters: A Guide for Teachers,"** **University of Illinois,** web.extension.uiuc.edu/disaster/teacher2/guide.html

Self-Help Reading Material

The more you read about PTSD, the better you understand both the disorder and the recovery process. The titles below can boost your knowledge about PTSD and a range of related problems:

- ✔ *The PTSD Workbook,* by Mary Beth Williams and Soili Poijula (New Harbinger Publications, 2002)

- ✔ *Recovering from the War: A Guide for All Veterans, Family Members, Friends and Therapists,* by Patience Mason (Patience Press, 1998)

- ✔ *Overcoming Anxiety For Dummies,* by Charles H. Elliott and Laura L. Smith (Wiley Publishing, 2002)

- ✔ *Anxiety & Depression Workbook For Dummies,* by Charles H. Elliott, Laura L. Smith, and Aaron T. Beck (Wiley Publishing, 2005)

- ✔ *Calming Your Anxious Mind,* by Jeffrey Brantley (New Harbinger Publications, 2007)

- ✔ *Depression For Dummies,* by Laura L. Smith and Charles H. Elliott (Wiley Publishing, 2003)

- ✔ *Addiction & Recovery For Dummies,* by Brian F. Shaw, Paul Ritvo, Jane Irvine, and M. David Lewis (Wiley Publishing, 2004)

- ✔ *Forgive for Good,* by Frederic Luskin (HarperOne, 2003)

- ✔ *The Post-Traumatic Gazette* (www.patiencepress.com/ptg.html)

  This outstanding publication offers articles for people experiencing PTSD after any form of trauma. Some issues of this newsletter are available online free of charge; others, for a small fee. The newsletter is no longer published, but all back issues are available. To order, visit the Web site or call 877-PATIENCE (877-728-4362) or 386-462-7210.

Books for Children and Teens

The following books, which offer a kid's-eye view of life crises, are excellent resources for children and teens who've experienced a trauma:

- ✔ *A Terrible Thing Happened,* by Margaret M. Holmes and Sasha J. Mudlaff (Magination Press, 2000), is a picture book for children ages 4–8 who've experienced a trauma.

- ✔ *What to Do When You're Scared and Worried: A Guide for Kids,* by James J. Crist (Free Spirit Publishing, 2004), is a reassuring self-help book for kids in grades five through eight.

- ✔ *When Molly Was in the Hospital: A Book for Brothers and Sisters of Hospitalized Children,* by Debbie Duncan (Rayve Productions, 1994), is a picture book for preschoolers and young elementary-aged children coping with the experience of a hospitalized sibling.

- ✔ *I Am a Survivor: A Child's Workbook About Surviving Disasters,* by Wendy Deaton and Kendall Johnson (Hunter House, 2002), offers activities to help children ages 9–12 to cope with the aftermath of a disaster.

- ✔ *Highs! Over 150 Ways to Feel Really, Really Good . . . Without Alcohol or Other Drugs,* by Alex J. Packer (Free Spirit Publishing, 2000), is an excellent resource for traumatized teens at risk for substance abuse.

- ✔ *I Miss You: A First Look at Death,* by Pat Thomas (Barron's Educational Series, 2001), is a sensitive picture book for children ages 4–8.

- ✔ *Chemo Girl: Saving the World One Treatment at a Time,* by Christina Richmond (Jones & Bartlett Publishers, 1996), is a positive book with a superhero theme for children ages 4–8 who are undergoing cancer treatment.

Documentaries on PTSD in Veterans

The following two programs offer insight into the challenges that soldiers or veterans with PTSD and their families face, as well as the help that's available for them. One caution: Both programs contain footage of combat scenes, so you may want to postpone watching them until you have your symptoms under control.

- ✔ *The Soldier's Heart,* a PBS *Frontline* documentary available free of charge at www.pbs.org/wgbh/pages/frontline/shows/heart/view, offers an in-depth look at the toll that PTSD takes on America's fighting forces.

- ✔ *Insights for Interventions: For Veterans and Families,* a documentary narrated by Jane Pauley, is available free of charge on the Web site of the National Center for Posttraumatic Stress Disorder at www.ncptsd.va.gov/ncmain/ncdocs/videos/emv_womenvet_vetfam.html. This program, which is one segment of a feature on women in the military, looks at the special problems of female veterans with PTSD and the treatment options that can benefit them.

Index

• N •

BUSINESS, CAREERS & PERSONAL FINANCE

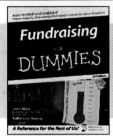

0-7645-9847-3

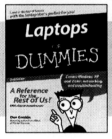

0-7645-2431-3

Also available:
- Business Plans Kit For Dummies
  0-7645-9794-9
- Economics For Dummies
  0-7645-5726-2
- Grant Writing For Dummies
  0-7645-8416-2
- Home Buying For Dummies
  0-7645-5331-3
- Managing For Dummies
  0-7645-1771-6
- Marketing For Dummies
  0-7645-5600-2

- Personal Finance For Dummies
  0-7645-2590-5*
- Resumes For Dummies
  0-7645-5471-9
- Selling For Dummies
  0-7645-5363-1
- Six Sigma For Dummies
  0-7645-6798-5
- Small Business Kit For Dummies
  0-7645-5984-2
- Starting an eBay Business For Dummies
  0-7645-6924-4
- Your Dream Career For Dummies
  0-7645-9795-7

HOME & BUSINESS COMPUTER BASICS

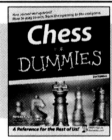

0-470-05432-8

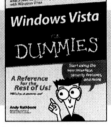

0-471-75421-8

Also available:
- Cleaning Windows Vista For Dummies
  0-471-78293-9
- Excel 2007 For Dummies
  0-470-03737-7
- Mac OS X Tiger For Dummies
  0-7645-7675-5
- MacBook For Dummies
  0-470-04859-X
- Macs For Dummies
  0-470-04849-2
- Office 2007 For Dummies
  0-470-00923-3

- Outlook 2007 For Dummies
  0-470-03830-6
- PCs For Dummies
  0-7645-8958-X
- Salesforce.com For Dummies
  0-470-04893-X
- Upgrading & Fixing Laptops For Dummies
  0-7645-8959-8
- Word 2007 For Dummies
  0-470-03658-3
- Quicken 2007 For Dummies
  0-470-04600-7

FOOD, HOME, GARDEN, HOBBIES, MUSIC & PETS

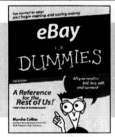

0-7645-8404-9

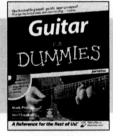

0-7645-9904-6

Also available:
- Candy Making For Dummies
  0-7645-9734-5
- Card Games For Dummies
  0-7645-9910-0
- Crocheting For Dummies
  0-7645-4151-X
- Dog Training For Dummies
  0-7645-8418-9
- Healthy Carb Cookbook For Dummies
  0-7645-8476-6
- Home Maintenance For Dummies
  0-7645-5215-5

- Horses For Dummies
  0-7645-9797-3
- Jewelry Making & Beading For Dummies
  0-7645-2571-9
- Orchids For Dummies
  0-7645-6759-4
- Puppies For Dummies
  0-7645-5255-4
- Rock Guitar For Dummies
  0-7645-5356-9
- Sewing For Dummies
  0-7645-6847-7
- Singing For Dummies
  0-7645-2475-5

INTERNET & DIGITAL MEDIA

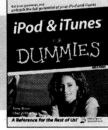

0-470-04529-9

0-470-04894-8

Also available:
- Blogging For Dummies
  0-471-77084-1
- Digital Photography For Dummies
  0-7645-9802-3
- Digital Photography All-in-One Desk Reference For Dummies
  0-470-03743-1
- Digital SLR Cameras and Photography For Dummies
  0-7645-9803-1
- eBay Business All-in-One Desk Reference For Dummies
  0-7645-8438-3
- HDTV For Dummies
  0-470-09673-X

- Home Entertainment PCs For Dummies
  0-470-05523-5
- MySpace For Dummies
  0-470-09529-6
- Search Engine Optimization For Dummies
  0-471-97998-8
- Skype For Dummies
  0-470-04891-3
- The Internet For Dummies
  0-7645-8996-2
- Wiring Your Digital Home For Dummies
  0-471-91830-X

* Separate Canadian edition also available
† Separate U.K. edition also available

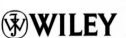 **WILEY**

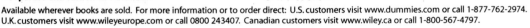
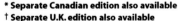

SPORTS, FITNESS, PARENTING, RELIGION & SPIRITUALITY

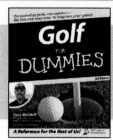

0-471-76871-5

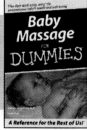

0-7645-7841-3

Also available:

- Catholicism For Dummies
  0-7645-5391-7
- Exercise Balls For Dummies
  0-7645-5623-1
- Fitness For Dummies
  0-7645-7851-0
- Football For Dummies
  0-7645-3936-1
- Judaism For Dummies
  0-7645-5299-6
- Potty Training For Dummies
  0-7645-5417-4
- Buddhism For Dummies
  0-7645-5359-3

- Pregnancy For Dummies
  0-7645-4483-7 †
- Ten Minute Tone-Ups For Dummies
  0-7645-7207-5
- NASCAR For Dummies
  0-7645-7681-X
- Religion For Dummies
  0-7645-5264-3
- Soccer For Dummies
  0-7645-5229-5
- Women in the Bible For Dummies
  0-7645-8475-8

TRAVEL

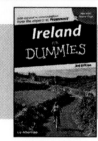

0-7645-7749-2

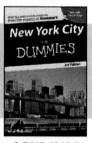

0-7645-6945-7

Also available:

- Alaska For Dummies
  0-7645-7746-8
- Cruise Vacations For Dummies
  0-7645-6941-4
- England For Dummies
  0-7645-4276-1
- Europe For Dummies
  0-7645-7529-5
- Germany For Dummies
  0-7645-7823-5
- Hawaii For Dummies
  0-7645-7402-7

- Italy For Dummies
  0-7645-7386-1
- Las Vegas For Dummies
  0-7645-7382-9
- London For Dummies
  0-7645-4277-X
- Paris For Dummies
  0-7645-7630-5
- RV Vacations For Dummies
  0-7645-4442-X
- Walt Disney World & Orlando
  For Dummies
  0-7645-9660-8

GRAPHICS, DESIGN & WEB DEVELOPMENT

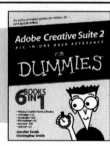

0-7645-8815-X

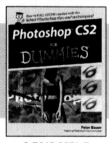

0-7645-9571-7

Also available:

- 3D Game Animation For Dummies
  0-7645-8789-7
- AutoCAD 2006 For Dummies
  0-7645-8925-3
- Building a Web Site For Dummies
  0-7645-7144-3
- Creating Web Pages For Dummies
  0-470-08030-2
- Creating Web Pages All-in-One Desk
  Reference For Dummies
  0-7645-4345-8
- Dreamweaver 8 For Dummies
  0-7645-9649-7

- InDesign CS2 For Dummies
  0-7645-9572-5
- Macromedia Flash 8 For Dummies
  0-7645-9691-8
- Photoshop CS2 and Digital
  Photography For Dummies
  0-7645-9580-6
- Photoshop Elements 4 For Dummies
  0-471-77483-9
- Syndicating Web Sites with RSS Feeds
  For Dummies
  0-7645-8848-6
- Yahoo! SiteBuilder For Dummies
  0-7645-9800-7

NETWORKING, SECURITY, PROGRAMMING & DATABASES

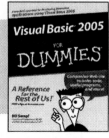

0-7645-7728-X

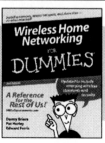

0-471-74940-0

Also available:

- Access 2007 For Dummies
  0-470-04612-0
- ASP.NET 2 For Dummies
  0-7645-7907-X
- C# 2005 For Dummies
  0-7645-9704-3
- Hacking For Dummies
  0-470-05235-X
- Hacking Wireless Networks
  For Dummies
  0-7645-9730-2
- Java For Dummies
  0-470-08716-1

- Microsoft SQL Server 2005 For Dummies
  0-7645-7755-7
- Networking All-in-One Desk Reference
  For Dummies
  0-7645-9939-9
- Preventing Identity Theft For Dummies
  0-7645-7336-5
- Telecom For Dummies
  0-471-77085-X
- Visual Studio 2005 All-in-One Desk
  Reference For Dummies
  0-7645-9775-2
- XML For Dummies
  0-7645-8845-1